The Logic of
Laboratory Medicine

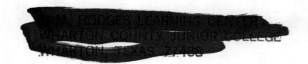

Principles for Use of the
Clinical Laboratory

The Logic of Laboratory Medicine

Dennis A. Noe, M.D.
The Johns Hopkins Hospital

With Contributions by

J. David Bessman, M.D.
Department of Medicine
The University of Texas Medical Branch at Galveston

James R. Carlson, Ph.D.
Departments of Pathology and Medicine
University of California, Davis, Medical Center

Daniel F. Cowan, M.D., C.M.
Department of Pathology
Temple University School of Medicine

Karen M. Kumor, M.D.
Addiction Research Center
National Institute on Drug Abuse

David G. Moore, Ph.D.
Department of Pathology and Laboratory Medicine
The University of Texas Medical School, Houston

68948

Urban & Schwarzenberg
Baltimore-Munich · 1985

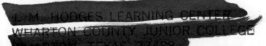

Urban & Schwarzenberg, Inc.
7 E. Redwood Street
Baltimore, Maryland 21202
USA

Urban & Schwarzenberg
Pettenkoferstrasse 18
D-8000 München 2
West Germany

NOTICES

The Editors (or Author(s)) and the Publisher of this work have made every effort to ensure that the drug dosage schedules herein are accurate and in accord with the standards accepted at the time of publication. The reader is strongly advised, however, to check the product information sheet included in the package of each drug he or she plans to administer to be certain that changes have not been made in the recommended dose or in the contraindications for administration.

The Publishers have made an extensive effort to trace original copyright holders for permission to use borrowed material. If any has been overlooked, it will be corrected at the first reprint.

Library of Congress Cataloging in Publication Data

The Logic of laboratory medicine.

Includes index.
1. Diagnosis, Laboratory.   2. Physiology, Pathological. I. Noe, Dennis
A.   [DNLM: 1. Diagnosis, Laboratory.
QY 4 L832
RB37.L74   1985   616.07′5   84-27106
ISBN 0-8067-1371-2 (pbk.)

Editor: Charles W. Mitchell
Copy editor: Starr Belsky
Production and design: Norman Och and Karen Babcock

ISBN 0-8067-1371-2 Baltimore

ISBN 3-541-71371-2 Munich

TABLE OF CONTENTS

Foreword by Robert C. Rock, M.D.
Preface
Introduction

Part I: ANALYTIC PRINCIPLES   1
1. Expressing Laboratory Results   3
    Classification and Quantification   3
    Expressing Quantitative Laboratory Results   4
    Interpretive Reporting   9
    Manipulation of Laboratory Results 10
    Appendix: Conversions Between Common and SI Units . 17
2. Variability in Laboratory Measurement 19
    Sources of Variability 19
    Frequency Distributions 23
3. Diagnostic Classification 31
    1. Study Performance 31
    Diagnostic Studies 31
    Study Performance 31
    Evaluation of Study Performance:
       Medical Journal Articles 39

Part II: ADVANCED ANALYTIC PRINCIPLES 53
4. Diagnostic Classification 55
    2. Study Performance: Further Considerations 55
    Optimal Study Performance 55
    Repeat and Combination Testing 64
    Multivariate Positivity Rules 72
5. Diagnostic Classification 79
    3. Individualizing Diagnoses 79
    Making Diagnoses 79
    The Likelihood of a Diagnosis 79
    Choosing Among Multiple Diagnostic Alternatives . . 94
    Likelihood Estimation using Multiple Study Results . 97

6. Diagnostic Classification 109
    4. The Selection and Ordering of Diagnostic Studies . . 109
      Selecting the Studies to Order 109
      Ordering Studies 121

Part III: PHYSIOLOGIC PRINCIPLES 127
7. Organ Function 129
    1. Synthesis and Clearance 129
      Measurement of Organ Function 129
      Physiologic Models: Marker Substances 129
      Synthesis and Clearance 131
      Organ Synthetic Rate 137
      Organ Clearance Rate 137
      Organ Clearance of Exogenous Substances 142
      Monitoring Synthetic Rate and Clearance Rate . . . 147
8. Organ Function 157
    2. Homeostatic Systems 157
      Homeostasis 157
      Classification of Endocrine Dysfunction 159
      Evaluation of Endocrine Gland Function 160
      Stimulation and Suppression Studies 164
9. Metabolism 171
    Dennis A. Noe, M.D. and J. David Bessman, M.D.
      Introduction 171
      Water and Abundant Metals 171
      Acid-Base Balance 177
      Trace Metals and Vitamins 187
      Plasma Proteins and Blood Cells 193
      Cellular Metabolism 194
10. Protein Binding in Plasma 201
      Physiologic Functions of Protein Binding 201
      Delivery Function 202
      Storage Function 205
      Buffer Function 205
      Laboratory Measurement 213
11. Tissue Injury 219
      Plasma Markers of Tissue Injury 219
      Detecting Tissue Injury — The Diagnostic Window . . 223
      Systemic Response to Tissue Injury 229
      Mediators of Tissue Injury 233

12. Neoplasia 239
    Daniel F. Cowan, M.D., C.M.
    Introduction 239
    Laboratory in Diagnosis 240
    Detection of Neoplasia in Asymptomatic People . . . 240
    Detection of Neoplasia in Symptomatic Patients . . 241
    Histopathologic Diagnosis 249
    Determining the Extent of a Neoplasm 252
    Recurrence After Treatment 254
    Conclusion 255
13. Therapeutic Drug Monitoring 257
    Karen M. Kumor, M.D.
    Philosophy 257
    Applying the Science to the Practice of
        Therapeutic Monitoring 262
    Other Considerations 277
    A Potpourri of Practical Points Providing
        Particularly Poignant Information 285
    Appendix: Timing of Blood Collection for
        Therapeutic Monitoring 293

Part IV: SELECTED ASPECTS OF LABORATORY PRACTICE 297
14. Clinical Microbiology 299
    James R. Carlson, Ph.D. and David G. Moore, Ph.D.
    Introduction 299
    Direct Visualization and Culture of
        Pathogenic Microorganisms 299
    Serologic Detection of Host Antibodies and
        Microbial Antigens in Body Fluids 310
15. Specimen Collection Procedures 315
    Introduction 315
    Venipuncture 315
    Arterial Puncture 318
    Fingerstick 321
    Heelstick 322
    Lumbar Puncture 324
    Thoracentesis 327
    Abdominal Paracentesis 330
    Urine: Random Voided Specimen 333
    Urine: Timed Voided Specimen 334

The Answers 337
Glossary 361

Wisdom is the principal thing;
therefore get wisdom
and with all thy getting get understanding.

Proverbs

To Paul and Robert,
Edmond and Alvan,
and Karen, Michael, and Sascha.

FOREWORD

One of the most troubling aspects of teaching the principles of laboratory medicine to medical students (as well as residents) has been the lack of a concise sourcebook to provide the basis for understanding the underlying analytical and quantitative principles of clinical laboratory measurements.

This text provides such a basis. Beginning with a discussion of the quantification of laboratory results, the author then presents several different approaches to the expression of quantitative laboratory data. My personal experiences with graduate physicians support the idea that many physicians try to interpret laboratory data without awareness of 1) the units of measurement, 2) interconversions between commonly used systems of units, or 3) distinctions between measured and calculated data.

The next major section establishes the basis for understanding the sources of variability in all laboratory measurements. This understanding is required to distinguish significant differences between laboratory data obtained longitudinally over time in the same subject (intraindividual variation) or in comparing data in any one subject from that of a reference population (interindividual variation).

Laboratory measurements can help the clinician in diagnostic classification, provided he has an understanding of the performance of the test in the clinical setting in which it is being used. The next section considers the criteria for evaluation of test performance (in terms of efficacy and predictive value) and helps the reader to apply these criteria in evaluating reports of diagnostic studies in the published medical literature.

Published studies of effective use of diagnostic procedures by experienced clinicians demonstrate the need to use the "right" test in parallel or in series with other "right" tests, in the "right" sequence for the clinical questions being asked. A major section on advanced analytic principles illustrates the "right" ways to optimize the efficacy of a study, alone or in combination, to help achieve an accurate diagnostic classification in an individual patient. In an environment in which the costs of medical care are being scrutinized, inappropriate use of laboratory studies needs to be reduced (whether over-utilization in the "shotgun" approach to diagnostic testing, or under-utilization of a test which permits earlier recognition of disease).

The next sections of the book illustrate the application of the physiologic principles underlying quantitative laboratory measurements of organ function (synthesis and clearance, as applied to assessment of hepatic and renal function, and homeostasis, as demonstrated by assessment of endocrine function). Metabolic processes are described in terms of laboratory evaluation of acid-base, water, and mineral metabolism.

Several sections consider the application of laboratory measurement to evaluate the pathophysiology of tissue injury and the development of neoplasia. Appropriate methods to reduce the risks of iatrogenic disease are presented in a section dealing with therapeutic drug monitoring, where many of the principles discussed in earlier chapters are reintroduced in applying clinical pharmacokinetics to the problems of drug therapy. The final chapters of the book deal with the selection of the appropriate laboratory methods for the laboratory evaluation of microbial infections and provide a useful compilation of procedures for correct specimen collection. Attention to the details of specimen collection helps to ensure that the final analytical result will be clinically valid.

Problems appear regularly throughout the book to help the reader apply the principles to clinical practice using actual laboratory data.

This book should serve both undergraduate medical students, who need a framework for developing rational approaches to diagnostic testing, and graduate physicians, who need to review the underlying principles of diagnostic testing in evaluating their own laboratory practice, particularly when deciding upon adoption of new diagnostic methods.

Robert C. Rock, M.D.
Director
Division of Laboratory Medicine
The Johns Hopkins School of Medicine
Baltimore, Maryland

PREFACE

"Truth," said a traveller,
"Is a rock, a mighty fortress;
"Often have I been to it,
"Even to its highest tower,
"From whence the world looks black."

"Truth," said a traveller,
"Is a breath, a wind,
"A shadow, a phantom;
"Long have I pursued it,
"But never have I touched
"The hem of its garment."

And I believed the second traveller;
For truth was to me
A breath, a wind,
A shadow, a phantom,
And never had I touched
The hem of its garment.

Stephen Crane

The absence of formal instruction in clinical reasoning constitutes a remarkable omission in the curricula of most medical schools. Clinical reasoning is, after all, the one unique aspect of medical practice. Of particular concern to me is the paucity of instruction in the application of analytical reasoning to laboratory use despite the fact that a large portion of the workday for most physicians consists of ordering and interpreting laboratory studies.

Although much has been made of recent efforts to improve the medical student's "fund of knowledge" concerning laboratory practice through courses in laboratory medicine, little, if any, time is devoted to discussions of medical logic. I am certain this is due in large part to the unavailability of a support text and the controversial nature of the topic owing to the lack of a consensus among laboratorians as to what constitutes the logical framework of laboratory medicine. This book has been written with the intent of eliminating the former obstacle and with the hope of contributing to the resolution of the latter.

I wish to express my gratitude to Denise Skidmore who was the manuscript and production typist on this project and to Joan Kuhar who was the illustrator. I also want to thank Doctors Karen Kumor and Robert Rock, who reviewed the manuscript for this

xv

textbook. Finally, I owe a special debt of thanks to the 1981–1982 sophomore class of the University of Texas Medical School, Houston, who faced the primitive ancestor of this textbook in the form of an introductory laboratory medicine course. I learned more from them than they learned from me, I fear. My hope is that I learned my lessons well. The reader will be the judge of that.

Dennis A. Noe
Baltimore

1984

INTRODUCTION

Everyone spoke of an information overload, but what
there was in fact was a non-information overload.

Richard Saul Wurman

LABORATORY MEDICINE

Medical studies may be defined as those procedures performed
upon patients, or upon specimens taken from patients, that provide clinical data beyond that which can be obtained by history-
taking and physical examination. Indeed, even a few components
of a modern physical examination, such as sphygmomanometry and
fundoscopy, are properly categorized as medical studies because
the techniques are instrument dependent. A laboratory study is
usually taken to mean a medical study performed in a laboratory
or supervised by laboratory personnel. In its broadest sense,
laboratory medicine is that branch of medicine concerned with the
performance and interpretation of laboratory studies.

If a laboratory study is conducted upon a specimen rather
than directly upon the patient, it is referred to as a clinical
laboratory study. These studies are usually done in the set of
laboratories known as the clinical laboratories, although sometimes they are performed by medical personnel in laboratories
near or associated with patient care facilities. In most cases
the clinical laboratories are under the administration of the
department of pathology. In some institutions, a division or
department of laboratory medicine runs the laboratories. Not
infrequently, laboratories operated by clinical divisions provide
specialized studies; this is usually so when collection of specimens requires special facilities (e.g., gastrointestinal function
studies). In most hospitals, radioactive isotope studies are
performed by the department of radiology through its division of
nuclear medicine.

This book is concerned primarily with laboratory medicine as
it pertains to clinical laboratory studies. Many fine texts
exist that discuss the theory and practice of diagnostic imaging,
laboratory electrophysiology, and the diverse other branches of
laboratory medicine. To these the reader is directed.

ORDERING LABORATORY STUDIES

Laboratory studies can be valuable, even invaluable, sources of information for the clinician in the care of his or her patients. To be of value, though, the studies must be requested and interpreted with the same thoughtfulness that the clinician shows in taking the medical history and performing the physical examination. Specifically, the clinician should ask the following questions before ordering a laboratory study:

1. What do I need to know beyond that which the history and physical examination have revealed?
2. What study(ies), if any, is (are) available that will provide this needed information?
3. Of these, which are the studies to order for this particular patient?

What Does a Clinician Need to Know?

A clinician needs information that will let him or her

1. detect and quantify the risk of future disease
2. detect subclinical disease in apparently healthy persons
3. establish and exclude diagnoses in patients
4. assess the severity of disease
5. establish prognoses for patients.

Of course, not all this information is required for each person seen by a physician. In addition, of the needed information much is derived from good history-taking and appropriate physical examination. The remainder, however, must come from laboratory studies. The analysis of diagnostic laboratory information is the topic of the chapters grouped under the heading "Analytic Principles."

What Laboratory Studies are Available?

Laboratory studies are available that can be used to

1. reveal the location and morphology of normal and abnormal anatomic structures
2. assess organ functional status
3. detect and quantify tissue injury
4. assess the body's metabolic function
5. monitor therapeutic agents
6. detect and monitor neoplasia
7. detect and identify infectious agents.

Studies available in the clinical laboratories can be used to achieve all but the first purpose.

It is the clinican's knowledge of pathophysiology that provides the insight into how a datum generated by a laboratory study represents information pertinent to one of the five clinical needs listed earlier. The aspects of normal and abnormal physiology of particular relevance to this exercise are considered in the chapters grouped under the heading "Physiologic Principles."

Which Are the Laboratory Studies to Order?

A direct answer to this query is beyond the scope of this book. The logic that underlies the ordering of laboratory studies is, however, very much the concern of this book.

The Logic of
Laboratory Medicine

PART I:

ANALYTIC PRINCIPLES

Chapter 1

EXPRESSING LABORATORY RESULTS

"When I use a word," Humpty Dumpty said, in
a rather scornful tone, "it means just what
I choose it to mean — neither more nor
less."
                                    Lewis Carroll

CLASSIFICATION AND QUANTIFICATION

Most laboratory studies are simply measurements. The information requested is of the type "How much, or many, of analyte x is present in this specimen?" As such, these studies are quantitative; that is, they quantify the analyte of interest. The level of quantification achieved varies depending upon clinical needs and the sophistication of the method of measurement.

Binary quantification characterizes **qualitative** studies. The analyte is reported as either "present" or "absent." Study results are arranged into grades or categories for **semiquantitative** studies. Results may, for example, be reported as "absent/trace/ moderate/marked" or "zone I/zone II/zone III." **Quantitative** studies use a scale of measurement graduated into regular divisions called units. For such studies results are expressed as a number followed by a unit. The unit identifies the magnitude of the reference measurement of the analyte, and the number indicates how many multiples of that reference measurement are contained in the specimen. For instance, the study result 123 milligrams per deciliter indicates that 123 multiples of the reference measurement, 1 milligram, are present in 1 deciliter of the plasma.

Laboratory studies may also be performed for the purpose of classification rather than quantification. They answer the question "What is present in this specimen?" For instance, tissue specimens submitted to the surgical pathology laboratory require a pathologic diagnosis. The specimen will be examined macroscopically and microscopically, and numerous observations will be made, sometimes including measurements such as specimen dimensions or number of cell mitoses seen per high power field. The pathologist will then render a pathologic diagnosis that represents his/her interpretation of the accumulated observations. Note that this diagnosis classifies the specimen, not the patient.

No laboratory study, with the possible exception of an autopsy, can satisfactorily answer the question "Given this specimen, what is the clinical state of the patient?" This is the province of clinical diagnosis. Such understanding comes only when all the pertinent clinical facts are available. Thus, these diagnoses remain the responsibility of the patient's physician.

EXPRESSING QUANTITATIVE LABORATORY RESULTS
(Lehmann and Lippert 1978; Lehmann 1979)

Five **base quantities,**

    time
    length
    mass
    amount of substance
    number of entities

and two **secondary quantities,**

    area = length squared
    volume = length cubed

form the basis of the **derived** quantities commonly measured in clinical medicine. They include the following:

Quantity	Derivation
flux	
volume flux	volume/time
mass flux	mass/time
substance flux	amount of substance/time
concentration	
mass concentration	mass/volume
substance concentration	amount of substance/volume (molarity)
	amount of substance/mass (molality)
catalytic concentration	(amount of substrate converted/time)/volume
number concentration	number/volume
pressure	$(\text{mass} \cdot \text{length}/\text{time}^2)/\text{area}$
fraction	
volume fraction	volume/volume
number fraction	number/number
quantity fraction	quantity/quantity

There are one or more units that serve as the basis of the scale of measurement for each quantity. Quantities and units in common use include

Quantity	Unit	Symbol
time	second	s
	minute	min
	hour	h
length	meter	m
mass	gram	g
amount of substance	mole	mol
	equivalent	eq
	osmole	osmol
catalytic activity	international unit	U
	(international unit =	
	micromole per minute)	
volume	liter	L
pressure	millimeter of mercury	mmHg

There exists an International System of Units (Système International d'Unités, abbreviated SI) advanced by the International Committee of Weights and Measures as the system of units to be adopted by all signatories of the Diplomatic Convention of the Meter (1875). From this system there has evolved a recommended system of units (Recommendation 1973) to be used in medicine. This system is based upon the SI, the use of substance quantities rather than mass quantities when possible, and the use of the liter as the preferred unit for volume (rather than m^3).

Recommendation 1973 is the product of the Clinical Chemistry Committee of the International Union of Pure and Applied Chemistry (IUPAC). It is supported by the International Federation of Clinical Chemistry, the International Committee for Standardization in Hematology, and the World Association of (Anatomic and Clinical) Pathology Societies. The medical community in the United States is not generally supportive of Recommendation 1973, but it is likely that laboratories and medical journals here will eventually accede to this international practice. Quantities and units advanced by Recommendation 1973 include

Quantity	Unit	Symbol
time	second	s
	note: minute, hour,	min,h,d,a
	day and year	
	may be used	
length	meter	m
mass	kilogram	kg
amount of substance	mole	mol
number of entities	[none]	
area	square meter	m^2
volume	cubic meter	m^3
	or liter	L

```
mass concentration        kilogram per liter          kg/L
substance concentration   mole per liter              mol/L
                          mole per kilogram           mol/kg
catalytic concentration   katal per liter             kat/L
                          (katal = mole per second)
pressure                  pascal                      Pa
                          (pascal = kilogram per
                                    meter per
                                    square meter)
fractions                 [none]
```

The flexibility of this system of units is increased by the use of magnitude prefixes. Rather than being restricted to using a scale graduated in unit divisions, measurements can be based upon divisions that are powers-often multiples of the standard unit. For example, a substance that is present in a concentration of $1.6(10^{-9})$ moles per liter can be described as having a concentration of 1.6 nanomoles per liter. The prefix nano- takes the place of the factor 10^{-9}. Similarly, large numbers can be avoided by using unit prefixes. A partial pressure of $6(10^{4})$ pascal becomes 60 kilopascal. Table 1-1 lists approved magnitude prefixes. Notice that for factors less than 10^{-3}, prefixes are available only for magnitude changes that are powers of 10^{-3}.

Table 1-1

Magnitude Prefixes for Units

Factor	Prefix	Symbol
10^{3}	kilo	k
10^{2}	hecto	h
10^{1}	deka	da
10^{-1}	deci	d
10^{-2}	centi	c
10^{-3}	milli	m
10^{-6}	micro	µ
10^{-9}	nano	n
10^{-12}	pico	p
10^{-15}	femto	f

The Appendix Table 1-1 to this chapter lists factors for converting between common and SI units for a number of frequently measured analytes.

The Problem of the Measurement of Concentration

The concentration of an analyte may be expressed in a variety of ways:

Expression	Commonly used units
mass concentration	grams per liter (g/L)
substance concentration	moles per liter (mol/L)
	equivalents per liter (eq/L)
	osmoles per kilogram water (osmol/kgH$_2$O)
catalytic concentration	international units per liter (U/L)

where

$moles$ = $mass$ $(g)/formula$ $weight$ of the $analyte$ in $atomic$ $mass$ $units$
$equivalents$ = $moles$ $\cdot$ $ionic$ $charge$ of the $analyte$
$osmoles$ = $moles$ of $discrete$ $particles$

Mass and substance concentrations are interchangeable expressions. A mass concentration can be converted to a substance concentration by dividing by the atomic weight of the analyte.

In general, the equivalent concentration of an analyte is greater than its electrochemical activity and the particle concentration exceeds the osmolality. This is so because in biologic fluids most species are present in free and complex-bound forms, thereby reducing the effective charge and decreasing the number of discrete particles:

$electrochemical$ $activity$ = γ $\cdot$ $equivalent$ $concentration$
$where$ γ = $activity$ $coefficient$ $\leq$ 1.0
$osmolality$ = ϕ $\cdot$ $particle$ $concentration$
$where$ ϕ = $osmotic$ $coefficient$ $\leq$ $1.0.$

When one wishes to quantify the concentration of an analyte participating in an electrochemical process, its electrochemical activity should be measured. If the activity coefficient of the analyte is large (probably greater than 0.6 is a good rule), the equivalent concentration is an adequate estimate of the electrochemical activity. This is so for sodium and potassium, for example. If the activity coefficient is small, the electrochemical activity of the substance should be measured directly. This is recommended for calcium.

If the analyte is participating in an osmotic process, its concentration is best measured as osmolality. It is not possible to measure directly the osmolality of a substance that is in solution with other substances. It is possible to measure the aggregate osmolality of a solution by direct osmometry, as is routinely done for plasma, serum, and urine. Since the physiologic processes of clinical interest depend upon aggregate rather than individual osmolality, solution osmolality is the laboratory determination of interest. For example, the rate of secretion of antidiuretic hormone depends upon total plasma osmolality, not upon the osmolality of any one of the constituent substances.

The plasma concentrations of binding proteins are sometimes expressed as binding capacities. The binding capacity of a protein is the concentration of ligand that can be bound by the protein present. This practice arises from the laboratory method used to quantify some of these proteins. An excess of ligand is mixed with the plasma sample, the bound ligand is separated from the free form, and the concentration of bound ligand is determined. The binding capacity can also be calculated by multiplying a protein's molar concentration times the number of binding sites on the protein.

Concentrations of enzymes are usually expressed as catalytic concentrations. Only occasionally, however, is the actual catalytic activity of an enzyme of clinical interest. Usually, enzyme concentrations are measured to estimate the release rate of intracellular enzymes into the body fluids. This intent would be achieved best by measuring a mass or substance concentration. The catalytic activity of an enzyme as measured in the laboratory depends not only upon the substance concentration of the enzyme but also upon the intactness of the enzyme's active site, the presence or absence of inhibitory substances, and the selection of substrate and reaction conditions. The greater the influence of one or more of the latter variables upon the measurement of enzyme activity, the greater the difference between the catalytic concentration and the substance concentration of the enzyme and, consequently, the less useful the determination. Despite these concerns experience has demonstrated the immense clinical utility of the measurement of enzyme as catalytic concentrations. In practice, very few enzymes are quantified as to mass or substance concentration.

INTERPRETIVE REPORTING

In an effort to ease the burden of data analysis for the clinician in this age of clinical data overload, some laboratories supplement the report of a study result with a brief interpretation. This is called **interpretive reporting**. A number of examples follow:

Factual report	Interpretive report
E. coli, $> 10^5$ organisms/ml urine	This patient has a urinary tract infection. Recommendation: singledose antibiotic therapy to delineate the anatomic site of infection.
175 mg glucose/dl plasma	Abnormal
175 mg glucose/dl plasma	This patient most likely has diabetes mellitus. Other diagnostic considerations include stress hyperglycemia, Cushing's syndrome, and pancreatitis.
8 µg gentamicin/ml plasma	Today's gentamicin level is twice that measured two days ago. If there has not been a change in the dosage regimen, drug accumulation may be occurring. Recommendation: measure creatinine clearance rate.

The appropriateness of this practice is questionable, though, for a number of reasons. First, such interpretations reduce the information content of a quantitative study to that of a semiquantitative or even a qualitative study. Thus interpretive reports are less informative than factual reports. Second, although interpretive reports are most often concerned with diagnostic classification, less than half of all laboratory studies performed are ordered for diagnostic purposes. The interpretations suggested for the glucose concentration in the preceding examples, for instance, are completely out of place when the glucose determinations are being used to monitor intravenous hyperalimentation. The interpretation suggested for the gentamicin concentration, on the other hand, is suited to monitoring purposes. Third, and perhaps most disturbing of all, diagnostic interpretations are rendered without reference to any additional clinical information. As will be discussed in subsequent chapters, this is <u>not</u> the way to integrate laboratory findings into the diagnostic process.

MANIPULATION OF LABORATORY RESULTS

Laboratory results are often transformed, or manipulated, to make them more informative to the clinician.

Scale (Unit) Conversion

Probably the most frequently performed manipulation of laboratory results is the changing of the reference magnitude (unit) of the scale of measurement. The formula for a unit conversion ($unit_1$ to $unit_2$) is

$$\begin{array}{ccc} number\ of\ multiples & = & number\ of\ multiples \quad \cdot \quad number\ of\ multiples \\ of\ unit_2 & & of\ unit_1 \qquad\qquad of\ unit_2\ in\ one\ unit_1 \end{array}$$

For example, consider the conversion of the whole blood hemoglobin concentration 16 g/dl to its SI expression.

$$SI\ unit\ of\ hemoglobin\ concentration = mol/L$$

and

$$\begin{array}{cc} number\ of\ multiples & = 10 \quad \cdot \quad \dfrac{1}{64,500} = 1.55\ (10^{-4}). \\ of\ mol/L\ in\ 1\ g/dl & \end{array}$$

$$\begin{array}{cc} conversion & conversion \\ of\ dl\ to\ L & of\ g\ to\ mole \end{array}$$

Thus,

$$\begin{array}{l} hemoglobin\ concentration = 16\ \cdot\ 1.55\ (10^{-4}) = 2.48\ mmol/L. \\ \quad in\ mol/L \end{array}$$

Normalizing Data

For certain quantitative studies, the interindividual biologic component of measurement variability (see Chapter 2) can be reduced by **normalization** of the study results. Consider Figure 1-1. The left panel depicts the values of a quantity, Y, found in a small group of individuals. Y ranges from y_1 to y_7. The right panel graphs the same results as a function of a variable X that is known to affect the value of Y. For given values of X, the range of values for Y is much smaller. At x_8, for instance, Y varies only between y_3 and y_4. Here normalizing the values of y for the concurrent values of X reduces the measurement variability.

Normalization is a two-step procedure. First, the value of the quantity to be normalized is adjusted to eliminate the effect

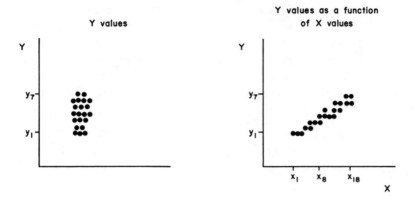

Fig 1-1   Reduction of Measurement
Variability by Normalization

of the recognized source of variability.   The usual adjustment is
a division:

   adjusted value = unadjusted value/value of normalizing quantity.

When there is a proportional relationship between the normalized
and normalizing quantities, i.e., when the value of one is a
multiple of the other, normalization by division yields a constant, the constant of proportionality.   Any difference between
the normalized value and the value of the constant is attributable to other sources of measurement variability, such as disease.   Second, the adjusted result is scaled to a normalization
standard by a unit conversion.   The unit for the normalized
measurement will indicate the normalization standard used.

   For example, measurement variability in the endogenous creatinine clearance rate is reduced substantially by normalizing for
body surface area.   The generally accepted normalization standard
is a surface area of 1.73 m^2.   For a female patient with a creatinine clearance of 50 ml/min and surface area of 1.2 m^2,

   adjusted clearance rate = 50/1.2 = 41.67 (ml/min)/m^2.

Unit conversion to the normalization standard yields

   normalized clearance rate = 41.67 · 1.73 = 72 (ml/min)/1.73 m^2.

                          conversion of
                          m^2 to 1.73 m^2

- 11 -

The unit expression indicates the unit of measurement, milliliters per minute, and the normalizing standard, 1.73 m^2. The
adjusted creatinine clearance rate in this patient differs from
the constant of proportionality between clearance rate and surface area, 55 (ml/min)/m^2, but is not outside of the range of
adjusted clearance rates in healthy adult females, 34-76
(ml/min)/m^2.

Calculated Values

When direct measurement of a quantity is impractical or impossible, its magnitude may be estimated by calculation. The
measurements used as quantitative input for these calculations
may describe quantities that have a theoretical relationship to
the unmeasured quantity, such as that among plasma bicarbonate
concentration in milliequivalents per liter (the unmeasured quantity), pH, and the partial pressure of dissolved carbon dioxide
(P_{CO2}) in millimeters of mercury:

$$log\ [HCO_3^-] = (pH - 6.1) + log\ 0.0301\ P_{CO2}.$$

Alternatively, a calculation may be based upon an empirical relationship between the unmeasured and measured quantities. The
calculation of body surface area using body height and weight is
an example.

Calculations can be performed in two ways. If a mathematical
formula is available, the value can be computed. This has become
particularly simple since the advent of inexpensive, powerful
handheld computers. Data presented as tables or diagrams and
graphic representations of mathematical equations, called nomograms, remove the need to make computations. For this reason
they are popular.

Surface area can be calculated from body weight and height,
for instance, using the formula of DuBois and DuBois (1916):

$$surface\ area\ (m^2) = 0.00784\ weight\ (kg)^{0.425} \cdot height\ (cm)^{0.725}.$$

Using this formula, a 20-year-old male who weighs 64 kg and is
145 cm tall has a surface area of 1.56 m^2. The DuBois and DuBois
formula is also available as a nomogram (Figure 1-2).

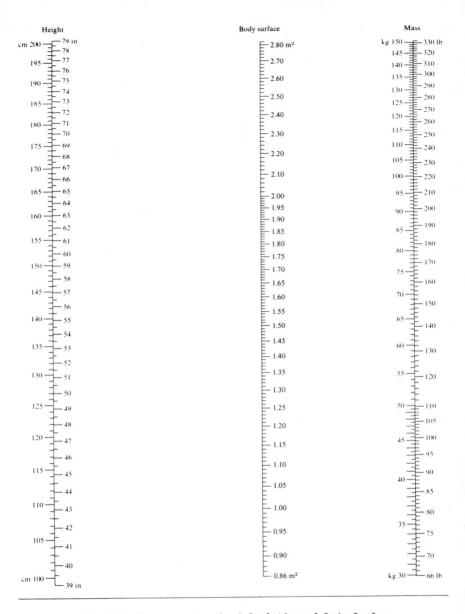

Fig 1-2   Nomogram for the Calculation of Body Surface
Area According to DuBois and DuBois (1916)
(From Lentner, C., ed. Geigy Scientific Tables, 8th
edition, volume 1, p. 227 © 1981, Ciba-Geigy, Basle)

To use the nomogram: Locate the weight in kilograms on the
right axis and the height in centimeters on the left axis.
Connect these two points with a straightedge. The point on
the center axis intersected by the straightedge is the body
surface area in square meters.

Gehan and George (1970) suggest that a somewhat different formula for body surface area is more accurate:

$$surface\ area\ (m^2) = 0.0235\ weight\ (kg)^{0.51456} \cdot height\ (cm)^{0.42246}.$$

Here the young man's surface area is found to be 1.65 m^2. The nomogram form of this formula is shown in Figure 1-3.

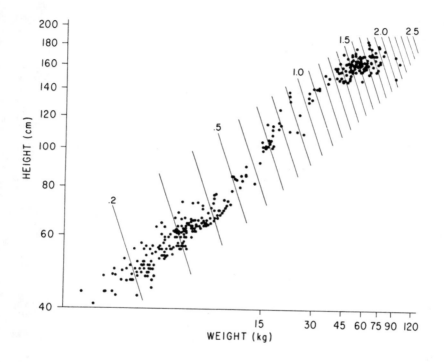

Fig 1-3 Nomogram for the Calculation of Body Surface
Area According to Gehan and George (1970)

To use the nomogram: Locate the weight in kilograms on the horizontal axis and the height in centimeters on the vertical axis (note: Because the scales are logarithmic, interpolated points are difficult to find accurately). Using a straightedge, construct two lines: one perpendicular to the horizontal axis, passing through the stipulated weight; the other perpendicular to the vertical axis, passing through the stipulated height. Locate the intersection of these two lines. The angled lines in the coordinate space are surface area isopleths (lines of equal measure). Identify the surface area rounded to the nearest tenth square meter.

Perform the following unit conversions:

1-1. 145 meq sodium/L to SI unit

1-2. 10 mg calcium/dl to eq/L

1-3. 14 U/L to SI unit

1-4. Present an argument in favor of establishing the mole per liter as the preferred unit for substance concentration. Present an argument against such a plan.

1-5. What is the normalized creatinine clearance for a 30-year-old female who weighs 50 kg, is 140 cm tall, and has a creatinine clearance of 110 ml/min?

1-6. An 18-year-old woman presents to your primary care clinic complaining of a swollen leg. Physical examination reveals a large, well circumscribed region of subcutaneous edema on one leg. She says that it started as a small bump where she hit her leg on a chair. Furthermore, other members of her family react to minor trauma in a similar fashion. You consider hereditary angioedema a possibility. Plasma complement (C1) esterase inhibitor, the deficiency of which causes hereditary angioedema, is present in normal concentration (20 mg/dl) as measured by radial immunodiffusion. The level determined by functional assay (40% normal activity) is reduced, however. Which result do you believe?

Mind-Expanding Exercise

1-7. Construct a nomogram for the calculation of plasma P_{CO2} (20-60 mmHg for multiples of ten) based upon plasma pH (7.2 to 7.6) and bicarbonate concentration (12 to 36 meq/L). Suggestion: Use the Gehan and George (1970) nomogram as a model.

REFERENCES

DuBois, D., DuBois, E.F. A formula to estimate the approximate surface area if height and weight be known. Arch. Intern. Med. 17:863, 1916.

Gehan, E.A., George, S.L. Estimation of human body surface area from height and weight. Cancer Chemother. Rep. 54:255, 1970.

Lehmann, H.P. SI units. CRC Crit. Rev. Clin. Lab. Sci. 8:147, 1979.

Lippert, H., Lehmann, H.P. SI Units in Medicine. Urban & Schwarzenberg, Baltimore, 1978.

APPENDIX

Conversions Between Common and SI Units

The following table lists the common units, SI units, and conversion factors for changing units for a number of analytes frequently measured in the clinical laboratory. Specific enzymes have not been included because the SI unit for catalytic activity, the katal, has not as yet been embraced by clinical laboratorians. In its stead the International Unit (U) remains the preferred unit.

Common Units, SI Units, and Conversion Factors

Analyte	Common unit	SI unit	Conversion factors Common unit to SI unit	Conversion factors SI unit to common unit
Albumin	g/dl	mmol/L	0.145	6.9
Ammonia	µg/dl	µmol/L	0.587	1.7
Bilirubin	mg/dl	µmol/L	17.1	0.058
Blood cell count	$10^3/\mu l$	$10^9/L$	10^6	10^{-6}
Carbon dioxide	meq/L	mmol/L	1	1
Calcium	mg/dl	mmol/L	0.25	4.0
Ceruloplasmin	mg/dl	umol/L	0.066	15.2
Chloride	meq/L	mmol/L	1	1
Cholesterol	mg/dl	mmol/L	0.0259	38.6
Copper	µg/dl	µmol/L	0.157	6.37
Cortisol	µg/dl	µmol/L	0.0276	36.2
Creatinine	mg/dl	µmol/L	88.4	0.011
Enzymes	U/L	nkat/L	16.67	0.06
Ferritin	µg/L	pmol/L	2.2	0.445
Fibrinogen	mg/dl	µmol/L	0.029	34.5
Folate	µg/dl	nmol/L	22.7	0.044
Glucose	mg/dl	mmol/L	0.0555	18.0
Haptoglobin	mg/dl	µmol/L	0.118	8.47
Hematocrit	%	[none]	0.01	100
Hemoglobin	g/dl	mmol/L	0.155	6.45
Iron	µg/dl	umol/L	0.179	5.59
Ketone bodies (as acetoacetate)	mg/dl	mmol/L	0.111	9.01
Lactic acid	mg/dl	mmol/L	0.111	9.01
Magnesium	mg/dl	mmol/L	0.411	2.43
Osmolality	mOsm/L	mK (milli degree Kelvin)	1.86	0.54
P_{CO2}	mmHg	kPa	0.133	7.5
P_{O2}	mmHg	kPa	0.133	7.5
Phosphorus	mg/dl	mmol/L	0.323	3.1
Potassium	meq/L	mmol/L	1	1
Red cell indices				
MCV	μm^3	fl	1	1
MCH	pg	pg	1	1
MCHC	%	[none]	0.01	100
Sodium	meq/L	mmol/L	1	1
Thyroxine	µg/dl	nmol/L	12.9	0.078
Transferrin	mg/dl	µmol/L	0.114	8.77
Triglycerides	mg/dl	mmol/L	0.0114	87.7
Urea nitrogen	mg/dl	mmol/L	0.714	1.4
Uric acid	mg/dl	mmol/L	0.0595	16.8
Vitamin B12	ng/dl	pmol/L	7.38	0.1355
Zinc	µg/dl	µmol/L	0.153	6.54

Abbreviations used: P_{CO2}, partial pressure of carbon dioxide; P_{O2}, partial pressure of oxygen; MCV, mean corpuscular volume; MCH, mean corpuscular hemoglobin; MCHC, mean corpuscular hemoglobin concentration.

Chapter 2

VARIABILITY IN LABORATORY MEASUREMENT

There is nothing in this world constant,
but inconstancy.

Jonathan Swift

SOURCES OF VARIABILITY
(Statland and Winkel 1977; Young 1979)

A laboratory measurement performed upon many different individuals or upon a single individual many times will show differences in the magnitude of the entity measured, that is, there will be **measurement variability**. This variability comes from a number of sources:

1. biologic variability
2. preanalytic variability
3. analytic variability
4. postanalytic variability.

Biologic Variability

Biologic variability is due to the heterogeneity of physiologic influences among individuals and in individuals over time. It is distinguished from other sources of variability in that it cannot be controlled to reduce its effect. The two components of biologic variability are

1. interindividual variability
2. intraindividual variability.

Interindividual variability alludes to differences in the magnitude of a laboratory measurement among individuals. Important sources of interindividual variability include

1. race
2. gender
3. age
4. body size.

Intraindividual variability refers to differences in a study result in one individual when determinations are made at different times. Important sources of intraindividual variability include
1. diurnal rhythms
2. circadian periodicity
3. the menstrual cycle
4. seasonal cycles
5. aging.

Typically, intraindividual variability is smaller than interindividual variability. Consequently, interindividual variability largely determines the total biologic variability. This finding is illustrated in Figure 2-1. For ten individuals, here numbered one through ten, the range of a set of replicate laboratory studies is shown. This range, one measure of total biologic variability, is separated into its component parts: the interindividual component, i.e., the range of average study results among the individuals, and the intraindividual component, i.e., the range of study results for each individual. Clearly, here the interindividual variability contributes more to the total

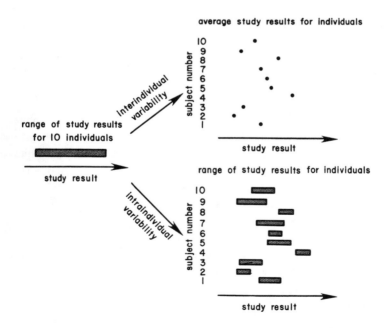

Fig 2-1   Separating Inter- from Intraindividual Variability

variability. Indeed, even if there were no intraindividual variability at all, the total range of study results would not be
lessened very much.

Preanalytic Variability

Preanalytic variability is due to physiologic influences that
can be controlled in the individual upon whom the measurement is
made. It also results from the effects of specimen collection
and handling, factors that can be controlled by the laboratory.

Important sources of physiologic preanalytic variability and,
therefore, important considerations in patient preparation include

1. food intake (including caffeine and ethanol-containing
   beverages)
2. physical exercise
3. drug therapy (including self prescribed drugs).

As a rule, it is recommended that laboratory studies be performed in the morning following an overnight fast. Strenuous,
stressful, or emotional physical activity should be avoided. If
drug therapy cannot be suspended, the laboratory results must be
interpreted with consideration of the influence of the therapy
upon the measurement. (Drugs may interfere with analytic methods
as well as alter the physiologic state of the patient.)

Important sources of variability due to specimen collection
and handling must be considered in reference to the type of
specimen. See Chapter 15 for further details.

Analytic Variability

Analytic variability is the variability in laboratory measurement that can be attributed to the analytic method generating
the measurement. The analytic method includes materials, equipment, procedures, and personnel. Variable performance of each of
these components contributes to the total analytic variability.
Analytic variability can be divided into

1. inaccuracy
2. imprecision

Inaccuracy is systematic error. It is measured as the difference between the mean of a set of replicate measurements and
the true or accepted value of the measurement. Imprecision is
the term applied to nonsystematic, that is random, error. It is
measured as the variability in a set of replicate measurements.

Analytic variability is kept within acceptable limits by both rigorous assessment and ongoing surveillance of the analytic method, using a **quality assurance program**. The definition of acceptable performance, i.e., tolerable limits of variability, for analytic methods is an area of intense current interest and controversy.

Postanalytic Variability

Postanalytic variability in laboratory measurement arises between the completion of the analytic method and the assimilation of the measurement by the clinician.

The major source of postanalytic variability is transcription error. Such errors may be made by laboratory personnel, laboratory clerks, ward clerks, medical students, resident physicians, or attending physicians. The opportunity for such error increases with increasing numbers of transcriptions. Therefore, the original laboratory report form is the most reliable source for the measurement.

The Clinician's Role in the Quality Assurance Program

Despite all the efforts to eliminate mistakes in the performance of laboratory studies, inevitably some study results that reach the clinician will harbor a laboratory error. The clinician must be vigilant for the evidence of such errors. At the same time, he or she must also remain open to the possibility that a study with a suspicious result was performed correctly and that the results, though surprising, are valid for the specimen received.

Laboratory error should be considered in each of the following three circumstances:

1. The study result is unreasonable, unphysiologic, or impossible.
2. The study result is inconsistent with previous results from the same patient or is incompatible with the results of other studies performed on the same specimen.
3. The study result differs from that expected on the grounds of the clinical impression. Here, the consideration of a laboratory error is appropriate, but re-evaluation of the clinical impression is equally necessary. It may even be advisable to confirm that the result really is inconsistent with the impression.

When a laboratory error is suspected, the clinician must act to confirm or refute the suspicion. It is not enough simply to ignore the result. If the result truly is in error, the laboratory must be made aware of the problem so that steps may be taken to prevent its recurrence. If the result is valid, the clinician must confront the unpleasant fact that either his or her interpretation of the study result was faulty or that his or her clinical impression may be incomplete or even frankly incorrect.

The clinician should evaluate the possible influences of known sources of biologic and preanalytic variability upon the laboratory study. Special attention should be paid to the effects of drug therapy upon both the physiologic state of the patient and the reliability of the laboratory study. If laboratory error is still suspected, he or she should request that the laboratory repeat the study upon the original specimen and, if possible, upon a new specimen. These actions, taken in the stated order, will detect the site of the error in almost all cases in which an error exists. Of equal importance, however, is that this regimen will also reveal the explanation for a puzzling but valid result and thereby facilitate patient care.

FREQUENCY DISTRIBUTIONS

When a laboratory study has been performed upon a number of individuals, a sample of a population, it is possible to construct a table or graph that relates the study results to their frequency of occurrence in the individuals studied. This relationship is called a **frequency distribution**. It characterizes the variability in measurement in the studied sample. The distribution may be used to estimate the probability of the occurrence of a particular study result in a person belonging to the same population. Conversely, the distribution may be used when estimating the probability that a studied individual belongs to the population from which the distribution was generated, based upon the study result in the individual. For both of these uses, the level of certainty of the estimate depends upon the number of persons in the sample from which the distribution was derived. The larger the sample size, the more reliable the estimate.

Frequency distributions may be discrete or continuous. Discrete distributions arise from qualitative and semiquantitative laboratory studies. Quantitative studies generate distributions that approach being continuous. Frequency distributions are graphed by plotting the frequency of occurrence of a study result versus the value of the study result. Figure 2-2 depicts two hypothetical frequency distributions. The discrete distribution arises from a five-category semiquantitative study.

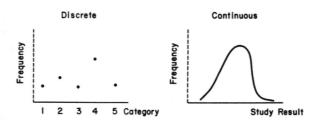

Fig 2-2   Two Frequency Distributions

Frequency distributions may be symmetric or asymmetric. Most biologic distributions are asymmetric. For a distribution with a single peak, i.e., one that is unimodal, if the bulk of the distribution lies to the left of the peak, the distribution is said to be "skewed to the left." If the bulk of the distribution lies to the right of the peak, the distribution is "skewed to the right." Distributions with more than one peak are called polymodal.

Frequency distributions can be presented in three ways:

1. Exhaustive listing — Each study result is listed with its associated frequency of occurrence; a graphic representation of a probability distribution is one form of exhaustive listing.

2. Percentiles — Study results are listed with the associated cumulative probability of that or a lesser study result.

3. Probability distribution functions — For some distributions, it is possible to express the relationship between the study results and the frequency of respective study results by use of a mathematical formula called a probability distribution function. The Gaussian (normal) and the log Gaussian probability distribution functions are of particular interest because the frequency distributions of many laboratory studies may be described by either one or the other.

Reference Frequency Distributions
(Gräsbeck and Alstrom 1981)

The central problem in the use of diagnostic laboratory studies is that of variability. A clinician must be able to decide if a given study is better explained by the presence of a certain disorder or by measurement variability in the study among persons free of the disease. To do this the clinician must have access to information regarding the distribution of study results in persons with and without the disorder. This is the function of **reference frequency distributions**.

A reference distribution is the frequency distribution that arises from the performance of a defined laboratory study upon a sample from a defined, or reference, subject population.

Establishing a Reference Distribution
(Gräsbeck et al. 1979; Ransohoff and Feinstein 1978)

The determination of a reference distribution for a laboratory study proceeds in five steps:

1. definition of the analytic procedure, equipment, and reagents that generate the measurement
2. definition of the reference population by specification of the criteria for subject inclusion and exclusion
3. solicitation of sample subjects and performance of the study
4. calculation of the study's frequency distribution
5. selection of the appropriate presentation of the probability distribution.

A satisfactory statement of the inclusion criteria for the population of individuals afflicted by the disease of interest is of paramount importance. These criteria, which amount to the basis for the diagnosis of the disease, must rely upon a universally accepted method for identifying the disease. Such methods are called reference methods or "gold standards." A related concern is that the stage or severity of the disease be considered when constructing the reference criteria.

The inclusion and exclusion criteria applied to populations free of the particular disease will determine the clinical settings in which these reference distributions will be useful. The criteria should define persons similar to those upon whom the laboratory study will be performed in practice. For instance, if the study is to be used to screen for a disease in the general population, a sample of the general population should be used. On the other hand, if the study is to be used exclusively to identify disease in a select subset of patients, the sample should consist of members of that subset. At the same time, the sample subjects should represent as broad a spectrum of biologic variability as is possible within the confines of the stipulated criteria. In particular, gender, age, and body size should be considered when defining the desired subject composition of the sample because these three characteristics contribute so much to the biologic variability of most laboratory studies. Alternatively, reference distributions may be constructed for each gender, for certain intervals of age, or for set intervals of body size. For a number of laboratory studies, this approach has been undertaken and has contributed greatly to the clinical usefulness of the reference distributions derived. In Figure 2-3 separate reference frequency distributions based upon gender are illustrated for the measurement of serum albumin concentration.

After the collection of the study results, the frequency distribution is calculated. Of course, because only a sample of the reference population has been studied, the calculated distribution is a sample distribution, that is, an estimate of the true reference distribution. The level of confidence in this estimate depends upon the number of subjects in the sample. The number required to assure a valid sampling of a reference population is a matter of some controversy and will not be discussed here. Suffice it to say that the number is large, certainly in the hundreds.

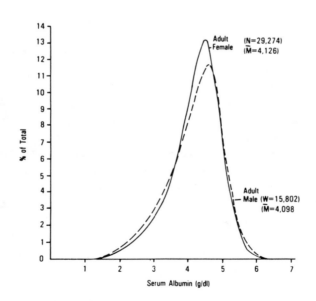

Fig 2-3   Frequency Distributions of Serum Albumin Concentration
(From Ritchie, R.F. Interpretation of serum protein
values. In: Ritzmann, S.E. (ed.) Physiology of
Immunoglobulins, p. 184 © 1982, Alan R. Liss, New York)

For those laboratory studies generating probability distributions that are well described by a Gaussian distribution function, the reference distribution can be described in terms of the distribution's mean and standard deviation. Data that do not fit a Gaussian distribution may become Gaussian following a mathematical transformation. For example, many plasma analytes have log Gaussian distributions. This means that the logarithms of the test results, though not the (untransformed) results themselves, distribute in a Gaussian manner.

If there is any doubt about the validity of a Gaussian description of a reference distribution, and there frequently is, the distribution should be recorded in its percentile form. Of course, the percentile presentation can also be used when the distribution fits the Gaussian form.

The Elusive Reference Population — Normals
(Feinstein 1974; Murphy 1966, 1972)

A persistent notion in clinical medicine is that of a reference frequency distribution based upon normal individuals, the so-called **normal range**. The identification of members of this reference population, and therefore the idea and use of normal ranges, is problematic, however.

What, for instance, is meant by the inclusion criterion "normal?" Murphy lists seven different ways in which the word normal is used (Table 2-1). For each use he proposes an alternative, preferable term. The paraphrase most nearly equivalent to the meaning of normal as it is used in laboratory medicine is number 3, "commonly encountered in its class," but the concept in number 4, that of "fittest," is often implied. For example, in some laboratories normal ranges are based upon the study results found in volunteers among the laboratory staff, the majority of whom are young and fit.

What are the exclusion criteria? Are there any? Some laboratories construct a normal range from values that arise from a study performed upon a sample of specimens submitted to the laboratory for other determinations. Some results are discarded on the basis of statistical rules, but no specimen, and therefore no sample subject, is excluded prior to the performance of the study.

Because of these and other conceptual difficulties inherent in identifying a normal population, the use of normal ranges is discouraged. In their stead, well characterized reference distributions should be used.

Table 2-1 Meanings for the Word Normal
(From Murphy, E.A. The Logic of Medicine, p. 125
© 1976, Johns Hopkins University Press, Baltimore)

Paraphrase	Domains of use	Preferable term
1. Having probability density function $$f(x) = \frac{1}{\sqrt{o^2 2\pi}} \exp\left[-\frac{1}{2}\left(\frac{x-\mu}{\sigma}\right)^2\right]$$	Statistics (predicated of a metrical character)	Gaussian
2. Most representative of its class	Descriptive science (biology, etc.)	Average, median, modal
3. Commonly encountered in its class	Descriptive science	Habitual
4. Most suited to survival and reproduction	Genetics, operations research quality control, etc.	Optimal or "fittest"
5. Carrying no penalty	Clinical medicine	Innocuous or harmless
6. Commonly aspired to	Politics, sociology, etc.	Conventional
7. Most perfect of its class	Metaphysics, esthetics, morals, etc.	Ideal

2-1. List examples of plasma analytes that show significant measurement variability due to each of the following:
1. gender
2. age
3. diurnal rhythm
4. analytic method.

2-2. Calculate the frequency distribution for the following study results. Present the distribution as an exhaustive listing, in percentiles, and in terms of its mean and standard deviation.

6	6	12
11	7	10
5	8	8
9	8	7
9	9	9
6	7	8
10	8	7
8	10	10
9	8	9
8	9	7

2-3. A young diabetic patient who in the past has had many keto-acidotic episodes is found to have a plasma glucose concentration of 360 mg/dl. His plasma potassium is also mildly elevated at 5.5 meq/L. He admits having skipped his last dose of insulin. Insulin is administered and 2 hours later the glucose level is 250 mg/dl, but the potassium concentration has increased to 6.0 meq/L. What do you do next?

2-4. Describe the appropriate reference populations, including clinical spectrums, for a laboratory study designed to detect acute myocardial infarction.

2-5. Discuss the sources of biologic variability that must be considered when constructing a frequency distribution for plasma cholesterol concentration in disease-free individuals.

Mind-Expanding Exercise

2-6. Find an example of a frequency distribution for which two or more sources of interindividual measurement variability have been taken into account.

REFERENCES

Feinstein, A.R. Clinical biostatistics. XXVII: The derange-
ments of the "range of normal." Clin. Pharmacol. Ther.
15:528, 1974.

Gräsbeck, R., Siest, G., Wilding, P., et al. Provisional recommendation on the theory of reference values. Part 1: The
concept of reference values. Clin. Chem. 25:1506, 1979.

Gräsbeck, R., Alstrom, T. Reference Values in Laboratory Medicine. John Wiley and Sons, New York, 1981.

Murphy, E.A. A scientific viewpoint on normalcy. Perspect.
Biol. Med. 9:33, 1966.

Murphy, E.A. The normal and the perils of the sylleptic argument. Perspect. Biol. Med. 15:566, 1972.

Ransohoff, D.F., Feinstein, A.R. Problems of spectrum and bias
in evaluating the efficacy of diagnostic tests. N. Engl. J.
Med. 299:926, 1978.

Statland, B.E., Winkel, P. Effects of preanalytical factors on
the intraindividual variation of analytes in the blood of
healthy subjects: Consideration of preparation of the subject
and time of venipuncture. CRC Crit. Rev. Clin. Lab. Sci.
8:105, 1977.

Young, D.S. Biologic variability. In: Brown, S.S., Mitchell,
F.L., Young, D.S. (eds.) Chemical Diagnosis of Disease.
Elsevier, Amsterdam, pp. 1-114, 1979.

Chapter 3

DIAGNOSTIC CLASSIFICATION

1. Study Performance

"Tracks," said Piglet, "Paw-marks."   He gave
a little squeak of excitement, "Oh, Pooh! Do
you think it's a-a-a Woozle?"

"It may be," said Pooh.   "Sometimes it is,
and sometimes it isn't. You never can tell
with paw-marks."
                                        A. A. Milne

DIAGNOSTIC STUDIES

A laboratory study that is designed, or discovered, to aid in
making a clinical diagnosis does so by improving the clinician's
ability to discriminate between persons suffering from the disease or condition of interest and persons free from the disease
or condition. This improved discrimination may be a result of
the study's superior ability to identify afflicted individuals,
its success in identifying unaffected persons, or a combination
of the two.

STUDY PERFORMANCE
(Galen and Gambino 1975; Griner et al. 1981)

The performance of a laboratory study as a diagnostic aid is
characterized by its **sensitivity** and **specificity**. The sensitivity of a study is the frequency with which the study indicates
the correct diagnosis in persons with the disease. The specificity is the frequency with which the study indicates the correct diagnosis in individuals who are disease free.

As an example, the data obtained in a clinical investigation
concerned with the laboratory diagnosis of iron deficiency in
1-year-old infants (Dallman et al. 1981) can be used to quantify
the performance of the study "transferrin saturation."   Plasma
transferrin saturation was determined in capillary blood specimens from 165 1-year-olds who were suspected of having iron
deficiency anemia.   Infants were classified as iron deficient if
the transferrin saturation was less than 10% and as iron replete
if the transferrin saturation was greater than 10%.   The study

Table 3-1

Classification Categories for Transferrin Saturation

Classification using transferrin saturation	Final diagnostic classification	
	Iron replete	Iron deficient
Iron replete	82	26
Iron deficient	28	29

Data from Dallman et al. (1981).

classifications, categorized according to the final diagnostic classification, are presented in Table 3-1. The numerical entries indicate the number of study subjects in each category.

The sensitivity of the study is calculated as the frequency of correct diagnosis in the iron deficient infants. In this case, the frequency is 29 divided by 55 which equals 0.53. A little better than one-half of the diseased infants are properly identified. The specificity is the frequency of correct diagnosis in the iron-replete subjects; here, it is 82 divided by 110 which equals 0.75. Three-quarters of the nondiseased infants are correctly identified. Notice that the denominators in the above calculations are found by adding the numbers in the respective columns of the category table.

A table of classification categories, as used in the example, can be constructed for any diagnostic study (Table 3-2). The

Table 3-2

Classification Categories for a Diagnostic Study

Study classification	Confirmed classification	
	Disease free	Disease
Disease free	True negative result	False negative result
Disease	False positive result	True positive result

designations true or false and positive or negative are usually assigned to the categories as shown.

From the table,

$$sensitivity = \frac{true\ positive\ results}{true\ positive\ results\ +\ false\ negative\ results}$$

and

$$specificity = \frac{true\ negative\ results}{true\ negative\ results\ +\ false\ positive\ results}$$

Because a study's sensitivity is determined by the frequency distribution of results in a single reference population, i.e., persons confirmed to have the disease, it will remain constant. There will be some variability in its measurement because the composition of the sample of subjects from which the measurement is made will vary by chance. But as long as the subjects are chosen at random from the same reference population, the estimates of the study's sensitivity will cluster around the value that would be found were the entire reference population to be studied. The same is true for specificity, which is determined by the frequency distribution of results in the reference population of persons known not to have the disease. It is clear, however, that both values will depend upon the inclusion and exclusion criteria that are stipulated when defining the reference populations and upon the spectrums of biologic variability in the samples of the populations. Therefore, it is absolutely essential to avoid the common practice of assuming that the values for a laboratory study's sensitivity and specificity as found in one reference population apply to a different clinical population. It would be ludicrous, for instance, to believe that the sensitivity and specificity of transferrin saturation for the diagnosis of iron deficiency would be the same for 1-year-old infants and for their mothers. For these two disparate populations, the performance of the study probably differs greatly. Although it may be less obvious, it is also improper to assume that the performance of a study in a select, i.e., nonrandom, sample of the reference population will be equivalent to the performance for the entire population. Laboratory studies almost always perform less well when they are applied to a nonselected, i.e. random, sample.

The Performance Characteristic Function
(McNeil et al. 1975; Metz 1978)

The findings obtained in any investigation of the performance of a diagnostic study depend upon the critical value. This is the study result that differentiates disease from freedom from disease. The critical value can be chosen, for example, to achieve a desired level of sensitivity for the study. The specificity of the study arising from this selection cannot then be arbitrarily set but instead is determined by the designated critical value and the frequency distribution of study results in the reference population of individuals free from the disease. An example of this is shown in Figure 3-1 in which the critical value A gives the study a sensitivity of 0.90. The corresponding specificity is 0.80 (Note: as depicted, the sensitivity of the study equals the area under the upper frequency distribution lying to the right of the critical value; the specificity equals the area under the lower frequency distribution lying to the left of the critical value.) Another common practice is to select the critical value so that a certain specificity is obtained. In that circumstance, the sensitivity of the test cannot be set, but rather is determined by the selected critical value and the frequency distribution of study results in the reference population of diseased individuals. In Figure 3-1 the critical value B has been chosen to give a study specificity of 0.95. The sensitivity is then 0.60. Notice that these different study performances came about merely from altering the critical value for the study.

The set of sensitivity and specificity pairs that are gener-

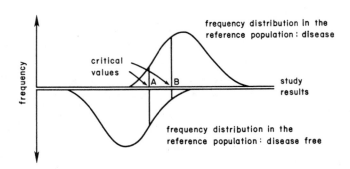

Fig 3-1   Reference Frequency Distributions
           for a Laboratory Study

ated by considering every possible critical value for a laboratory study constitute the **performance characteristic function.**
This function completely defines the performance of the study
when applied to a given pair of reference frequency distributions. Consequently, it is the most informative way to record
the findings from an investigation of the study's performance.
Using it, one can identify the critical value that generates a
desired pairing of sensitivity and specificity.

A performance characteristic function for transferrin saturation can be obtained by again referring to the data reported by
Dallman et al. (1981). The authors include in their article
histograms indicating the distribution of study values in the two
reference populations. Study values are categorical, being of
the form "less than a% but greater than b%." In Figure 3-2 the
data are recast as frequency distributions.

To construct the performance characteristic function, first
select an extreme study value (here 0% is a likely choice) and
calculate the sensitivity and specificity that would result were
this the critical value. No iron deficient subject has a transferrin saturation less than 0% so the sensitivity is 0. All the
iron replete subjects have saturations greater than 0% so the
specificity is 1.0. Then, repeat the calculations using the next
permissible value of the study, 5%, as the critical value. Since

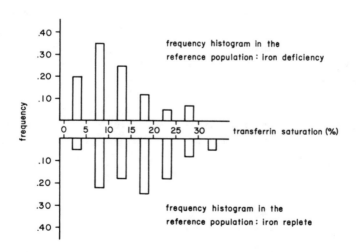

Fig 3-2   Reference Frequency Histograms
for Transferrin Saturation
[Data from Dallman et al. (1981)]

Table 3-3

Performance Characteristic Function
for Transferrin Saturation

	Critical value						
	0%	5%	10%	15%	20%	25%	30%
Sensitivity	0	0.20	0.53	0.76	0.87	0.93	1.00
Specificity	1.00	0.96	0.75	0.55	0.32	0.13	0.04

Data from Dallman et al. (1981).

0.2 of the iron-deficient infants have transferrin saturations below 5%, the sensitivity is 0.2. Of the iron replete subjects, 0.04 have saturations less than 5% so only 0.96 of these subjects are correctly identified. Thus, the specificity is 0.96. This procedure is repeated until all the possible critical values have been considered. The results for these data are shown in Table 3-3. When 10% is used as the critical value, which is the case in the article, the specificity and sensitivity values are 0.75 and 0.53, respectively, as was found earlier.

Performance characteristic functions are often presented in their graphic form. These are called **performance characteristic curves** or, for historic reasons, **receiver operating characteristic curves**. Figure 3-3 shows the performance characteristic curve for transferrin saturation.

Efficacy

The **efficacy** of a diagnostic study in a clinical setting, defined as the overall frequency of correct diagnostic classification, is determined by three factors:

1. the sensitivity of the study
2. the specificity of the study
3. the relative number of diseased versus disease-free persons in the clinical population.

The term usually applied to the third parameter is disease **prevalence** or simply **prevalence**, which is the fraction of persons in the clinical population suffering from the disease. The fraction of persons free from the disease is then one minus the

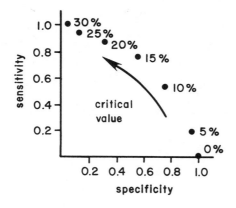

Fig 3-3   Performance Characteristic Curve
for Transferrin Saturation
[Data from Dallman et al. (1981)]

prevalence. Prevalence is a term also used in epidemiologic
studies.   There the denominator used in the calculation of
disease prevalence is the number of persons in a specified
demographic population.   When the demographic population is the
same as the clinical population of interest, the prevalences are
identical.

The effects of disease prevalence upon study efficacy are
indicated by rewriting the definition of efficacy,

$$efficacy = \frac{true\ positive\ results\ +\ true\ negative\ results}{total\ number\ of\ study\ results}$$

in terms of sensitivity, specificity, and prevalence.   For instance, the number of true negative results equals the number of
individuals free of the disease times the specificity of the
study:

$$(1 - prevalence) \cdot N \cdot specificity$$

where N is the total number of subjects studied.   Substituting
the alternative expressions for each of the components of the
efficacy formula yields

$$efficacy = prevalence \cdot sensitivity + (1 - prevalence)\ specificity.$$

This formula reveals the validity of a number of intuitive insights regarding the behavior of study efficacy. First, when the disease prevalence is low, the efficacy of the study is determined largely by its specificity. Second, when the disease prevalence is high, the efficacy of a study is determined largely by its sensitivity. Third, as disease prevalence increases, the efficacy of a study will increase only if its sensitivity is greater than its specificity.

Predictive Value

Another way to assess study efficacy is to calculate the frequency with which a study classification is correct. This is called the **predictive value of a study result**. The formulas for the predictive values are

$$
\text{predictive value of a positive result} = \frac{\textit{true positive results}}{\textit{total number of positive study results}} =
$$

$$
\frac{\textit{prevalence} \cdot \textit{sensitivity}}{\textit{prevalence} \cdot \textit{sensitivity} + (1 - \textit{prevalence})(1 - \textit{specificity})}
$$

and

$$
\text{predictive value of a negative result} = \frac{\textit{true negative results}}{\textit{total number of negative study results}} =
$$

$$
\frac{(1 - \textit{prevalence}) \, \textit{specificity}}{(1 - \textit{prevalence}) \, \textit{specificity} + \textit{prevalence} \, (1 - \textit{sensitivity})}
$$

The formulas, as well as good sense, reveal that the predictive value of a positive study result increases with increasing disease prevalence and with increasing study sensitivity and specificity. When the disease prevalence is low, the frequency with which positive study results are correct is small, unless the study specificity is nearly one. The predictive value of a negative study result increases with decreasing disease prevalence and with increasing study sensitivity and specificity. When the disease prevalence is low, the frequency of correct negative study results is high even when the diagnostic performance of the study is poor. Consider two laboratory studies. The

Table 3-4

Predictive Values of Study Results

Prevalence	Study 1		Study 2	
	Predictive value positive result	Predictive value negative result	Predictive value positive result	Predictive value negative result
0.05	0.84	0.999	0.05	0.95
0.01	0.50	0.9999	0.01	0.99
0.001	0.09	0.99999	0.001	0.999
0.0001	0.01	0.999999	0.0001	0.9999

first has a sensitivity and a specificity of 0.99. The sensitivity and specificity of the second are 0.50. Table 3-4 shows the predictive values of these studies over a range of disease prevalences. Despite being highly sensitive and specific, at low disease prevalences study 1 has a low predictive value of a positive study result. On the other hand, at low disease prevalences, the predictive value of a negative result for study 2, even with its poor performance characteristics, is nearly equal to that of study 1.

Improving Study Performance

Diagnostic uncertainty exists only for study results that lie in the interval of overlap of the competing reference distributions (review Figure 3-1). It is in this interval that diagnostic misclassification occurs. Therefore, the frequency of misclassification can be decreased, and study performance improved, if the overlap interval is made smaller. This can be accomplished by reducing the controllable sources of measurement variability, i.e., the preanalytic and analytic components, when performing the study.

EVALUATION OF STUDY PERFORMANCE: MEDICAL JOURNAL ARTICLES
(Dept. of Clinical Epidemiology and Biostatistics 1981;
Zweig and Robertson 1982)

> It is astonishing with how little reading a doctor
> can practice medicine, but it is not astonishing how
> badly he may do it.
> Sir William Osler

Clinicians learn about diagnostic laboratory studies from the investigations of study performance reported in medical journals. Because errors and shortcomings in the design, execution, and description of such evaluations are frequently encountered, it is necessary to be an astute and thoughtful reader. Which is to say that one must read with two intentions: to learn the results of the performance evaluation and to judge the quality of the evaluation based upon the description given in the report. The degree of confidence in the results should correspond to the level of satisfaction with the evaluation's quality.

Components of a Performance Evaluation
(Metz 1978; Ransohoff and Feinstein 1978)

A complete description of a performance evaluation includes the following:
1. definition of the diagnostic classes
2. definition of the analytic procedure
3. definition of the reference method for diagnostic classification
4. description of the reference populations
5. description of the performance
6. validation of the findings.

Definition of the Diagnostic Classes

The necessary start to any report of performance evaluation, and a crucial consideration in the design of the evaluation, is a clear statement of the diagnostic classes meant to be distinguished by use of the diagnostic study. This statement should indicate the disease of interest, the clinical setting in which the study is to be used, and the manner in which the study is to be incorporated into the diagnostic evaluation, in particular if it is meant to be part of a study series or combination. The nondisease class should be defined explicitly in the description of the clinical setting.

Definition of the Analytic Procedure

Although often little attention is given to the description of the analytic procedure used to make a study measurement, the procedure chosen affects the reliability and clinical applicability of a performance evaluation. Reliable evaluations are based upon accurate and precise analytic methods. The use of inaccurate methods, especially those suffering from poor analytic specificity, or imprecise methods results in underestimates of study performance. Analytic methods should also be performed "blind." When a method is not performed "blind," that is, when the presumed diagnosis is known to the individual performing the study, and when such knowledge can influence the result reported, there is a risk that, consciously or unconsciously, results may be biased in favor of agreement with the diagnoses. This kind of investigation bias, called test-review bias, leads to overestimates of study performance. A discussion of the accuracy and precision of the methods and an assurance that the study determinations were performed "blind" should appear in the definition of the analytic procedure.

The clinical applicability of an evaluation depends upon the extent to which its analytic procedure can be reproduced in the clinical setting. Specifically, patient preparation, the manner of specimen collection and handling, and the analytic methodology, including instrumentation, need to be comparable to those in the evaluation. It is necessary, therefore, that the definition of the procedure include these details.

Definition of Reference Method for Diagnostic Classification

Ideally, the reference or gold standard diagnostic method used in a performance evaluation should be a perfect diagnostic classifier. In reality, of course, reference methods fall short of perfection. The point of describing the reference method in the evaluation report is to allow the readers to judge by how much the method differs from the ideal.

Most often reference diagnostic methods are specific but not completely sensitive. This is true for nearly all methods based upon pathologic examination of the subjects' tissues: mild forms or small foci of a disorder can be missed, but detection of the disorder means the subject unarguably has the disease. It can be shown that specific reference methods permit an accurate estimation of the sensitivity of the particular diagnostic study but lead to underestimation of its specificity.

Sometimes reference methods that are neither completely specific nor sensitive are utilized. This is usually the case when the diagnostically specific methods are unduly invasive, painful, expensive, or inconvenient. The estimates of study specificity and sensitivity found in a performance evaluation using such reference methods are subject to systematic error and thus must be considered, at best, rough approximations. The reference method description should explain the selection of such a reference method and state its performance characteristics in the populations studied. Needless to say, the worse the performance of the reference technique, the more suspect the performance estimates of the study under investigation.

It is also important to learn from the reference method description whether the results of the study contributed to the reference diagnostic classifications. If so, the classifications will be biased in favor of agreement with the results, which will result in overestimation of study performance. This form of investigation bias is called **diagnostic-review bias.**

Description of the Reference Populations

The reference populations should consist of persons who satisfy the stipulated definitions of the diagnostic classes. This is rarely a problem with the diseased population, but it is a frequent concern with the disease-free population. Rather than utilizing disease-free individuals for whom the study is appropriate, i.e., patients who have illnesses similar to the disease of diagnostic interest, often patients with completely unrelated disorders or even healthy persons are used. False positive results are less likely in these populations, so study specificity is overestimated.

For both populations the spectrum of biologic variability should be as broad as possible. Patients with mild and early forms of the disease of interest should be included in the diseased population, as should patients presenting with unusual clinical features. The diseased population should not consist entirely of patients with advanced disease. That will lead to overestimation of the sensitivity of the study. Similarly, the study sensitivity will be overestimated if the population consists of subjects selected because their chances of having the particular disease were great enough to justify the use of an invasive or painful reference method for diagnostic classification. This form of investigation bias is called **work-up bias.**

The disease-free population should consist of individuals with the various illnesses that can be confused with the disease under investigation. Ideally it should include many patients in whom diagnoses cannot be rendered without use of the reference classification method. In addition, the disease-free individuals should represent a diverse sample in terms of biologic attributes, such as age and gender. Failure to assemble a population with an adequate clinical or biologic spectrum usually results in overestimation of study specificity.

Table 3-5

The Effects of Common Errors in the Design
and Execution of Performance Evaluations
upon the Estimates of Sensitivity and Specificity

Errors	Sensitivity estimate	Specificity estimate
Inaccurate or imprecise analytic method	Under	Under
Test-review bias	Over	Over
Imperfect reference method (specificity = 1; sensitivity < 1)	Correct	Under
Displaced reference method (specificity < 1; sensitivity < 1)	Incorrect	Incorrect
Diagnostic-review bias	Over	Over
Inappropriate population	-	Over
Inadequate spectrum	Over	Over
Work-up bias	Over	Under

Table 3-5 summarizes the effects that the errors in the design and execution of performance evaluations have upon the
estimates of study sensitivity and specificity.

Description of the Performance

It is still uncommon to see the complete performance data for
a study evaluation. Instead, the sensitivity (often called "true
positive rate") and specificity ("true negative rate") of the
study at a single critical value are reported. This is fine as
long as the critical value used is the one appropriate for the
clinical setting in which the study is to be used. But sometimes
it is not.

For evaluations based upon a specific critical value, the
performance description should state explicitly the basis for the
author's selection of the critical value. The three most commonly cited criteria are that the critical value

    1. is used by other researchers

    2. yields a specificity of 0.95

    3. yields maximum efficacy among the subjects studied.

Use of the first criterion allows the results of the evaluation to be compared to those reported by others. However, it may not permit ready comparison of the performance of the particular study with that of alternative diagnostic studies. Use of the second criterion does permit performance comparisons among alternative studies also evaluated at a specificity of 0.95. Neither of these desirable properties is found with use of the third criterion, which, therefore, must be viewed as much inferior to the first two.

When reported, complete performance data can be presented in either of two ways: as reference frequency distributions or as performance characteristic curves. An example of the presentation of reference frequency distributions is shown in Figure 3-4. Actually these histograms are simple result distributions because

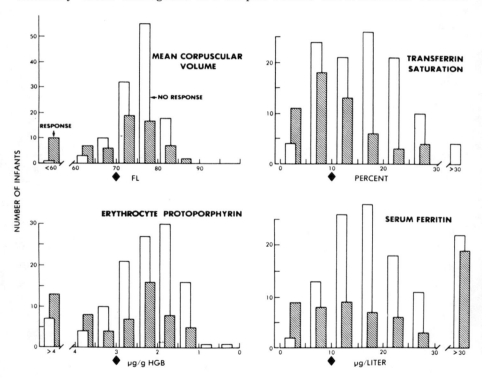

Fig 3-4   Reference Result Distributions for Four Tests
of Body Iron Stores.
(From Dallman, P.R., Reeves, J.D., Driggers, D.A., Lo, E.Y.T. Diagnosis of iron deficiency: the limitations of laboratory tests in predicting response to iron treatment in 1-year-old-infants. J. Pediatr. 99:376, 1981 © C.V. Mosby Company, St. Louis.)

Response = iron deficiency; no response = iron replete.

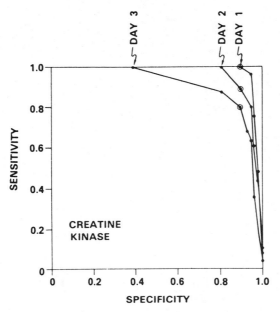

Fig 3-5   Performance Characteristic Curves for Serum
Creatine Kinase Concentration Used as a Marker of Acute
Myocardial Infarction.   Curves are shown for application
of the study on the first, second, and third days
following the onset of the chest pain.
(Reprinted with permission from Werner, M. Brooks, S.H.,
Mohrbacher, R.J., Wasserman, A.G.   Diagnostic performance of enzymes in the discrimination of myocardial
infarction.   Clin. Chem. 28:1297, 1982 © American Association for Clinical Chemistry, Inc., Washington, D.C.)

the height of the bars corresponds to the number of infants with
each study result.   They can be converted to the frequency distributions for each diagnostic group by dividing by the total
number of infants studied in the group.

A presentation of performance characteristic curves is shown
in Figure 3-5.   The method for graphing performance characteristic curves has not yet been standardized in the medical literature.   In the example, the horizontal and vertical axes are,
respectively, specificity and sensitivity.   This agrees with the
convention used in this book.   Graphs in which the horizontal
axis is one minus specificity (usually called the "false positive
rate") and the vertical axis is sensitivity are often found.
They give curves that are left-to-right mirror images of those
obtained when the horizontal axis is specificity.

Both forms of presentation are useful.   As discussed in the
following chapters, reference frequency distributions are needed

when estimating disease likelihood in individual patients, and
performance characteristic curves are the means to determine
optimal critical values and to select among alternative diagnostic studies. Furthermore, performance characteristic curves
are a convenient way to compare the diagnostic performance of
studies.

The statistical treatment of performance results should
include calculation of the confidence intervals for the performance estimates and, for evaluations based upon a specified critical value, verification of the significance of the performance
results.

A confidence interval is the range of values within which, to
a certain level of confidence (usually 0.95), the true sensitivity or true specificity of the study lies. For proportions,
such as sensitivity and specificity, confidence intervals are
found using the cumulative binomial distribution. Oftentimes
confidence intervals are not reported, so a graph for their calculation is reproduced here (Figure 3-6).

Verification of the significance of the performance results
for a specified critical value amounts to asking the statistical
question: at a certain level of confidence (usually 0.95), are
the number of diagnostic misclassifications at the critical value
less than what would be expected on the basis of chance alone?
If the critical value has been specified prior to reviewing the
performance data, the appropriate statistical instruments are the
Fisher exact test, for small sample numbers, and the chi-square
test, for large sample numbers. If, however, the critical value
has been selected after examining the data, as when it is chosen
to maximize efficacy among the subjects studied, a significance
test such as the one developed by Gail and Green is required
(Gail and Green 1976).

In addition to reporting the sensitivity and specificity of
the diagnostic study under investigation, many researchers also
calculate its efficacy and the predictive values for positive and
negative study results. Sometimes these calculations are based
upon the appropriate epidemiologic estimates of the prevalence of
the disease studied, but more often they are derived using the
disease's prevalence among the investigational subjects. The
prevalence is usually much greater among the subjects than in the
clinical setting, however, because researchers typically seek out
individuals with the disease in order to study a large number of
them. Not infrequently half of the subjects have the particular

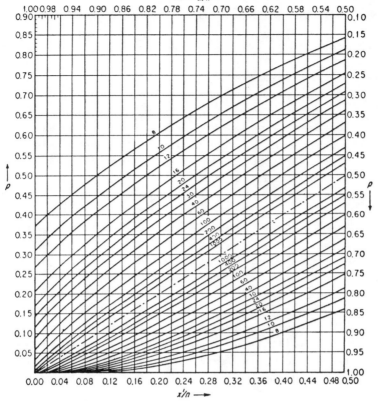

Fig 3-6   Confidence Limits for Performance Estimates;
            Confidence Coefficient = 0.95.
(Reprinted with permission from Beyer, W.H. ed. Hand-
book of Tables for Probability and Statistics, 2nd
   edition, p. 220 © CRC Press, Inc., Boca Raton, FL)

To use the figure: Find the performance estimate on the
horizontal axes: estimates up to 0.50 are on the lower
axis, and estimates greater than 0.50 are on the upper
axis.   Locate the intersections of the vertical line
corresponding to the estimate with the two oblique lines
labeled with the number of subjects in the reference
population. Using a straightedge, construct horizontal
lines from the points of intersection to the vertical
axis: on the left for estimates less than 0.50, on the
right for estimates greater than 0.50.   Identify the
            indicated confidence limits.

disease while the other half serve as disease-free controls. Obviously, when study efficacy and predictive value are based upon such inflated prevalence measurements, they are meaningless. Conversely, if the study evaluation has been designed to include an epidemiologic inquiry into disease prevalence, the reported estimates of efficacy and predictive value will be useful.

Validation of the Findings

The most convincing way to demonstrate the validity of performance evaluation findings is to perform identical investigations in new samples of subjects and arrive at the same performance estimates. This task is usually left to other researchers, but not always. The simplest technique for self-validation, and that most often seen in the medical literature, is to perform the evaluation using one half of the subjects, having selected them at random. The evaluation is then repeated using the other half. Concurrence of the performance estimates in the two groups indicates that the findings are valid.

Another way to demonstrate the validity of a performance evaluation is to show that the findings do not change as a consequence of reasonable variation in the analytic and reference procedures or in the composition of the reference populations. Such an analysis may be provided for as part of the evaluation design (for example, using a design that permits evaluation of the effects of inter- and intraobserver variability), or it may be performed retrospectively (for example, using regression analysis to evaluate the effects of demographic variables). This form of validation should be a part of every performance evaluation.

The components of a performance evaluation and the commonly encountered errors in the design, execution, and description of the components are listed in Table 3-6. The table also indicates where in the evaluation report to look for the description of the components.

Table 3-6

Common Errors in the Design, Execution and Description of Performance Evaluations

Component of performance evaluation	Where to look for description	Errors
Definition of diagnostic classes	Introduction	Failure to define nondisease class
Definition of analytic procedure	Methods	Inadequate description Inaccurate or imprecise method Test-review bias
Definition of reference method for diagnostic classification	Methods	Imperfect method
Description of reference populations		
Diseased population	Methods and results	Inadequate spectrum of disease Work-up bias
Disease-free population	Methods and results	Inappropriate population Inadequate clinical spectrum Work-up bias
Description of performance		
Single critical value	Results	Selection of inappropriate critical value Inappropriate statistical analysis
Complete	Results	Lack of statistical analysis
Validation of findings	Results	No validation

EXERCISES

3-1. The performance characteristics for transferrin saturation discussed in this chapter apply to infants who have low blood hemoglobin concentrations (i.e., screen-positive infants). How might the diagnostic performance of this study change were it performed in an unscreened infant population?

3-2. What are the predictive values of a positive and a negative result for transferrin saturation (critical value 10%) in a screen-positive infant? Assume a disease prevalence of 0.33 in this population. What is its efficacy?

3-3. Using the data from the article by Dallman et al. (1981), construct the performance characteristic curve for serum ferritin concentration as a marker of iron deficiency in screen-positive infants.

3-4. Which study is a better diagnostic tool, transferrin saturation or serum ferritin concentration?

3-5. When a study's sensitivity and specificity are calculated from a fourfold classification table (e.g., Table 3-2), the following formulas are used:

$$sensitivity = \frac{true\ positive\ results}{true\ positive\ results\ +\ false\ negative\ results}$$

and

$$specificity = \frac{true\ negative\ results}{true\ negative\ results\ +\ false\ positive\ results}$$

Confirm that the estimates of sensitivity and specificity found by using these formulas are not influenced by the prevalence of the disease in the population studied.

Mind-Expanding Exercises

3-6. Select a medical journal article reporting the performance evaluation for a diagnostic laboratory study. Assess the design, execution, and description of each component of the evaluation.

3-7. In a paper discussing the measurement of the discriminatory performance of diagnostic studies, Feinstein (1975: Section B, summary indexes) uses an example for which the calculation of sensitivity and specificity is problematic because there are more than two diagnostic categories. His example is inappropriate. Why?

REFERENCES

Dallman, P.R., Reeves, J.D., Driggers, D.A., Lo, E.Y.T. Diagnosis of iron deficiency: The limitations of laboratory tests in predicting response to iron treatment in 1-year-old infants. J. Pediatr. 99:376, 1981.

Department of Clinical Epidemiology and Biostatistics, McMaster University Health Sciences Centre. How to read clinical journals. II: To learn about a diagnostic study. Can. Med. Assoc. J. 124:703, 1981.

Feinstein, A.R. Clinical biostatistics. XXXI: On the sensitivity, specificity, and discrimination of diagnostic tests. Clin. Pharmacol. Ther. 17:104, 1975.

Gail, M.H., Green, S.B. A generalization of the one-sided two-sample Kolmogorov-Smirnov statistic for evaluating diagnostic tests. Biometrics 32:561, 1976.

Galen, R.S., Gambino, S.R. Beyond Normality: The Predictive Value and Efficiency of Medical Diagnoses. Wiley, New York, 1975.

Griner, P.F., Mayewski, R.J., Mushlin, A.I., et al. Selection and interpretation of diagnostic tests and procedures. Principles and applications. Ann. Intern. Med. 94:553, 1981.

McNeil, B.J., Keeler, E., Adelstein, S.J. Primer on certain elements of medical decision making. N. Engl. J. Med. 293:211, 1975.

Metz, C.E. Basic principles of ROC analysis. Semin. Nucl. Med. 8:283, 1978.

Ransohoff, D.F., Feinstein, A.R. Problems of spectrum and bias in evaluating the efficacy of diagnostic tests. N. Engl. J. Med. 299:926, 1978.

Zweig, M.H., Robertson, E.A. Why we need better test evaluations. Clin. Chem. 28:1271, 1982.

PART II:

ADVANCED ANALYTIC PRINCIPLES

Chapter 4

DIAGNOSTIC CLASSIFICATION

2. Study Performance: Further Considerations

> "Pooh!" cried Piglet. "Do you think it is another
> Woozle?"
> "No," said Pooh, "because it makes different
> marks. It is either Two Woozles and one, as it
> might be, Wizzle, or Two, as it might be, Wizzles
> and one, if so it is, Woozle ...."
>
> A. A. Milne

OPTIMAL STUDY PERFORMANCE
(Noe 1983)

The clinical usefulness of a diagnostic study depends upon the importance, or value, of the diagnostic classifications it renders and upon the accuracy with which these classifications are made. The critical value that is used as the criterion for making these diagnostic classifications will determine the study's performance and should be selected to maximize the study's usefulness in the given clinical setting. The critical value that accomplishes this maximization is called the optimal critical value.

Maximizing Expected Efficacy

To maximize study efficacy means to maximize the rate of correct diagnostic classification or, conversely, to minimize the rate of diagnostic misclassification. When the number of critical values from which to choose is small, the maximum efficacy is revealed by calculating of the efficacy associated with each of the possible critical values of the study.

For example, the transferrin saturation data from the paper by Dallman et al. (1981) give the following results:

Critical value	Efficacy
0%	0.67
5%	0.71
10%	0.68
15%	0.62
20%	0.50
25%	0.40
30%	0.36

using the prevalence of iron deficiency found in the studied infants, 0.33 (22/165). The maximum efficacy is 0.71, which arises from the selection of 5% as the critical value for transferrin saturation.

When the number of potential critical values is great, the burden of computing the efficacies is excessive. In these cases, the optimal critical value can be identified from the performance characteristic curve for the study. It can be shown that diagnostic efficacy is maximized at the point on the performance characteristic curve with slope equal to

$$\frac{prevalence - 1}{prevalence} \cdot$$

The optimal critical value for the study is the study value corresponding to that coordinate.

The optimal performance coordinate can be identified easily using a graphic technique. A number of lines with slopes equal to (prevalence-1)/prevalence are drawn. The one that is tangent to the performance characteristic curve passes through the optimal coordinate.

This technique can be used as well when the performance characteristic curve is constructed from a limited number of performance coordinates, as in the example. Figure 4-1 shows the performance characteristic curve for transferrin saturation. For

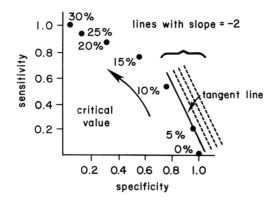

Fig 4-1   Performance Characteristic Curve
for Transferrin Saturation: Maximizing Expected Efficacy
[Data from Dallman et al. (1981)]

the clinical population investigated, the study's efficacy is maximized at the coordinate with the slope

$$\frac{0.33 - 1}{0.33} = -2 \quad .$$

The tangent line with slope -2 passes through the coordinate (0.20,0.96). That corresponds to the use of 5% as the critical value for transferrin saturation.

Maximizing Expected Value

Although the selection of 5% transferrin saturation maximizes the efficacy of this diagnostic study, it may not be the proper choice to maximize its clinical usefulness. That depends upon the importance, or value, of the diagnostic classifications that are made, as well as upon the efficacy of the study. For instance, one is often willing to sacrifice accurate identification of a relatively unimportant diagnostic class in order to increase the rate of correct identification of a more important class. In other words, there is a trade-off between efficacy and diagnostic value. A study's maximum usefulness is obtained when the performance is selected to maximize the study's net value when it is applied to the clinical population.

The first step is to rank the classification categories. Which is the most clinically valuable or desirable category? For the example study, surely it is the true positive result. Here asymptomatic but diseased infants are identified, permitting the institution of iron repletion therapy and thereby eliminating the potentially deleterious effects of infantile iron deficiency. True negative results, which merely serve to confirm iron repleteness in asymptomatic infants, are not as valuable. The least desirable, or stated differently, most costly category is the false negative result. Such a result will lead to the withholding of needed iron therapy. False positive results are much less costly in that a course of iron repletion therapy, even though unneeded, is unlikely to harm the child. Thus, the classification categories, ranked from most valuable to most costly, are

1. true positive result
2. true negative result
3. false positive result
4. false negative result.

To deal quantitatively with the trade-off between study efficacy and classification value, the category ranking must now be
scaled and each category must be assigned a value on the scale.
This is by far the most difficult step in the value maximization
process — and also the most controversial. The scaling technique
described here is that of relative exchange values. Although it
is by no means the only possible value scale for diagnostic
studies, it does represent a good paraphrase of how medical value
judgments are made. In addition, it is fairly easy to use. What
follows is a hypothetical clinical conversation concerned with
value assessment using the relative exchange value scale.

The clinician responsible for selecting the critical value
that maximizes the expected clinical value of the study serves as
the respondent, i.e., the value assessor, in the dialogue.

Guide: As you realize, the diagnostic performance of a
              laboratory study can be altered by a change in
              the critical value of the study. By critical
              value, I mean that study result that differen-
              tiates disease from the absence of disease. If
              the critical value is adjusted to increase the
              number of true positive study results, the
              number of true negative results will lessen and
              the number of false positive results will in-
              crease. Conversely, if the critical value is
              set so that the number of false positive results
              is decreased, the number of true positive
              results will be less and the number of false
              negative results will increase. Assume that I
              can reset the critical value to increase or
              decrease the number of study results in each one
              of the diagnostic categories. I want to find
              out what rate of exchange you feel is appro-
              priate when trading study results in one diag-
              nostic category for study results in another
              category.

Clinician: Alright.

Guide: We have already determined your ranking of the
              classification categories. It is listed above.
              Let us consider the category you rank highest,
              true positive results. Say that I offer you a
              trade — you can identify one additional iron-
              deficient infant, but in doing so you must

accept not identifying some of the iron-replete infants. How many true negative results would you exchange for one additional true positive result? Don't worry about which classification the iron-replete infants enter. The diagnostic study will simply be withheld from them. So, how many true negative results would you exchange for one true positive result?

Clinician: Well ... I really don't feel that identification of an iron replete infant is very important at all, so I would trade a large number ... uh, 20 or 30. It's hard to quantify.

Guide: That's fine. An exact number is not necessary. In fact, I shall write down "large" as your response. That will be adequate. Next question: how many iron replete infants are you willing to treat unnecessarily in order to identify one additional iron-deficient infant?

Clinician: (pause) ... I have a different kind of problem here. I am definitely willing to treat two infants unnecessarily to achieve this trade, but I cannot see increasing the number by three.

Guide: That's no problem. Let me rephrase the question. In order to identify two additional cases of iron deficiency, how many iron replete infants could you accept treating?

Clinician: Now I have it. Five for two. Five iron-replete infants for two iron-deficient ones. And I see how you resolved the problem. By using increasing integer values for your side of the trade, eventually I can select an integer value for my side. That way we don't have to trade fractions.

Guide: Exactly. Now let us consider the least desirable category. In order to reduce by one the number of iron-deficient infants missed, how many iron-replete infants would you tolerate treating?

Clinician: (pause) The answer is again five for two. I would treat five iron-replete infants in order to avoid missing two iron-deficient infants. I

	was able to do the entire calculation in my head, you'll notice.
Guide:	Yes, I noticed. My last question is this: How many iron replete infants are you willing not to identify in order to reduce by one the number of iron-deficient infants not identified?
Clinician:	Here, again, I think a large number.
Guide:	Fine. I shall again enter "large". I now have enough information to place a value on each of the diagnostic categories we have considered. To begin, let me draw a scale, a relative exchange value scale, extending from -∞ to +1.

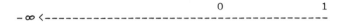

I shall assign the classification category true positive a value of +1. It is positive because this category results in a benefit. The category true negative also has a positive value so its magnitude must be between 0 and 1. Because you said you were willing to trade a "large number" of true negative results for one true positive result, the value of a true negative result must be very small. I shall give this category a value of 0 as an approximation.

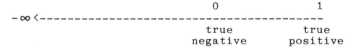

I shall now consider the negative portion of the scale where the values for false positive and false negative results will appear. You stated that you would accept five false positive results for two additional true positive results. That means that the value of a false positive result is two fifths that of a true positive result, or -0.4. Finally, you said that you were willing to accept five false positive results in order to eliminate two false negative results. Therefore, the value of a false nega-

tive must be 2.5 times that of a false positive
result, or -1.

<pre>
              -1   -0.4   0   1
   - ∞ <---
              false   false   true   true
              negative positive negative   positive
</pre>

All four classification categories have now been
assigned values on the relative exchange value
scale. But we are left with one as yet unused
exchange evaluation, that is, true negative
results for false negative results. The relative value you assessed for that exchange can be
used as a check upon the value assignments already made. You said that a large number of
true negative results could be tolerated in a
trade for one less false negative result. The
value of a true negative result must be a very
small positive number. This agrees with the
evaluation assessed earlier and validates the
category scaling.

This dialogue has been used to reveal the elements and mechanism of value assessment when using the relative exchange value
scale. The process is summarized below:
1. Briefly describe the task to be undertaken.
2. Establish the exchange rates between the most valuable
    diagnostic category and each of the two competing diag-
    nostic categories. If the top-ranked category is true
    positive results, exchange for true negative and false
    positive results; if it is true negative results, ex-
    change for false negative and true positive results.
3. Establish the exchange rates between the most costly
    diagnostic category and each of the two competing diag-
    nostic categories.
4. Construct a relative exchange value scale with a value of
    +1 given to the most valuable diagnostic category.
5. For the appropriate two competing categories, assign
    values equal in magnitude to the inverse of their ex-
    change rates with the most valuable category. True
    classifications are positive, false classifications are
    negative.

6. For the two appropriate competing categories, assign values equal in magnitude to the inverse of their exchange rates with the most costly category.

7. One category will have two valuations. These should show reasonable agreement. If not, consider redoing the assessment.

The final steps in the value maximization process are to identify the study performance that will yield the maximum value when the study is applied to the defined clinical population.

Just as for efficacy, when the number of critical values to be considered is manageable, the maximum value can be identified by calculation of the net expected value for each of the possible critical values of the study. Net value is calculated using the formula,

net value = the sum of the products of the fraction of individuals in each classification category multiplied by the relative exchange value assigned to the study result comprising that category.

Otherwise, the optimal critical value can be identified from the study's performance characteristic curve. In this case, it can be shown that the net value is maximized at that point on the performance characteristic curve with slope

$$\frac{prevalence - 1}{prevalence} \cdot \frac{U_{TN} - U_{FP}}{U_{TP} - U_{FN}}$$

where

U_{TN} = *relative exchange value of a true negative result*

U_{FP} = *relative exchange value of a false positive result*

U_{TP} = *relative exchange value of a true positive result*

U_{FN} = *relative exchange value of a false negative result* .

The optimal critical value is the one corresponding to that performance coordinate. Here also the graphic technique for identifying this coordinate may be used.

This approach can be applied readily to our clinical example. Using 0.33 for the prevalence of iron deficiency and the value scaling decided upon in the imaginary dialogue, the slope at the optimal performance coordinate is

$$\frac{0.33 - 1}{0.33} \cdot \frac{0 + 0.4}{1 + 1} = -0.4$$

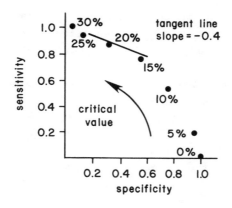

Fig 4-2   Performance Characteristic Curve
for Transferrin Saturation: Maximizing Expected Value
[Data from Dallman et al. (1981)]

Figure 4-2 shows the performance characteristic curve for transferrin saturation. The tangent line with slope -0.4 passes
through the coordinate (0.32, 0.87). That corresponds to the use
of 20% as the critical value for transferrin saturation. Notice
that the optimal critical value, 20%, is not equal to the efficacy-maximizing critical value, 5%. This is because, instead of
study efficacy, study value has been maximized.

Because of the concavity of performance characteristic
curves, when net value is maximized, larger slopes call for
increased study specificity and decreased sensitivity. Smaller
slopes indicate that higher sensitivity and lesser specificity
are needed. Therefore, high study specificity should be sought
when the disease prevalence is low, when the clinical value of
true negative classifications is large, and when the cost of
false positive results is small. Study sensitivity should be
high when the disease prevalence is high, when true positive
results are highly valued, and when false negative results have a
large cost. These findings are quite in keeping with good
clinical sense, as well they must be.

Suboptimal Study Performance
    The identification of the optimal critical value for a quan-
titative diagnostic study depends upon two conditions that, re-
gretably, are not frequently met:
    1. The performance characteristic curve for the study is
        available.

2. The reference populations from which the performance characteristic curve was generated are comparable to the patient populations in the specific clinical setting in which the study is to be used.

This means that, more often than not, the critical value is selected by a procedure that cannot assure that the optimal value will be chosen. Suboptimal study performance is the result — adequate performance, perhaps, but, nevertheless, suboptimal.

The procedure most often used to select critical values relies entirely upon the frequency distribution of a study's results in a reference population of individuals believed to be healthy. (Notice the unsettling suggestion of a normal reference population?) Two critical values are chosen: one corresponding to the 2.5th percentile of the reference frequency distribution and the other to the 97.5th percentile. The study results bounded by these two critical values constitute a **reference interval.** Study results within the reference interval are negative for disease, those outside of the reference interval are positive.

In the reference population used to define the reference interval, the specificity of the interval is 0.95. In a clinical setting, however, the specificity can be quite different because of the very different composition of the reference population of disease-free persons. In the example cited, for instance, the reference interval for transferrin saturation is bounded by the value 10% saturation, so the specificity is 0.75. The associated sensitivity is 0.53. As has been shown, the use of 10% saturation as a critical value neither minimizes misclassification nor maximizes net clinical value. In this case the popular procedure for selecting critical values has led to suboptimal study performance.

REPEAT AND COMBINATION TESTING

Another approach to improving the performance of a diagnostic study is to repeat the study, perhaps a number of times, or to use the study in combination with one or more other studies known to have diagnostic capacities on their own. The performance that results from such multiple testing depends largely upon two new considerations: the **positivity rule** used to make the ultimate diagnostic classifications and the **classification correlation** between repeated tests or among combinations of tests.

Repeat Testing

(Cebul et al. 1982; Cornell 1978; Politser 1982)

The two most frequently used positivity rules for repeat testing are illustrated in the following example.

The single test diagnostic performance of transferrin saturation at the critical value of 10% saturation recommended by Dallman et al. (1981) consists of a sensitivity of 0.53 and a specificity of 0.75. What happens if the study is repeated in the same patients? If there is no classification correlation between the initial and repeat study, that is, if the partition of patients into subgroups according to the initial diagnostic classifications does not affect the performance of the study, the repeat study results will be as shown in Figure 4-3. For the 82 iron replete patients initially classified correctly, 62 will

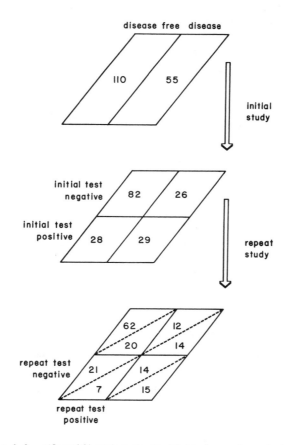

Fig 4-3   Classification Performance for a Repeated
Transferrin Saturation Study

- 65 -

have true negative results with the repeat study (62/82 = 0.76 = specificity), but 20 will have false positive results (20/82 = 0.24 = 1 - specificity). For the 29 patients with true positive results from the first test, 15 will be classified correctly by the repeat study (15/29 = 0.52 = sensitivity) and 14 incorrectly (14/29 = 0.48 = 1 - sensitivity). And so on for the other categories.

One way to categorize these patients clinically is to decide that the test series is positive if either the initial or repeat study result is positive. This positivity rule is designated "believe the positive." The diagnostic performance resulting from this rule is indicated in the left panel of Figure 4-4. Forty-three iron-deficient patients will have at least one positive test result, so the sensitivity of the series is 0.78 (43/55). Of the patients who are iron replete, sixty-two will have both results negative and will therefore be appropriately categorized. The specificity is therefore 0.56 (62/110). Another way to categorize the patients is to consider the test series positive only if both study results are positive. Predictably, this positivity rule is referred to as "believe the negative." Its performance, as demonstrated in the right panel of Figure 4-4, is a sensitivity of 0.27 and a specificity of 0.94.

As shown in the example, the believe-the-positive positivity rule leads to an increased sensitivity and a decreased specificity compared to a single application of the study. This is

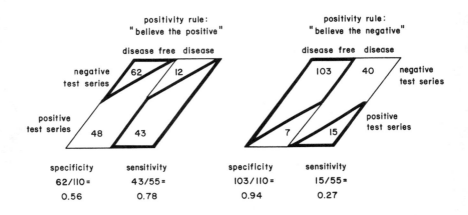

Fig 4-4   Application of Different Positivity Rules
to a Repeated Transferrin Saturation Study

because diseased individuals have two opportunities to be detected while those who are disease free have two chances to be misclassified. In contrast, use of the believe-the-negative positivity rule results in decreased sensitivity but increased specificity. With this rule diseased patients have two opportunities to be misclassified while those who are disease free have two chances to be correctly identified. With additional repetitions of the study, the performance of the series is removed further still from that of the single study, as shown in Figure 4-5 for series of up to five studies. Optimal series strategies for the stipulated critical study value are also indicated. The performance pair that minimizes diagnostic misclassification at a disease prevalence of 0.33 is that corresponding to a single test repetition and application of the believe-the-negative positivity rule. The net value of a test series is maximal when four studies are performed and the believe-the-positive rule is applied.

All of the foregoing calculations have been based upon the condition that there is no classification correlation between repeat studies. In reality, classification correlation usually exists. A repeat study in an individual is likely to yield a result close to a previous result and, therefore, to give a

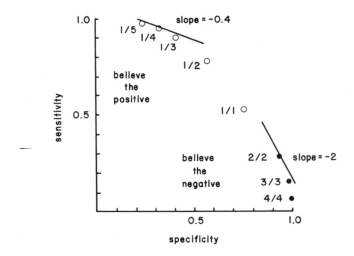

Fig 4-5   Performance of Repeat Testing with Transferrin Saturation.
Critical Value: 10% Saturation
Numerator: minimum number of positive study results
needed to establish the diagnosis
Denominator: number of studies performed

similar diagnostic classification, even if it is a misclassification. As a consequence, the actual diagnostic performance of a test series will differ from that computed under the assumption that the classification correlation is zero. For the believe-the-positive rule, the actual sensitivity will be less than that expected and the actual specificity will be greater; for the believe-the-negative rule, the actual sensitivity will be greater than predicted and the actual specificity will be less. Unfortunately, as far as the example considered in this section is concerned, repeat series were not conducted, so the disparity between actual and predicted performance cannot be examined.

Combination Testing
(Cebul et al. 1982)

Two popular positivity rules for combination testing are identical to those used for repeat testing. The rule "any test positive," for which the test combination is considered positive if any of the constituent study results are positive, is the same as the believe-the-positive rule. The "all tests positive" positivity rule is equivalent to the believe-the-negative rule for repeat testing. And just as for repeat testing, the first rule leads to an increased sensitivity and decreased specificity compared to the individual studies in the combination, and the second rule results in decreased sensitivity but increased specificity. This is shown in Figure 4-6 for the combination of transferrin saturation and ferritin concentration as comarkers of iron deficiency. Transferrin saturation has a sensitivity of 0.53 and a specificity of 0.75, and ferritin concentration has a sensitivity of 0.28 and a specificity of 0.87 [again using the data in the article by Dallman et al. (1981)]. Depending upon which of the above positivity rules is used, if there is no classification correlation between the studies, the performance of the test combination shows a sensitivity of 0.65 and a specificity of 0.65 or a sensitivity 0.15 and a specificity 0.97.

The actual performance of a number of positivity rules for combination testing with transferrin saturation, ferritin concentration, mean red cell volume, and red cell protoporphyrin

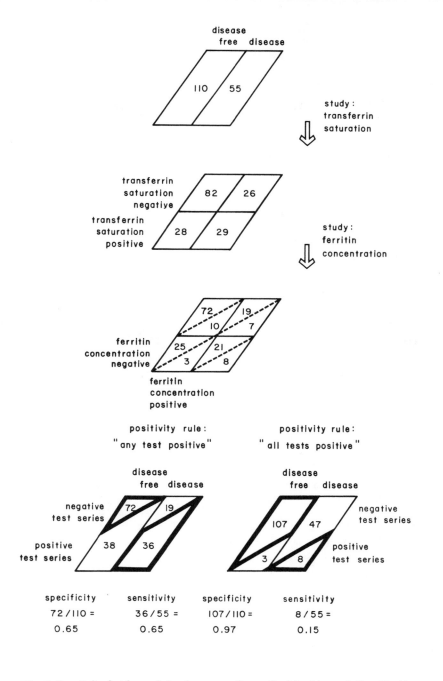

Fig 4-6   Calculation of Performance for a Combination of Two Studies:
Transferrin Saturation and Ferritin Concentration

Table 4-1

Performance of Individual Studies

Study	Specificity	Sensitivity	Author's critical value
Transferrin saturation	0.75	0.53	<10%
Ferritin concentration	0.88	0.28	<10 µg/L
Mean red cell volume	0.89	0.34	<70 fl
Red cell protoporphyrin concentration	0.82	0.41	>3.0 µg/g hemoglobin

Data from Dallman et al. (1981).

concentration is reported in the article by Dallman et al. (1981). Table 4-1 shows the performance of the individual studies, and Table 4-2 shows the performance of the test combinations. Four test combination positivity rules are considered: the any-test-positive rule (number of positive study results $\geq$ 1); the all-tests-positive rule (number of positive study results $=$ 4); and two intermediate rules (number of positive study results $\geq$ 2 and $\geq$ 3). The effect of classification correlation is well demonstrated by the differences between the

Table 4-2

Performance of the Combination of All Four Studies
Using Various Positivity Rules

Positivity rule (number of positive study results)	Specificity		Sensitivity	
	Expected	Observed	Expected	Observed
$\geq$1	0.48	0.45	0.88	0.87
$\geq$2	0.88	0.70	0.51	0.45
$\geq$3	0.986	0.86	0.16	0.32
4	0.999	0.98	0.02	0.23

Data from Dallman et al. (1981).

expected and observed sensitivities of the combination testing. For the strict positivity rules the observed sensitivities exceed those predicted on the assumption of no correlation. For the lenient positivity rules, the observed sensitivities are less than expected, although, it must be admitted, not by much for the any-test-positive rule. The specificity findings are not so satisfying. In the presence of classification correlation, the observed specificity with the any-test-positive rule should have been greater, not less than, that expected. The performance of the other rules is consistent with classification correlation, however.

Multiphasic Health Screens

A frequently employed form of combination testing is the so-called multiphasic health screen. These are combinations of 12, 18, 24, and sometimes more laboratory determinations performed upon a single blood sample for the purpose of detecting silent disease in asymptomatic individuals. The presence of a study result outside of the reference interval for the analyte is supposed to identify persons who should be evaluated further for subclinical disease. The diagnostic specificity of such testing is low, however. Very low!

For one laboratory study with a reference interval based upon a specificity of 0.95, the chance that a healthy person will have a test result outside of the reference interval is 0.05. For a combination of j uncorrelated laboratory studies, each of which has a reference interval chosen to give a specificity of 0.95, the chance of a positive result in a healthy individual is $(0.95)^j$. The chances of encountering a test result outside its reference interval increase with an increasing number of tests. The consequences are shown in Table 4-3.

Table 4-3

Specificity of Multiphasic Health Screens

Number of tests	Probability of abnormal result	Specificity
12	0.46	0.54
18	0.60	0.40
24	0.71	0.29

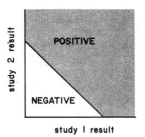

positivity rule: multivariate reference space	positivity rule: multivariate discriminant function

Fig 4-7   Multivariate Positivity Rules:
Bivariate Case

MULTIVARIATE POSITIVITY RULES

(Solberg 1978; Winkel et al. 1972)

The positivity rules for combination testing discussed in the preceding section rely upon the positivity rules, i.e., critical values, of the constituent studies. These rules, in turn, are derived from univariate (one study) frequency distributions for the reference populations. A different and rather more imaginative approach to defining test combination positivity is found in multivariate positivity rules. These rules are constructed with consideration for multivariate (multiple study) frequency distributions for the reference populations. Two multivariate positivity rules, as applied to the case of a two-study test combination, are illustrated in Figure 4-7.

In the left panel of Figure 4-7 the multivariate equivalent of a reference interval, called a multivariate reference space, is depicted. The reference space consists of the result combinations that give rise to the central 0.95 of the multivariate frequency distribution for the nondisease reference population. For the bivariate (two-study) case, if the frequency distribution of study results is Gaussian, an ellipse delimits the reference space, as pictured here. In the right panel, negative result combinations are separated from positive result combinations by a line. The equation of the line is

$$study\ 2\ result = a + b\ (study\ 1\ result)$$

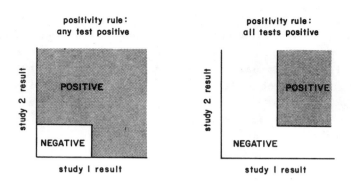

Fig 4-8   Combined Univariate Positivity Rules:
           Bivariate Case

where a is the vertical axis intercept and b is the slope of the
line.   For positive result combinations,

$$study\ 2\ result\ -\ b\ (study\ 1\ result)\ >\ a$$

and for negative result combinations,

$$study\ 2\ result\ -\ b\ (study\ 1\ result)\ <\ a.$$

The linear combination of study results,

$$study\ 2\ result\ -\ b\ (study\ 1\ result)$$

is called a **multivariate discriminant function**.   The critical
value for the function is a.

For contrast, Figure 4-8 shows the diagnostic spaces that
result from the use of combined univariate positivity rules,
again for the case of a two-study test combination.

Diagnostic Ratio

Diagnostic ratios are a popular approach to test combination
interpretation when only two laboratory studies are concerned:

$$diagnostic\ ratio\ =\ value\ study\ 2\ /\ value\ study\ 2.$$

They have proved most useful when the values of the studies change in opposite directions in response to disease. The ratio of the two magnifies the changes and thereby increases the diagnostic resolution. Transferrin saturation, which is the ratio of serum iron concentration to serum total iron-binding capacity, is a more reliable marker of iron deficiency than either measure taken separately because as the serum iron concentration declines with iron deficiency, the total iron-binding capacity increases. Consequently, the ratio of the two diminishes markedly.

Taking the natural logarithm (ln) of the diagnostic ratio reveals that the ratio has the form of a multivariate discriminant function,

$$ln \ (value \ study \ 2) - ln \ (value \ study \ 1).$$

Unlike a discriminant function, however, the coefficients of the terms are constrained: one is 1 and the other is -1. These coefficients are, in general, not the ones that will give the greatest diagnostic accuracy. Rather, a discriminant function has the more general form,

$$ln \ (value \ study \ 2) - b \ ln \ (value \ study \ 1)$$

where the coefficient b can be set to achieve the maximum separation of diagnostic classes. Taking the antilogarithm of this equation shows that a discriminant diagnostic ratio would have the form,

$$value \ study \ 2 \ / \ (value \ study \ 1)^{b}.$$

Because of their superior accuracy, discriminant ratios are preferable to diagnostic ratios for use as bivariate positivity rules.

4-1. Using the frequency distributions for ferritin concentra-
      tion from Dallman et al. (1981), identify the critical
      value that will maximize diagnostic efficacy in screen-
      positive infants. Assume that in this population the
      prevalence of iron deficiency is 0.33.
4-2. What is the maximum efficacy?
4-3. What is the diagnostic efficacy achieved by use of the
      reference interval < 10 µg/L?
4-4. Assume the role of a pediatrician concerned with selecting
      the optimal critical value to use with transferrin satu-
      ration when diagnosing iron deficiency in infants. Rank
      the classification categories according to your sentiments.
      Assign values to the categories using the relative exchange
      value scale. Assuming a disease prevalence of 0.33 in
      screenpositive infants, determine the optimal critical
      value for transferrin saturation. What is the net value of
      using the study given this critical value?
4-5. An asymptomatic 30-year-old male is found to have two study
      results outside of their reference intervals on a 12-test
      multiphasic health screen. What is the probability of this
      happening even though the individual is completely healthy?
4-6. Assume that the prevalence of iron deficiency in an un-
      screened population of infants is one-tenth that of the
      screened population, i.e., 0.033. If transferrin satura-
      tion shows no classification correlation and has the same
      performance characteristics in this population, how many
      test repetitions are needed for a believe-the-negative
      positivity rule to achieve maximum efficacy?

Mind-Expanding Exercises

You are a clerk on the oncology service. The attending physician
laments the difficulty she has in differentiating osteoporosis
from early metastatic disease in her elderly patients. Both
diseases can show elevations of markers of bone turnover, the
serum concentration of the bone isoenzyme of alkaline phosphatase
(BP), and the daily urinary excretion of hydroxyproline (UH). A
bright resident suggests that the ratio of UH to BP may be a
helpful diagnostic index. An even brighter medical student (in
all modesty, yourself) thinks that a multivariate discriminant

function will probably do a better job. You find an article in the medical literature pertinent to this question (Stepan et al. 1978).

4-7. What is the discriminant diagnostic ratio and what is its critical value?

4-8. What is the efficacy of the discriminant diagnostic ratio in the patients reported in the article?

4-9. What is the maximum efficacy achievable by the diagnostic ratio UH/BP?

REFERENCES

Cebul, R.D., Hershey, J.C., Williams, S.V. Using multiple tests: Series and parallel approaches. Clinics in Laboratory Medicine 2:871, 1982.

Cornell, R.G. Sequence length for repeated screening tests. J. Chronic Dis. 31:539, 1978.

Dallman, P.R., Reeves, J.D., Driggers, D.A., Lo, E.Y.T. Diagnosis of iron deficiency: The limitations of laboratory tests in predicting response to iron treatment in 1-year-old infants. J. Pediatr. 99:376, 1981.

Noe, D.A. Selecting a diagnostic study's cutoff value by using its receiver operating characteristic curve. Clin. Chem. 29:571, 1983.

Politser, P. Reliability, decision rules, and the value of repeated tests. Medical Decision Making 2:47, 1982.

Solberg, H.E. Discriminant analysis. CRC Crit. Rev. Clin. Lab. Sci. 9:209, 1978.

Stěpán, J., Pacovský, V., Horn, V., et al. Relationship of the activity of the bone isoenzyme of serum alkaline phosphatase to urinary hydroxyproline excretion in metabolic and neoplastic bone diseases. Eur. J. Clin. Invest. 8:373, 1978.

Winkel, P., Lyngbyte, J., Jorgensen, K. The normal region — a multivariate problem. Scand. J. Clin. Lab. Invest. 30:339, 1972.

Chapter 5

DIAGNOSTIC CLASSIFICATION

3. Individualizing Diagnoses

"It's like this," he said. "When you go
after honey with a balloon, the great thing
is not to let the bees know you're coming.
Now, if you have a green balloon, they might
think you were only part of the tree, and not
notice you, and if you have a blue balloon,
they might think you were only part of the
sky, and not notice you, and the question is:
which is most likely?"

A. A. Milne

MAKING DIAGNOSES

How does a clinician use the results of laboratory studies to
arrive at a diagnosis? The critical values and positivity rules
discussed in the preceding chapters apply to the performance of
studies in populations of patients and are selected using the
classification values of physicians. In contrast, when making a
diagnosis, the central considerations are the likelihood of disease in the patient and the classification values of the patient.
In individuals study results are used to arrive at the estimates
of disease likelihood upon which diagnoses are based.

THE LIKELIHOOD OF A DIAGNOSIS
(Diamond and Forrester 1983)

There is usually some degree of uncertainty in the diagnostic
classification of a patient. This uncertainty is of two kinds.
The first kind is that which arises from an inability to separate
completely the presence of a disease from its absence on the
basis of clinical or laboratory findings. Diagnostic studies are
inaccurate. This means that the presence of the disease can be
expressed only as a likelihood: "It is quite likely you are
affected," "There is a fifty-fifty chance you have this disorder," "You could be suffering from," and so forth. When
expressed quantitatively, disease likelihood has a value between
zero, which means the disease is definitely not present, and one,
which means the disease is unarguably present. The second kind
of uncertainty arises from variability in the diagnostic per-

formance of clinical and laboratory studies. Diagnostic studies
are imprecise. This means that any statement of disease likelihood is merely an estimate. The actual likelihood may be
greater or less in proportion to the imprecision of the study.
The magnitude of this uncertainty can be expressed quantitatively
as a confidence interval around the likelihood estimate. In
practice only uncertainty due to study inaccuracy is explicitly
considered in the diagnostic process. The clinician must be
mindful of uncertainty due to study imprecision, though. It
distinguishes studies that are reliable from those that are not.

Formal approaches exist for estimating the likelihood of
disease and for establishing rules by which these estimates are
used to make diagnoses. Two of these, the Bayesian approach to
likelihood assessment and the threshold likelihood approach for
accepting or rejecting diagnoses, have informal counterparts in
the diagnostic decision-making of many, if not most, clinicians.
These two approaches provide a framework for diagnostic decision
making that is practicable even in its formal realization.
Because of this they are the most common methods used in
computer-based medical decision support. They will be discussed
in some detail in this chapter.

It should be noted that voices have been raised against the
clinical use of Bayesian likelihood assessment and value theory
[for example, Feinstein (1979) and Bursztajn (1982)]. Before
becoming an advocate of one or the other side in this controversy, the reader is cautioned to become familiar with the arguments offered by both.

Assessing Prior Likelihood
(Feinstein 1972)

The **prior likelihood of disease** in a patient is the estimate
of the disease likelihood arrived at prior to the performance of
diagnostic studies. It is based upon the symptoms elicited by
history-taking, the signs revealed by physical examination, and
additional pertinent historic and demographic data such as age,
gender, disease history, disease exposure, and, in the evaluation
of heritable disorders, family history and genetic stock. For
example, in a retrospective review of 3627 patients with chest
pain referred to their medical center for cardiac catheteriza-
tion, Pryor et al. (1983) found that the prevalence of coronary
artery disease varied widely among patients grouped according to

various characteristics. Figure 5-1 (their Figure 1, page 773), shows the prevalence of coronary disease in each of the different groups. Those characteristics associated with a disease prevalence greater than the overall prevalence are referred to as **risk factors**; those associated with prevalences less than the overall prevalence are **protective factors**. Notice, for instance, that although the average prevalence of disease was 0.66, in those patients with chest pain considered nonanginal the prevalence was only 0.21, whereas in those with typical anginal chest pain the prevalence was 0.87. Therefore, the prior likelihood of coronary artery disease based solely upon pain type is 0.87 for patients with typical anginal pain and 0.21 for those with nonanginal pain. Were the overall prevalence of 0.66 to be used as an estimate of the prior probability of coronary artery disease in a patient with nonanginal pain, subsequent calculations of disease likelihood would be substantial overestimates; for a patient with typical angina, underestimates would result.

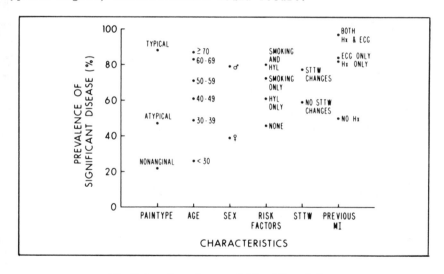

Fig 5-1   Prevalence of Significant Coronary
Artery Disease by Patient Characteristics
(From Pryor, D.B., Harrell, F.E., Lee, K.L.,
Califf, R.M., Rosati, R.A. Estimating the like-
lihood of significant coronary artery disease.
Am. J. Med. 75:771, 1983 © American College of
Physicians, Philadelphia.)

ECG = electrocardiographic evidence
Hx. = history
HYL = hyperlipidemia
MI   = myocardial infarction
STTW = ST-T wave changes

Using the data from this study, it is possible to establish the prior likelihood of coronary artery disease based upon combinations of characteristics. Indeed the authors were able to categorize patients into groups for which the prior likelihood of significant coronary artery disease varied from 0.025 to 0.99.

Assessing Posterior Likelihood
(Horbar 1983; McNeil et al. 1975)

Diagnostic laboratory studies are ordered with the intent of adjusting the estimate of the likelihood of disease in a patient based upon the study results. The revised estimate of disease likelihood based upon the result of the diagnostic study is called the **posterior likelihood of disease.** The method of adjusting likelihood estimates to be discussed here is based upon Bayes' formula for inverting a conditional probability. The method possesses a great intuitive appeal, and in addition, the formulation is rigorously provable from the axioms of probability theory.

Consider the case of a 55-year-old woman who is suspected of having coronary artery disease because she complains of typical anginal chest pain. Her prior likelihood of significant disease is 0.35 [using the nomogram supplied by Pryor et al. (1983)]. She undergoes an electrocardiographic exercise test that reveals a maximum ST-segment depression of 1.0 mm. What is the posterior likelihood of disease? Examination of Figure 5-2, the reference

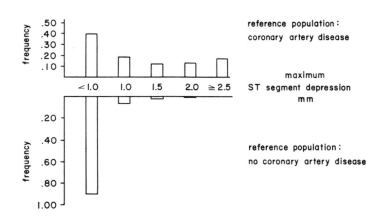

Fig 5-2   Reference Frequency Histograms
for Exercise Electrocardiography
[Data from Bartel et al. (1974)]

frequency histograms for exercise electrocardiography [construc-
ted from data in Bartel et al. (1974)], indicates that if she has
significant coronary disease, the chances of her having a maximum
ST-segment depression of 1.0 mm are 0.18. The chances of that
study result are 0.065 if she does not have coronary disease.
Thus she is 2.8 times (0.18/0.065) more likely to have a 1.0-mm
ST-segment depression if she has coronary artery disease than if
she does not. Conversely, given the study result, she is that
much more likely to have coronary disease, i.e., the likelihood
of disease is increased by the factor 2.8 relative to the likelihood of freedom from disease. The prior likelihoods of disease
and freedom from disease are 0.35 and 0.65, respectively, so the
relative posterior likelihoods are 0.98 (2.8 - 0.35) and 0.65,
respectively. When the relative posterior likelihoods are scaled
so that their sum will equal one (because the patient either does
or does not have coronary artery disease), the absolute posterior
likelihoods are obtained, 0.60 and 0.40. The posterior likelihood of disease in this patient is 0.60.

This case serves as an example of the application of Bayes'
formula for the calculation of a posterior likelihood:

$$\begin{array}{l}\textit{posterior likelihood} \\ \textit{of disease}\end{array} = \dfrac{\left(\begin{array}{c}\textit{prior likelihood} \\ \textit{of disease}\end{array}\right)\left(\begin{array}{c}\textit{likelihood} \\ \textit{ratio}\end{array}\right)}{\left(\begin{array}{c}\textit{prior likelihood} \\ \textit{of disease}\end{array}\right)\left(\begin{array}{c}\textit{likelihood} \\ \textit{ratio}\end{array}\right) + \left(\begin{array}{c}\textit{1-prior likelihood} \\ \textit{of disease}\end{array}\right)}$$

where the prior likelihood was 0.35 and the likelihood ratio,
which is the ratio of the frequency of a study result in persons
with the disease to the frequency of the result in persons free
of the disease, was 2.8. The formula states that the likelihood
of disease is increased if a study result is more common in
disease (likelihood ratio > 1) and is decreased if the result is
more common in the absence of disease (likelihood ratio < 1).

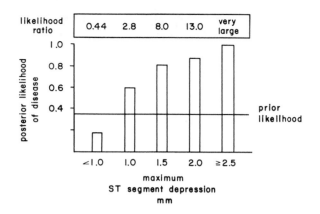

Fig 5-3   Likelihood Ratios and Posterior Likelihoods
of Disease for Exercise Electrocardiography
(Prior Likelihood of 0.35)

The likelihood ratios and posterior likelihood calculations at each value of ST-segment depression, given a prior likelihood of 0.35, are shown in Figure 5-3. For depressions equal to or greater than 1 mm, the likelihood ratios are greater than the prior likelihood. For a depression less than 1 mm, the likelihood ratio is less than one and the posterior likelihood is less than the prior likelihood.

It is of utmost importance to remember that the application of Bayes' formula is valid only if the likelihood ratio used is derived from frequency distributions in reference populations comparable to the patient populations in the clinical setting. Likelihood ratios will usually vary widely among different reference populations. Careless application of a likelihood ratio that is not appropriate to the actual clinical situation can be expected to result in erroneous posterior likelihood calculations and subsequent diagnostic inaccuracy.

Sometimes, however, the performance of a diagnostic study is essentially constant among various clinical populations. Electrocardiographic exercise testing for coronary artery disease is such a study. The graphic representation of Bayes' formula for a positive qualitative test result (ST-segment depression $\geq$ 1 mm) over the entire range of prior likelihood is shown in Figure 5-4 [from Rifkin (1977)]. Note that for a positive qualitative study the likelihood ratio is 7.42. The smooth line shows the curvi-

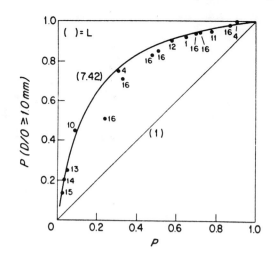

Fig 5-4   Posterior Likelihood of Coronary
Artery Disease as a Function of Prior Likelihood
of Disease and the Result of Qualitative
Electrocardiographic Exercise Testing
(Reprinted with permission from Rifkin, R.D.,
Hood, W.B. Bayesian analysis of electrocardio-
graphic exercise stress testing.   N. Engl. J.
Med. 297:681, 1977 © New England Journal of
Medicine, Boston.)

P = prior likelihood
P(D/O) = posterior likelihood
L = likelihood ratio

linear relationship that exists between prior and posterior likelihood if the likelihood ratio is a constant. Note that the most
substantial changes in the magnitude of the likelihood estimates
occur at intermediate values of prior likelihood; only small
increments in likelihood are to be had at the extreme values of
prior likelihood.   The prior and posterior likelihood pairs reported in a number of clinical investigations are also shown in
Figure 5-4.   The excellent fit of the curve to the data indicates
that constancy of the likelihood ratio is indeed a feature of
this diagnostic study.

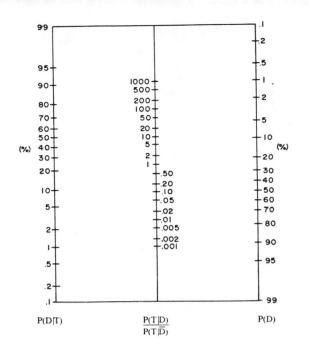

Fig 5-5   Nomogram for Bayes' Formula
(Reprinted with permission from Fagan, T.J.
Nomogram for Bayes' theorem. N. Engl. J. Med.
293:257, 1975 © New England Journal of Medicine,
Boston.)

To use the nomogram: the prior likelihood of
disease, P(D), and the likelihood ratio,
P(T/D)/P(T/D̄), must be known. Locate the prior
likelihood on the right-hand scale and the likelihood ratio on the middle scale. Connect the
two points with a straightedge. The straightedge
crosses the left-hand scale at the posterior
likelihood, P(D/T).

A nomogram for Bayes' formula has been published (Fagan 1975)
and is reproduced in Figure 5-5.

Threshold Likelihoods for Accepting and Rejecting Diagnoses

Diagnostic decisions are binary. A patient is either treated
as having or not having a particular disease. He/she cannot
receive partial therapy in proportion to the likelihood of the
diagnosis. The task for the diagnostician is to decide if, at a
certain level of likelihood, the acceptance of a diagnosis is
justified, if rejection of the diagnosis is prudent, or if further diagnostic evaluation is necessary. The approach to indi-

vidualized diagnostic classification described here is that of threshold likelihood rules based upon the diagnostic classification values of the patient. Threshold likelihood rules can also be derived from the physician's classification values, and probably frequently are in routine practice, but ideally the patient's values take precedence over those of the clinician. (This is sometimes a hard pill to swallow!)

In the presence of uncertainty, decisions are made by balancing expectations. For instance, I always carry an umbrella when it looks like rain. I also carry one when the skies are clear if there is a chance of showers later. How great a chance? That depends upon what I'm wearing. If I have on a suit even the hint of rain convinces me to take protection. If I'm dressed for gardening, precipitation must be a near certainty. In both cases I have balanced expectations: the expected benefit of having an umbrella should it rain against the expected inconvenience of carrying the umbrella through a dry day. The expected benefit is the product of the magnitude of the benefit times its likelihood. In the first instance the benefit is large but the likelihood of experiencing the benefit is small. In the second, the benefit is small but the likelihood is great. The expected inconvenience is the product of the magnitude of the inconvenience times its likelihood (which is one minus the likelihood of receiving a benefit). I carry an umbrella when the likelihood of rain is such that the expected benefit of an umbrella exceeds the expected inconvenience, or, to express it differently, when the sum of the expected benefit and the expected cost, i.e., the net expected value, is positive. The net expected value of a diagnostic decision is the sum of the expected value of the correct diagnostic classification plus the expected cost of the complementary incorrect classification.

The net expected value of accepting a diagnosis is the expected value of a true positive classification plus the expected cost of a false positive classification. The threshold likelihood for accepting a diagnosis is that likelihood of disease at which, in the mind of the patient, the net expected value of making the diagnosis is zero. At all greater levels of likelihood the net expected value of making the diagnosis is positive, so the diagnosis should be accepted. At all lesser levels of likelihood the net expected value of making the diagnosis is negative, so the diagnosis should not be made (not "rejected" but rather, "not accepted").

The threshold likelihood is easily calculated by rearrangement of the linear relationship of net expected value to disease likelihood:

$$
\begin{aligned}
\text{net expected value of} \\
\text{accepting the diagnosis}
\end{aligned}
=
\begin{pmatrix} likelihood\ of \\ disease \end{pmatrix}
\begin{pmatrix} value\ of \\ true\ positive \end{pmatrix}
$$
$$
+ \begin{pmatrix} 1\text{-}likelihood\ of \\ disease \end{pmatrix}
\begin{pmatrix} value\ of \\ false\ positive \end{pmatrix}
$$

Because at the threshold likelihood the net expected value is zero,

$$
\begin{aligned}
\text{threshold likelihood for} \\
\text{accepting the diagnosis}
\end{aligned}
= \frac{value\ of\ false\ positive}{value\ of\ false\ positive - value\ of\ true\ positive}
$$

$$
= \frac{1}{1 - \dfrac{value\ of\ true\ positive}{value\ of\ false\ positive}}
$$

A similar calculation yields the **threshold likelihood for rejecting a diagnosis**:

$$
\begin{aligned}
\text{net expected value of} \\
\text{rejecting the diagnosis}
\end{aligned}
=
\begin{pmatrix} 1\text{-}likelihood\ of \\ disease \end{pmatrix}
\begin{pmatrix} value\ of \\ true\ negative \end{pmatrix}
$$
$$
+ \begin{pmatrix} likelihood\ of \\ disease \end{pmatrix}
\begin{pmatrix} value\ of \\ false\ negative \end{pmatrix}
$$

At the threshold likelihood net expected value is zero, so

$$
\begin{aligned}
\text{threshold likelihood for} \\
\text{rejecting the diagnosis}
\end{aligned}
= \frac{value\ of\ true\ negative}{value\ of\ true\ negative - value\ of\ false\ negative}
$$

$$
= \frac{1}{1 - \dfrac{value\ of\ false\ negative}{value\ of\ true\ negative}}\ .
$$

In both cases the threshold likelihoods are determined by the ratio of the value of the correct (true) diagnostic classification to the value of the incorrect (false) classification. The larger this ratio, the smaller the magnitude of the threshold likelihood for accepting a diagnosis. This agrees with the intuitive notion that a diagnosis should be made or treatment begun at lower levels of diagnostic certainty when the benefits of action far outweigh the possible detrimental consequences (e.g., antibiotic therapy of meningitis is usually initiated prior to confirmation of a bacterial etiology). The smaller the value ratio, the smaller the magnitude of the threshold likelihood for rejecting a diagnosis. This means that the exclusion of a diagnosis demands increasing diagnostic certainty as the cost of the false negative classification increases relative to the benefit of the true negative designation; this is again an intuitively appealing conclusion (e.g., pigmented skin lesions are deemed benign only after confirmation by histopathologic examination, the most reliable diagnostic study available).

Figure 5-6 portrays a graphic approach to the determination of critical likelihoods. A hypothetical set of patient classification values is displayed on the value axis. The line representing the net expected value of accepting the diagnosis crosses the likelihood axis at the threshold likelihood for

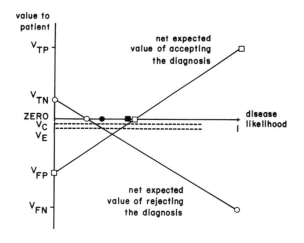

Fig 5-6   Critical Likelihoods for Accepting ($\square$, $\blacksquare$)
and Rejecting (0, ●) a Diagnosis

V_C = cost of confirming a diagnosis
V_E = cost of excluding a diagnosis

net expected value = (likelihood) V_{TP} + (1-likelihood) V_{FP}
of accepting the diagnosis

net expected value = (1-likelihood) V_{TN} + (likelihood) V_{FN}
of rejecting the diagnosis

accepting the diagnosis (□) because, at that point, the net expected value is zero. Similarly, the threshold likelihood for rejecting the diagnosis (O) is identified by the intersection of the likelihood axis and the line representing the net expected value of rejecting the diagnosis. The interval on the likelihood axis that lies between these two threshold likelihoods is the range of disease likelihoods for which further diagnostic evaluation is indicated. Also shown in Figure 5-6 is the effect that the costs of laboratory testing — physical, psychologic, and financial — have upon the calculation of the critical likelihoods. When confirming the presence of a disease has a cost, the threshold likelihood for accepting the diagnosis (■) is that likelihood at which the net expected value of accepting the diagnosis equals the cost of confirmation, i.e., the intersection of the net expected value line and the confirmation value line. This likelihood is always less than that which obtains when confirmation has no appreciable cost. Which is to say that a somewhat lesser level of certainty justifies making a diagnosis if the patient considers the diagnostic work-up to be costly. When excluding a diagnosis has a cost, the threshold likelihood for rejecting the diagnosis (●) is that likelihood at which the net expected value of rejecting the diagnosis equals the cost of exclusion. This likelihood is always greater than that found when excluding the diagnosis has no cost. Here a lesser level of certainty of the absence of disease is permitted in consideration of a costly diagnostic procedure.

Although the costs of diagnostic procedures are taken into account when calculating critical likelihoods, study performance is not [for a contrary opinion see Pauker and Kassirer (1980)]. It is in the selection of diagnostic studies that study performance is considered, as will be discussed in the following chapter.

Eliciting Threshold Likelihoods from the Patient

Rather than trying to compute a threshold likelihood based upon classification values elicited from the patient, a simpler method is to ascertain the threshold likelihood directly. This approach is also almost certainly more reliable because most patients (as well as their physicians) are unable to quantify their classification values accurately using explicit value scaling techniques. We seem much better able to express our values implicitly in terms of net expected value. We can usually state with confidence whether the net expected value of a choice is positive, i.e., to our liking; negative, i.e., not acceptable; or indistinguishable from zero, i.e., a matter of indifference.

What follows is a contrived conversation wherein a clinician elicits a patient's threshold likelihood for accepting a diagnosis (in this case, a provisional diagnosis). In this depiction the patient is unusually articulate and cooperative, so the creativity and patience of the clinician are not put to the test. In addition, the patient is not uncomfortable participating in the clinical decision process. Many patients are. For such patients, a much more subtle and circumspect approach must be taken.

Clinician: As you realize, the chest pain you have been experiencing could be a symptom of heart disease. In particular it has us worried about coronary artery disease, which is the type of heart disease where the arteries supplying blood to the heart become narrowed. This is a dangerous disease because a blood clot can develop in a narrowed artery and completely block the flow of blood to that part of the heart, causing a heart attack. Fortunately, a surgical procedure called coronary artery bypass — you may have heard of it — can be used to treat this disease. Before we would consider surgery, though, we would need to confirm that you do indeed have coronary artery disease. To do this we must perform coronary angiography, which is a special kind of x-ray procedure. Because there are risks involved in angiography, we want to find out how certain you want us to be that you have heart disease before we recommend that you undergo angiography. We know that this will not be easy for you to do, but it is necessary.

Patient: I want to help but I don't really think I can answer your question.

Clinician: I think that I can help you. First, let me describe coronary angiography in more detail. The object of the procedure is to inject a small amount of dye into the arteries of your heart while we take x-rays. By examining the x-ray pictures of the vessels, we can determine if they are narrowed or not. In order to get the dye into the heart's arteries, a plastic tube has to be put into a leg artery - in this hospital we use the one under the skin here (gesture) - and then threaded along the artery all the way back to the heart. The tip of the tube is then put into the opening of the artery supplying the heart and the dye is injected. While the procedure is being performed, patients are lightly sedated, and, of course, local anesthesia is used at the incision site on the leg. If there are no complications, the patient can resume his of her normal activities within a day. Now, as for complications, they are uncommon but can be serious. Two patients in a thousand suffer a stroke or heart attack as a result of the procedure and one person in a thousand dies. Less significant complications occur a bit more frequently, at a rate of one patient in twenty. This includes bleeding or injury to the artery at the puncture site, abnormal heartbeat pattern, fainting due to low blood pressure, and allergic reactions to the x-ray dye. Lastly, in approximately 2% of the cases, the study is inconclusive and needs to be repeated.

Patient: Tell me this, I'm not very old and otherwise I'm in pretty good shape; does that mean I'm less likely to have a complication?

Clinician: It may lessen your risks somewhat; I can't actually give you numbers. It does not eliminate the possibility of a complication, though.

Patient: I see ... well, the procedure itself doesn't sound too bad but I have to say that I am worried about complications, even if they are unusual.

Clinician: We worry about them, too. That's why we're asking you to help us make this decision.

Patient: Okay, but I still don't have an answer.

Clinician: That's what we're going to work on now that you know something about the procedure. Remember, what we want is to determine how certain you want us to be that you have heart disease before we recommend angiography. If you actually do have coronary artery disease, angiography is needed before we can undertake treatment. If you do not have coronary

	disease, undergoing angiography will cause you un- necessary pain and inconvenience and expose you needlessly to the risk of complications. With that in mind, let me offer you some hypothetical choices. If I told you that there were a one in ten chance that you had heart disease, would you want us to go ahead with angiography?
Patient:	No, I think not.
Clinician:	Okay. If your chances were fifty-fifty, would you choose angiography?
Patient:	No ... still no.
Clinician:	Fine. What if the chance that you didn't, that's didn't now, have heart disease were one in twenty?
Patient:	Hmm ... one in twenty that I don't have heart disease. In that case I'd choose angiography, even with the possibility of a complication.
Clinician:	It's going to get harder now. What if the chance that you didn't have heart disease were one in ten?
Patient:	I'd still go with angiography.
Clinician:	If the chance were one in five?
Patient:	That's tough. I'd probably still chose angiography, though.
Clinician:	If the chance were one in four? That means a 25 percent chance you don't have heart disease.
Patient:	(pause) Now I'm leaning toward not having the procedure, but not strongly.
Clinician:	We're considering a 75% chance that you have coronary disease. You would choose not to undergo angiography?
Patient:	Yes ... yes, that's right.
Clinician:	That's fine. We're done now. Thank you. Your answers to my questions indicate that we should consider angiography only if the other diagnostic studies we are going to perform point to an 80% chance of your having coronary artery disease.

This dialogue has been presented as an example of the method of identifying a critical diagnostic likelihood by direct patient inquiry. The process is summarized as follows:

1. Briefly describe the purpose and process of the interview.

2. Describe the medical action that will be taken in response to the diagnostic classification being considered.

Table 5-1

Consequences of Medical Actions

Medical Action	Consequences	
	Without disease	With disease
Discharge	Clean bill of health	Persistent symptoms; unaltered prognosis
Therapeutic intervention	Unnecessary mental and social anguish	Benefits of intervention upon symptoms and prognosis
	Risk of morbidity and mortality from intervention	Risk of morbidity and mortality from intervention
	Expense of intervention	Expense of intervention

3. Indicate the consequences of the stipulated medical action and other pertinent considerations depending upon whether the diagnostic classification is correct or incorrect (Table 5-1).

4. Establish the likelihood of disease at which the patient is indifferent to the correctness of the classification.

5. If appropriate, evaluate the patient's perception of the cost of studies for the confirmation or exclusion of the diagnosis.

CHOOSING AMONG MULTIPLE DIAGNOSTIC ALTERNATIVES

Although in the preceding section diagnostic classification was treated as a binary process — is the disease present or absent? — more often than not clinicians must choose among a multiplicity of diagnostic alternatives - which of these diseases does the patient have? This is obviously a more challenging decision.

In the evaluation of coronary artery disease, for instance, it is important to distinguish among one-, two-, and three-vessel disease. Figure 5-7 shows the reference frequency histograms for these three diagnostic categories based upon the results of exercise electrocardiography (Bartel et al. 1974). A result of 1.0-mm maximum ST-segment depression, for example, occurred in approximately 12% of patients with one-vessel disease, 24% of patients with two-vessel disease, and 19% of patients with three-vessel disease. For the hypothetical patient discussed earlier

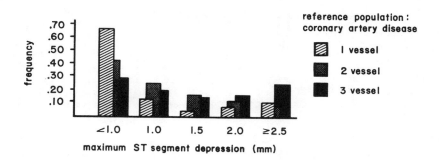

Fig 5-7   Reference Frequency Histograms
for Exercise Electrocardiography;
Number of Diseased Coronary Vessels Distinguished
[Data from Bartel et al. (1974)]

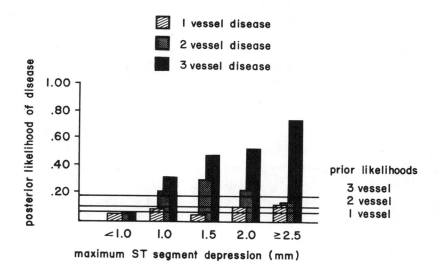

Fig 5-8   Posterior Likelihoods of Disease for
Exercise Electrocardiography;
Number of Diseased Coronary Vessels Distinguished

in the chapter, the prior likelihood of one-vessel disease is 0.07, of two-vessel disease is 0.10, and of three-vessel disease is 0.18. If the frequency data is used, the posterior likelihood for each diagnostic category can be calculated. Figure 5-8, which shows the posterior likelihoods of the categories calculated for each value of ST-segment depression, reveals that the patient is most likely to have three-vessel disease.

A more general form of Bayes' formula has been used to make these calculations:

$$\text{posterior likelihood of a diagnostic alternative} = \frac{\left(\begin{array}{c}\text{prior likelihood}\\\text{of the alternative}\end{array}\right)\left(\begin{array}{c}\text{frequency of the study}\\\text{result in the alternative}\end{array}\right)}{\sum_{\text{all } i}\left(\begin{array}{c}\text{prior likelihood}\\\text{of alternative } i\end{array}\right)\left(\begin{array}{c}\text{frequency of the study}\\\text{result in alternative } i\end{array}\right)}$$

where $\sum$ stands for "the sum of."

Note that if only two alternatives, disease and the absence of disease, are considered this formula is the same as the Bayesian formula introduced earlier in the chapter.

Determining threshold likelihoods for competing diagnoses is very similar to identifying the threshold likelihoods in choosing between disease and nondisease. As for the disease-versus-nondisease case, the acceptance or rejection of a diagnosis must be evaluated on its own merits and also in terms of the complementary decision for the diagnostic alternative. In the case of competing diagnoses, accepting one of the diagnoses means rejecting the others and vice versa.

The classification values that underlie the balancing of the patient's expectations for two diagnostic alternatives are demonstrated in Figure 5-9. A true positive classification of one disease is equivalent to a true negative classification of the second; a false positive classification for the one is the same as a false negative classification of the other (the lines of complementary net expected value are mirror images). The threshold likelihoods for accepting or rejecting the diagnosis of one disease are, therefore, one minus the threshold likelihoods for rejecting or accepting the other.

The presence of multiple diagnostic alternatives significantly increases the computational burden of interpreting study results and making diagnoses. An additional challenge for the clinician is the selection of the laboratory study that maximally separates the diagnostic categories and thereby leads to the optimal overall diagnostic performance. Of course, clinicians are rarely constrained to order only a single diagnostic study. This is fortunate because there are no pandiagnostics just as there are no panaceas. Instead, multiple studies are usually needed. The clinical challenge, therefore, is actually the selection and interpretation of the series or combination of laboratory studies that permits optimal diagnostic performance.

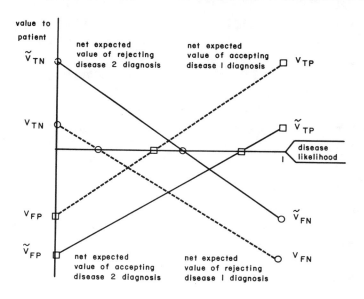

Fig 5-9   Critical Likelihoods for
Accepting and Rejecting Competing Diagnoses

V_{TP}, $\tilde{V}_{TP}$ = value of true positive classification
for diseases 1 and 2, respectively

V_{FP}, $\tilde{V}_{FP}$ = value of false positive classification
for diseases 1 and 2, respectively

V_{TN}, $\tilde{V}_{TN}$ = value of true negative classification
for diseases 1 and 2, respectively

V_{FN}, $\tilde{V}_{FN}$ = value of false negative classification
for diseases 1 and 2, respectively

LIKELIHOOD ESTIMATION USING MULTIPLE STUDY RESULTS
(Albert 1982; Russek 1983)

Most clinical information is processed sequentially. First, certain facts are uncovered by the history and physical; next, the results of the preliminary laboratory studies are obtained; and then, over a period of hours to weeks, the results of additional laboratory studies ordered by the clinician become available. As each new study result is received, the clinician is able to reassess the likelihood of the competing diagnoses using Bayes' formula. The posterior likelihood calculated from the preceding study result serves as the prior likelihood for the computation of disease likelihood based upon the current study result.

This technique is correct as long as there is no result correlation among the studies, that is, as long as the segregation of patients into subgroups according to study results does not affect the result frequency distributions and, hence, likelihood ratios, for any one of the studies. When there is appreciable result correlation — and there often is — this approach will generate likelihood estimates that are exaggerated. Low likelihood estimates will be too low, high likelihood estimates will be too high. Indeed, as the number of study results becomes large, the likelihood estimates will approach either one or zero even though intermediate likelihoods, in fact, exist. Consequently, diagnoses will be accepted or rejected erroneously.

In the presence of result correlation, conditional likelihood ratios must be used in Bayes' formula. A conditional likelihood ratio is the likelihood ratio for a study result calculated from the result frequency distributions arising from those persons in the reference populations who have identical results for the preceding studies. This ratio may be greater than, less than, or equal to the ratio that would be calculated from the entirety of the reference population.

If multiple study results are available concurrently, the following form of Bayes' formula can be used:

$$posterior\ likelihood\ of\ disease = \frac{\left(\begin{array}{c} prior\ likelihood \\ of\ disease \end{array}\right) \prod\limits_{all_i} \left(\begin{array}{c} likelihood\ ratio \\ for\ result\ i \end{array}\right)}{\left(\begin{array}{c} prior\ likelihood \\ of\ disease \end{array}\right) \prod\limits_{all_i} \left(\begin{array}{c} likelihood\ ratio \\ for\ result\ i \end{array}\right) + \left(\begin{array}{c} 1-prior\ likelihood \\ of\ disease \end{array}\right)}$$

where $\prod$ stands for "the product of."

When study correlation is present, the joint likelihood ratio should be used in the equation instead of the product of the likelihood ratios. The joint likelihood ratio is the ratio of the frequency of the combination of study results in the presence of disease to that in the absence of disease. The frequency of a result combination is called a joint frequency.

Figure 5-10 depicts the joint frequency distributions for two hypothetical diagnostic studies. The likelihood ratio for a result pair is the ratio of the corresponding joint frequencies. For example, for the result combination indicated by the dotted lines, the ratio of the corresponding joint frequencies, shown darkened, is one. Therefore the likelihood ratio for this result pair is one.

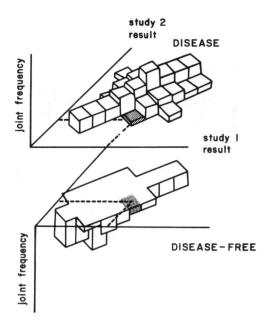

Fig 5-10   Joint Frequency Distributions
for Two Hypothetical Diagnostic Studies

A Multivariate Approach

(Solberg 1978)

Although the calculation of joint likelihood ratios is simple
in the case of two diagnostic studies, as the number of studies
increases, the computational burden becomes significant.   More
importantly, tabulation of the ratios for their ready use clinically becomes nearly impossible, although the growing availability of computer databases may soon make it achievable.

One method for circumventing these difficulties is to
construct univariate frequency distributions based upon the joint
frequency distributions and then to calculate the likelihood
ratios according to these distributions.   The univariate frequency distributions best suited to this purpose are the ones
defined by the multivariate discriminant function for the study
combination.   This is so because the discriminant function has
the singular property that the frequency distributions it generates maximally separate the diagnostic classes.

As mentioned in the preceding chapter, a multivarite discriminant function is a linear combination of study results.
Consequently, many different result combinations will give the

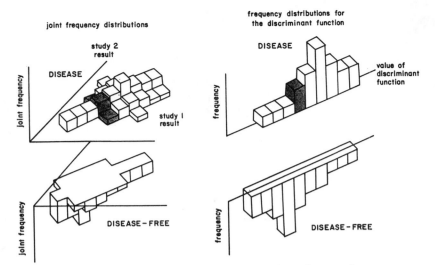

Fig 5-11   Joint Frequency Distributions for Result
Combinations and Frequency Distributions
for the Discriminant Function

same function value. The frequency of a function value will,
therefore, equal the sum of the joint frequencies of the result
combinations yielding that value. In this way, for each diagnostic class, the frequency distribution for the discriminant
function is constructed from the joint frequency distribution of
the study combinations in the class.

The right panel of Figure 5-11 shows the frequency distributions for the discrimination function based upon the joint
frequency distributions shown both in Figure 5-10 and in the left
panel of Figure 5-11. The darkened frequency in the distribution
for the discriminant function, for instance, equals the sum of
the three darkened frequencies in the joint distribution.

The likelihood ratios for the frequency distributions of the
discriminant function are shown in the right panel of Figure
5-12. The darkened likelihood ratio, for example, is the ratio
of the frequency of the indicated value of the discriminant
function in disease to that in persons free from disease. These
are the darkened frequencies in the frequency distribution histograms in the left panel. Because of inaccuracies in the frequency distributions resulting from the limited number of subjects
studied and the vagaries of the sampling process, the empirical
likelihood ratio histogram, or curve, is often irregular, as in
the figure. This problem is overcome by the use of a smoothing

function, called the **logistic function**, which produces a regular likelihood curve. The form of the logistic function is

$$likelihood\ ratio = constant \cdot e^j$$

where j represents the value of the discriminant function.
The logistic function for the example data is also shown in the right panel of Figure 5-12.

It is important to note that the likelihood ratio for a study result combination found by using the discriminant function is only an approximation of the corresponding joint likelihood ratio. This is because joint likelihood ratios are computed using individual joint result frequencies, whereas the likelihood ratios for the discriminant function are calculated using the sums of joint frequencies. This is the price paid for making multivariate data tractable.

Clinical Algorithms
(Feinstein 1973/1974)

An non-Bayesian approach to the interpretation of multiple test results is the **clinical algorithm**. An algorithm is a set of step-by-step instructions that, when followed, allows a problem to be solved. The clinical algorithms of interest here are those designed to direct the diagnostic process. Almost all are written as flowcharts with instruction nodes and directed outlet branches. The diagnostic path one follows is determined at each instruction node encountered. Say, for instance, that a particular laboratory study has been ordered in compliance with the

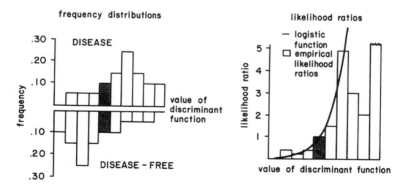

Fig 5-12   Frequency Distributions and Likelihood
Ratios for the Discriminant Function

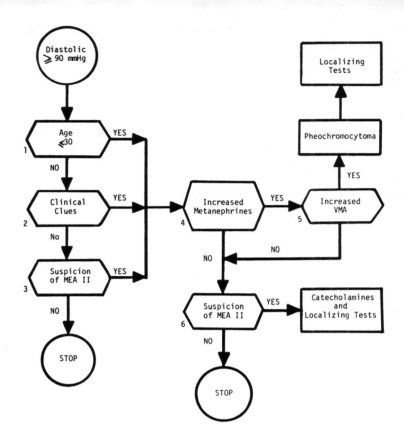

Fig 5-13   Diagnostic Algorithm for Pheochromocytoma
(Reprinted with permission from Burke, M.D.
Hypertension: Diagnostic test strategies.
CRC Crit. Rev. Lab. Sci. 12:279, 1980
© CRC Press, Inc., Boca Raton, FL.)

instruction at an instruction node. The result from that study
will dictate which outlet branch is to be followed from the node:
perhaps branch 1 if the result is greater than 80 mmol/L, branch
2 if it is between 80 and 20 mmol/L, and branch 3 if it is less
than 20 mmol/L. Each of the branches will direct the diagnostic
work-up along a portion of a diagnostic path. At the end of a
path is a diagnosis.

The diagnostic algorithm for pheochromocytoma illustrated in
Figure 5-13 is a good example. The problem to be solved is:
does this patient have a pheochromocytoma? The chart indicates
at the entry point that patients with diastolic blood pressures
above 90 mmHg constitute the clinical population for whom the

algorithm is efficacious. The first instruction (implicit in the flowchart) is: determine the patient's age. If he/she is 30 years old or less, the YES branch should be followed; if he/she is older than 30 years, the NO branch should be taken. For the young patient the next instruction is: determine the daily urinary excretion rate of metanephrines. If the rate is "increased above normal," the clinician is directed to the node instructing that the daily urinary vanillylmandelic acid excretion rate be determined. If the rate is "normal," the next instruction is to decide if the multiple endocrine adenomatous II syndrome is suspected. And so on. Eventually, the diagnosis is either excluded or confirmed.

The diagnostic performance of a clinical algorithm can be expressed in terms of its sensitivity and specificity. As with a diagnostic study, a certain level of performance is required for an algorithm to be useful clinically. The characteristics that improve the performance and applicability of clinical algorithms are

1. Completeness — Are the instructions and directions unambiguous?

2. A defined domain of applicability — Is it easy to decide if a particular clinical problem will be solved by the algorithm? Do the stopping points provide solutions to the problem?

3. Transportability — Are the decision values for the stipulated studies applicable in the given clinical setting?

4. Practicability — Can the studies called for be performed? Are the demands for time and personnel and the expense of the studies reasonable?

A fifth characteristic is also highly desirable:

5. Robustness — Can the algorithm be employed even if some of the requested data cannot be obtained? If the work-up of the patient is stopped short, can the information already gathered be used to make a diagnosis?

<u>EXERCISES</u>

A 40-year-old white woman presents to her internist with symptoms that suggest systemic lupus erythematosus (SLE).   He documents five of the six criteria of SLE.   He is a strict Bayesian interested in minimizing diagnostic misclassification, so he does <u>not</u> make the diagnosis of SLE.   He does, however, refer the patient to a world-renowned academic rheumatologist.   The rheumatologist confirms the same five criteria of SLE and, being a devoted Bayesian concerned with minimizing misclassification, diagnoses SLE.

   5/6 criteria sensitivity 0.632
   for SLE: specificity 0.995

   prevalence   women aged 15-64 140/100,000
   of SLE:

          patients of full-time
          academic rheumatologists 10,080/100,000

5-1. What is the likelihood of SLE in the patient as calculated by the clinic internist?

5-2. What is the likelihood of SLE in the patient as calculated by the rheumatologist?

5-3. Why the difference?

5-4. Common things occur commonly.   When you hear hoofbeats, think of horses, not zebras.   Place your bets on uncommon manifestations of common conditions rather than common manifestations of uncommon conditions.   Comment.

5-5. Determine your threshold likelihoods for accepting and rejecting a diagnosis of significant coronary artery disease. If you had typical anginal pain and were 20 years older, what would be your likelihood of having coronary disease? [Consult Pryor et al. (1983).]   If you underwent exercise electrocardiography that revealed a 1.0-mm ST-segment depression, what would then be your likelihood of having significant coronary disease?   Would you accept the diagnosis, reject it, or desire to undergo further diagnostic evaluation?   What are your feelings regarding the cost of coronary angiography?

5-6. Demonstrate for a pair of study results that the posterior likelihood of disease computed by the sequential application of Bayes' formula is identical to that calculated by the formula for the result combination. Assume that there is no result correlation between the studies. This finding is true for any number of study results.

5-7. The cerebrospinal fluid immunoglobulin G (IgG) index is a laboratory study that has been found useful in distinguishing patients with multiple sclerosis from those with other neurologic disorders. The computation of the likelihood ratios for this diagnostic separation has been made simpler by the availability of a logistic function (Hische et al. 1982):

likelihood ratio = $e^{(-4.28 + 5.9 \text{ IgG index result})}$.

What is the likelihood of multiple sclerosis in a patient with a prior likelihood of 0.3 and an IgG index of 0.8?

5-8. Using the clinical algorithm discussed in this chapter, what is the proper disposition of the following case? A 25-year-old man comes to your office complaining of excessive sweating. The family history reveals that his mother has a parathyroid adenoma, that other members of his mother's family have had what he has been told are unusual tumors, and that his father has hypertension. The physical examination is remarkable only in that his resting diastolic blood pressure is 100 mmHg. A 24-hour urine specimen is collected and assayed for metanephrines (present in normal amounts) and vanillylmandelic acid (present in increased amount).

Mind-Expanding Exercise

5-9. Determine the 90% confidence interval for the likelihood of coronary artery disease in an asymptomatic 55-year-old man who has 1 mm of ST-segment depression during exercise electrocardiography. [Hint: consult Diamond and Forrester (1983).]

Albert, A. On the use and computation of likelihood rations in clinical chemistry. Clin. Chem. 28:1113, 1982.

Bartel, A.G., Behar, V.S., Peter, R.H. Graded exercise stress tests in angiographically documented coronary artery disease. Circulation 49:348, 1974.

Bursztajn, H., Hamm, R.M. The clinical utility of utility assessment. Medical Decision Making 2:161, 1982.

Diamond, G.A., Forrester, J.S. Metadiagnosis. An epistemologic model of clinical judgment. Am. J. Med. 75:129, 1983.

Fagan, T.J. Nomogram for Bayes' theorem. N. Engl. J. Med. 293:257, 1975.

Feinstein, A.R. Clinical biostatistics. XV. The process of prognostic stratification (part 1). Clin. Pharmacol. Ther. 13:442, 1972.

Feinstein, A.R. An analysis of diagnostic reasoning. Yale J. Biol. Med. 46:212, 1973 (part 1); 1:5, 1974 (part 2).

Feinstein, A.R. Clinical biostatistics. XXXIX. The haze of Bayes, the aerial palaces of decision analysis, and the computerized Ouija board. Clin. Pharmacol. Ther. 21:482, 1979.

Hische, E.A.H., van der Helm, H.J., van Walbeck, H.K. The cerebrospinal fluid immunoglobulin G index as a diagnostic aid in multiple sclerosis: A Bayesian approach. Clin. Chem. 28:354, 1982.

Horbar, J.D. Revising ranked probabilities: A Bayesian approach to incomplete knowledge. Comput. Biomed. Res. 16:367, 1983.

McNeil, B.J., Keeler, E., Adelstein, S.J. Primer on certain elements of medical decision making. N. Engl. J. Med. 293:211, 1975.

Pauker, S.G., Kassirer, J.P. The threshold approach to clinical decision making. N. Engl. J. Med. 302:1109, 1980.

Pryor, D.B., Harrell, F.E., Lee, K.L., Califf, R.M., Rosati, R.A. Estimating the likelihood of significant coronary artery disease. Am. J. Med. 75:771, 1983.

Rifkin, R.D., Hood, W.B. Bayesian analysis of electrocardiographic exercise stress testing. N. Engl. J. Med. 297:681, 1977.

Russek, E., Kronmal, R.A., Fisher, L.D. The effect of assuming independence in applying Bayes' theorem to risk estimation and classification in diagnosis. Comput. Biomed. Res. 16:537, 1983.

Solberg, H.E. Discriminant analysis. CRC Crit. Rev. Clin. Lab. Sci. 9:209, 1978.

Chapter 6
DIAGNOSTIC CLASSIFICATION

3. The Selection and Ordering of Diagnostic Studies

> "I think the bees suspect something!"
> "What sort of thing?"
> "I don't know. But something tells
> me that they're suspicious!"
>
> A. A. Milne

SELECTING THE STUDIES TO ORDER

In the previous chapter the individualization of the diagnostic process was discussed as it pertains to interpretation of study results. This chapter addresses the individualization of test ordering — how to identify tests that will be useful and how to order them so that patient care is expeditious and economical.

The first step in study selection is recognition of the diagnostic possibilities in the patient based upon clinical examination and preliminary laboratory studies. Diagnostic studies will then be chosen from among those that are pertinent to the possibilities. If a patient is thought to have viral hepatitis, he or she should not be subjected to studies designed to detect multiple sclerosis and vice versa.

The selection of appropriate studies or study combinations from the sometimes extensive list of pertinent tests depends largely upon the level of clinical suspicion (i.e., the magnitude of the prior probability). If a diagnosis is likely, confirmation is sought. Important but unlikely alternatives must be excluded. Diagnoses of intermediate likelihood require substantiation from evidential studies. Diseases in their clinically silent stage must be detected in asymptomatic individuals. Different tests will usually be needed to achieve these different clinical ends. Which studies serve which needs is revealed by a consideration of the performance characteristics necessitated by each.

Performance Characteristics of Confirming and Excluding Studies

A confirming laboratory study is one that raises the likelihood of a suspected diagnosis past the level of the threshold likelihood for acceptance of the diagnosis. This means that the posterior likelihood of disease given a positive result for the study must at least equal the threshold likelihood. What that means in terms of necessary performance characteristics can be appreciated by reviewing the formula for posterior likelihood, given a positive test result:

$$\frac{(prior\ likelihood)(sensitivity)}{(prior\ likelihood)(sensitivity)+(1-prior\ likelihood)(1-specificity)}.$$

For this expression to achieve values near one, in the vicinity of which the threshold likelihoods of many diseases lie, the term (1-prior likelihood)(1-specificity) must approach zero. Thus, the specificity of a confirming study should be high, the closer to one the better. In addition, the cause is helped greatly if the prior probability of the diagnosis is already fairly high. The greater the prior probability, the less the specificity required of the study.

An **excluding** laboratory study is one for which a negative test result lowers the likelihood of a diagnosis below the threshold likelihood for rejection of the diagnosis. The posterior likelihood of disease given a negative test result is

$$\frac{(prior\ likelihood)(1-sensitivity)}{(prior\ likelihood)(1-sensitivity)+(1-prior\ likelihood)(specificity)}.$$

Because the threshold likelihood for rejection is usually small, an excluding study should have performance characteristics that cause the posterior likelihood to approach zero. Inspection reveals that this is achieved when the sensitivity of the study approaches one. Here, the closer the sensitivity is to one, the better.

As an example of the use of confirming and excluding studies, consider a patient who on routine physical examination is found to have a palpable thyroid nodule. Is it benign or malignant? If the clinician's mindset is to prove that it is benign, he or she will want to order an excluding study. If a diagnosis of malignancy is sought so that early treatment can be instituted, a confirming study is needed. Let the threshold likelihood for the performance of excisional surgery be 0.5 and that for rejection of the diagnosis 0.04, i.e., on average 1 patient in 25 left untreated will actually harbor a cancer. The performance characteristics of the laboratory studies relevant to this problem have

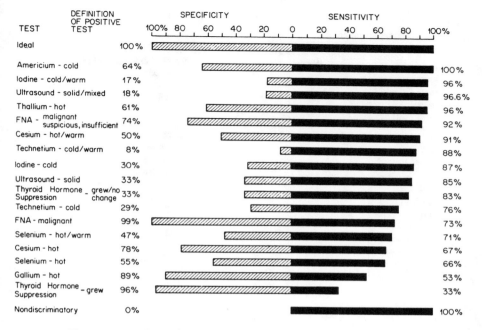

TEST	DEFINITION OF POSITIVE TEST		
Ideal	100%		
Americium - cold	64%		100%
Iodine - cold/warm	17%		96%
Ultrasound - solid/mixed	18%		96.6%
Thallium - hot	61%		96%
FNA - malignant suspicious, insufficient	74%		92%
Cesium - hot/warm	50%		91%
Technetium - cold/warm	8%		88%
Iodine - cold	30%		87%
Ultrasound - solid	33%		85%
Thyroid Hormone Suppression - grew/no change	33%		83%
Technetium - cold	29%		76%
FNA - malignant	99%		73%
Selenium - hot/warm	47%		71%
Cesium - hot	78%		67%
Selenium - hot	55%		66%
Gallium - hot	89%		53%
Thyroid Hormone Suppression - grew	96%		33%
Nondiscriminatory	0%		100%

Fig 6-1   Performance Characteristics of Studies Used to
Differentiate Benign from Malignant Thyroid Nodules
(From Ashcraft, M.W.   Analysis of techniques to
evaluate thyroid nodules.   In van Herle, A.J.
moderator.   The thyroid nodule.   Ann. Intern. Med.
96:221, 1982 © American College of Physicians,
Philadelphia.)

FNA = fine needle aspiration

been summarized by Ashcraft (1982) and are reproduced in Figure
6-1.   The tests are treated as dichotomous, although many are
trichotomous.   Those tests that are trichotomous have been
divided in two: In one case, positive and equivocal results
define the positive diagnostic category; in the other, only positive results are considered as diagnostic.

Using a prior probability of malignancy of 0.18 in this clinical setting, the posterior likelihood of malignancy for positive
and negative test results can be calculated using Bayes' formula.
The results are shown in Figure 6-2.   [This figure is a reworking
of Figure 8 from Ashcraft (1982).]

There are four studies that can be used as excluding studies:
americium scan (negative result: hot), fine needle aspiration
(negative result: not malignant), thallium scan (negative result:
cold), and cesium scan (negative result: cold).   For these, the

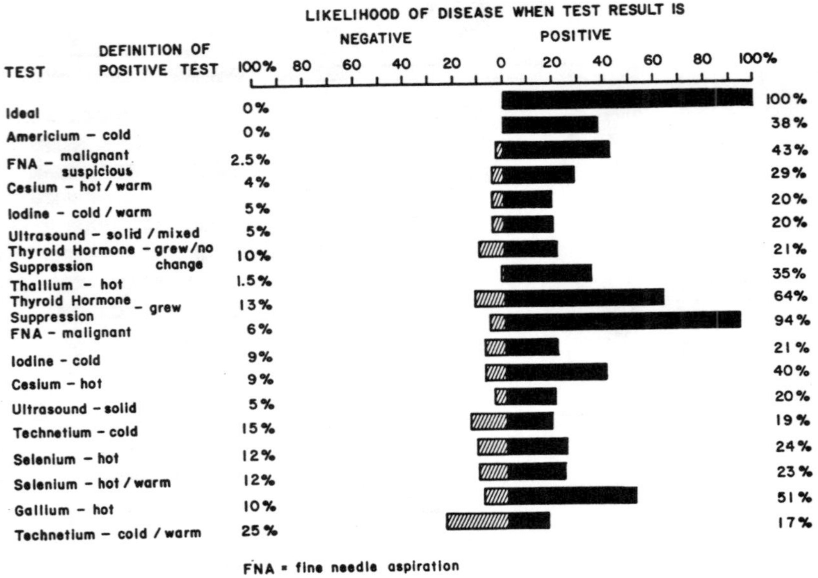

LIKELIHOOD OF DISEASE WHEN TEST RESULT IS

TEST	DEFINITION OF POSITIVE TEST	NEGATIVE	POSITIVE
Ideal	0%		100%
Americium – cold	0%		38%
FNA – malignant suspicious	2.5%		43%
Cesium – hot / warm	4%		29%
Iodine – cold / warm	5%		20%
Ultrasound – solid / mixed	5%		20%
Thyroid Hormone – grew/no change Suppression	10%		21%
Thallium – hot	1.5%		35%
Thyroid Hormone – grew Suppression	13%		64%
FNA – malignant	6%		94%
Iodine – cold	9%		21%
Cesium – hot	9%		40%
Ultrasound – solid	5%		20%
Technetium – cold	15%		19%
Selenium – hot	12%		24%
Selenium – hot / warm	12%		23%
Gallium – hot	10%		51%
Technetium – cold / warm	25%		17%

FNA = fine needle aspiration

Fig 6-2   Probabilities of Thyroid Malignancy
Given the Indicated Study Results
[Data from Ashcraft (1982)]

FNA = fine needle aspiration

posterior likelihood of disease is less than the threshold likelihood for rejecting the diagnosis, which has been set at 0.04.
Three studies satisfy the requirements for a confirming study:
thyroid hormone suppression test (positive result: nodule grows),
fine needle aspiration (positive result: malignant), and gallium
scan (positive result: hot). They produce likelihoods of disease
in excess of 0.5. Notice that fine needle aspiration could be
used as either a confirming or a excluding study given either
definition of a positive study if the threshold likelihoods were
to be relaxed somewhat.

        Of course, a quantitative laboratory study can also be used
as a confirming or an excluding study as long as there exist
values of the likelihood ratio that raise or lower the likelihood
of the diagnosis above or below the respective threshold likelihood. Thus, for confirming results,

$$\frac{\left(\begin{array}{c}prior\\likelihood\end{array}\right)\left(\begin{array}{c}likelihood\ ratio\\for\ acceptance\end{array}\right)}{\left(\begin{array}{c}prior\\likelihood\end{array}\right)\left(\begin{array}{c}likelihood\ ratio\\for\ acceptance\end{array}\right)+\left(\begin{array}{c}1-prior\\likelihood\end{array}\right)} > \begin{array}{l}threshold\ likelihood\\for\ accepting\\the\ diagnosis\end{array}$$

This rearranges to

$$\text{likelihood ratio for acceptance} > \frac{\left(\dfrac{1 - prior}{likelihood}\right)\left(\begin{array}{c}threshold\ likelihood\\ for\ acceptance\end{array}\right)}{\left(\dfrac{prior}{likelihood}\right)\left(\begin{array}{c}1 - threshold\ likelihood\\ for\ acceptance\end{array}\right)}$$

Substitution of the values used in the prior example yields

likelihood ratio for acceptance > 4.55.

Figure 6-3 shows the performance characteristic curves (actually points) for the diagnostic techniques used to differentiate benign from malignant thyroid nodules. Some of the methods have only one possible performance pair, but most have two: a half-shaded circle indicates that the positive diagnostic classification is defined as a positive test result; a full-shaded

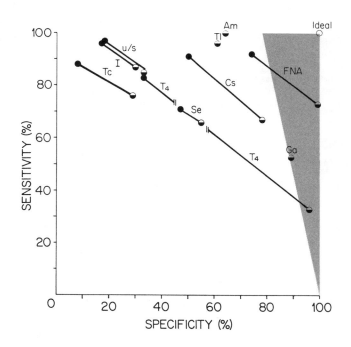

Fig 6-3   Performance Characteristic Curves for Studies
Used to Differentiate Benign from Malignant Thyroid Nodules;
Confirming Performances in Gray Region
(Modified from Ashcraft, M.W.   Analysis of tech-
niques to evaluate thyroid nodules.   In van Herle,
A.J. moderator.   The thyroid nodule. <u>Ann. Intern.
Med.</u> 96:221, 1982 © American College of Physicians,
Philadelphia.)

circle means that positive and equivocal results both are considered diagnostic.

To use the performance characteristic curves, the relationship,

likelihood ratio for acceptance = sensitivity/(1-specificity)

is used to recast the likelihood ratio inequality into a performance characteristic inequality,

(1/likelihood ratio for acceptance) sensitivity + specificity > 1.

The region of the performance characteristic surface that satisfies this inequality for a likelihood ratio for acceptance of 4.55 is shown in gray. Study results associated with performance pairs within this region are confirmatory. The studies identified earlier are indicated as satisfactory here also: thyroid hormone suppression test (narrow definition), fine needle aspiration (narrow definition), and gallium scan.

A similar approach gives

$$\text{likelihood ratio for rejection} < \frac{\left(1 - \frac{prior}{likelihood}\right)\left(\begin{array}{c}threshold\ likelihood\\ for\ rejection\end{array}\right)}{\left(\frac{prior}{likelihood}\right)\left(1 - \begin{array}{c}threshold\ likelihood\\ for\ rejection.\end{array}\right)}$$

and

sensitivity + (likelihood ratio for rejection) (specificity) > 1.

The excluding studies that satisfy this performance inequality for the values used in the example fall within the gray region indicated in Figure 6-4. Americium and thallium scans (both narrow definition), cesium scan (broad definition), and fine needle aspiration (broad definition) are identified. It can be seen that radioiodine scan and ultrasonography (both broad definition) come close to achieving the performance requirements.

In both cases more than one technique was found to be satisfactory for the intended diagnostic purpose. Which should be ordered? First, assume that the different studies are roughly equivalent in their value (i.e., cost) to the patient. As was shown in the preceding chapter, the expected value from diagnostic confirmation increases with increasing likelihood of the diagnosis, and the expected value from rejection of a diagnosis increases with decreasing disease likelihood. The maximum value to the patient is thereby obtained by selecting the study with

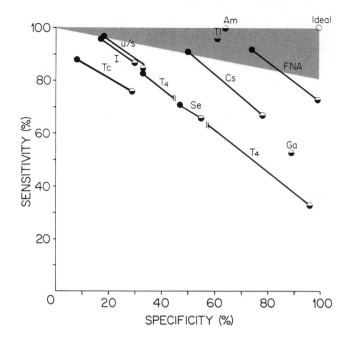

Fig 6-4   Performance Characteristic Curves for Studies
Used to Differentiate Benign from Malignant Thyroid Nodules;
Rejecting Performances in Gray Region
(Modified from Ashcraft, M.W.   Analysis of tech-
niques to evaluate thyroid nodules.   In van Herle,
A.J. moderator. The thyroid nodule. Ann. Intern.
Med. 96:221, 1982 © American College of Physicians,
Philadelphia.)

which the posterior likelihood can be maximized, if for confirmation, or minimized, if for rejection.   The posterior likelihood is maximized by choosing the performance pair with the
largest likelihood ratio.   This is easily done graphically as
follows: place a straightedge so as to connect the performance
pairs (specificity = 1.0, sensitivity = 1.0) and (specificity =
1.0, sensitivity = 0); pivoting at the point on the specificity
axis, rotate the straightedge into the coordinate space.   The
first point encountered is the performance pair with the maximum
likelihood ratio and, therefore, the maximum posterior likelihood.   In the current example, fine needle aspiration with a
narrow definition of malignancy is the preferred confirming
study. The minimum posterior likelihood arises from the performance pair with the smallest likelihood ratio.   Connect the per-

formance pairs (specificity = 1.0, sensitivity = 1.0) and (specificity = 0, sensitivity = 1.0) with a straightedge; pivoting at
the point on the sensitivity axis, rotate the straightedge into
the coordinate space. The first point encountered is the performance pair with the minimum likelihood ratio and minimum
posterior likelihood. Americium scan is the preferred excluding
study.

When there are gross differences in value to the patient
among the available satisfactory studies, maximum value may come
from selecting the study with the least personal cost rather than
utilizing the one that achieves the most desirable posterior
likelihood.

Performance Characteristics of Screening Studies

A screening laboratory study is one used to detect a serious,
treatable disease in persons afflicted with the disorder but who
have no clinical findings suggestive of the disease. Such clinically silent disease is sometimes labeled "occult." Feinstein
(1967) calls patients with silent disease "lanthanic," which
means noncomplaining.

Because the object of screening tests is to detect disease,
they must be sensitive. But they must also be specific or else
prohibitive numbers of disease-free individuals will be subjected
to postscreening clinical and laboratory evaluation. A reasonable goal to set for overall test performance is that the sensitivity and specificity be such that, given a positive study
result, the posterior likelihood of disease exceeds the threshold
likelihood for excluding the disease. Further evaluation is then
clearly justified. Of the studies available for screening for a
particular disease, the one that satisfies the performance criteria and has the greatest sensitivity should be preferred.

Therefore, the necessary study performance is

$$\frac{\left(\begin{smallmatrix}prior\\likelihood\end{smallmatrix}\right)\ sensitivity}{\left(\begin{smallmatrix}prior\\likelihood\end{smallmatrix}\right)sensitivity\ +\ \left(\begin{smallmatrix}1\text{-}prior\\likelihood\end{smallmatrix}\right)\left(1\text{-}specificity\right)} > \begin{smallmatrix}threshold\ likelihood\\for\ rejecting\\the\ diagnosis.\end{smallmatrix}$$

The prior likelihood of disease here is simply the prevalence of
the disease in similar individuals, i.e., in lanthanic individuals sharing similar risk or protection factors. In coronary
heart disease, for instance, males in their fifties share two
risk factors: male gender and late middle age. Females in their

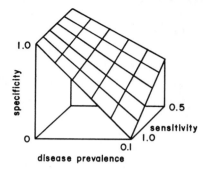

threshold likelihood for rejection of diagnosis = 0.1

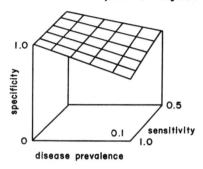

threshold likelihood for rejection of diagnosis = 0.25

Fig 6-5   Graphic Representation of Performance Criteria
for a Screening Study (Prevalence < 0.1)

thirties have two common protective features: female gender and
early middle age.   The prevalence of coronary heart disease in
these dissimilar groups is dramatically unequal.   Therefore, the
appropriate estimate for disease prevalence must be used to quantify prior likelihood.

The graphic representation of the performance criteria for a
screening study are shown in Figure 6-5 for two values of the
threshold likelihood for rejecting a diagnosis.   The minimal
acceptable performance pairings are indicated by the gridwork
surfaces.

Some generalizations that apply to the performance characteristics of screening studies are readily appreciated from
inspection of the figure:

1.   The greater the sensitivity of the study, the less the
demands upon the specificity.

2.   The lower the prevalence of the disease screened for, the
greater the study specificity required; if the prevalence

is very low, the specificity must approach unity.

3. The larger the critical likelihood for rejection of a diagnosis, the greater the specificity necessary.

The third generalization is somewhat unexpected because it states that the less critical the clinician is about excluding a certain disease, the better the performance required of a screening test. Such a conclusion is at odds with the intuitive notion that less serious illnesses can be screened for casually, with studies of mediocre quality. But in fact, evidence from a study of high quality is needed to convince a clinician to abandon an impression of health, which is after all the alternate hypothesis in a lanthanic patient, in favor of the pursuit of a disorder of little clinical moment.

There are diseases for which there are no laboratory studies available that possess the performance characteristics required of a screening study. Screening for these diseases may still be possible, however, by the use of repeat testing. When the object of repeat testing is to increase the sensitivity of a screening study, the believe-the-positive positivity rule should apply. When specificity needs to be augmented through repeat testing, the believe-the-negative rule is appropriate. In either case, clinical studies need to be performed to confirm that the stipulated testing regimen and the accompanying positivity rule actually achieve the desired diagnostic performance.

Interval Screening

Confirming and excluding laboratory studies are performed upon patients who, being ill, are in need of a diagnosis and therapy. There is very little question as to the appropriate timing for obtaining a study — the disease has made itself manifest and demands attention. This contrasts with the very real problem of establishing guidelines for the administration of screening studies. Which individuals need to be studied? When and how often should a lanthanic individual be studied?

Screening studies should be performed only upon those persons for whom there is a reasonable expectation that the disease could be present: Menopausal women are screened for endometrial carcinoma; screening for sickle cell hemoglobinopathy is conducted among blacks. Gender (endometrial carcinoma) and geographic ancestry (sickle cell hemoglobinopathy) are charactertistics frequently used to distinguish persons who need screening from those who do not. A family history of a heritable or a transmissible disorder detectable in its lanthanic stage is another indication for screening studies.

Inherited and acquired diseases alike are looked for when the lanthanic individual is at risk for harboring subclinical disease. One is certainly at risk when some of the members of one's risk cohort, i.e., persons with similar risk characteristics, show overt disease. The recommended ages for beginning clinical and laboratory screening for many forms of cancer have been selected on the basis of such a rule. For certain diseases, it is clear that the subclinical stage is long-lived, and individuals are at risk for silent disease long before the age when overt disease begins to appear. Coronary artery disease is an example of this kind of disorder. Unfortunately, there are currently no reliable noninvasive screening studies for detecting this disease while it is subclinical and, presumably, more treatable. The inborn errors of metabolism, i.e., genetic diseases such as homocystinuria and sickle hemoglobinopathy, are present from conception although they may not become manifest for years. Screening studies, if performed, are usually done early in life.

The frequency with which a lanthanic individual is screened for a particular disease depends in large measure upon the natural history of the disease and upon the performance of the available screening study. To demonstrate this, imagine a disorder for which the treatable subclinical stage lasts 3 to 6 years. A screening study exists that can detect the disease during its final 1 1/2 years of reversible development, even in the most rapidly evolving cases. Here "detect" means that the peformance characteristics of the study satisfy the criteria discussed in the preceding section of the chapter. A negative screen indicates either that the tested individual is truly free from subclinical disease or that the subclinical disease has not yet developed to the point of detectability. Those persons with undetected subclinical disease will experience progression of their disease, but at least for 1 1/2 years they will remain treatable. After 1 1/2 years, though, some of those persons who at the time of the first screening study had subclinical disease that was just slightly too underdeveloped for detection will suffer irreversible progression of their disease. Therefore, a second screening study should be administered 1 1/2 years after the first. Similar reasoning leads to the conclusion that all persons at risk should be screened every 1 1/2 years. But what if a better screening study becomes available, say one that can detect disease at any time during the subclinical stage? Using this study a negative screen means that a person is disease free. The disease can arise and progress to incurability in as little as 3 years, so the screening study should be repeated every 3 years.

In general, if the study is insensitive to early disease, the interval between successive screening studies should be the length of time the subclinical disease is detectable by the screening study. If the study can detect early disease, the minimum duration of the treatable subclinical stage should be the screening interval. Because repeated testing will alter the performance characteristics of a screening study, it is imperative to confirm by clinical studies that implementation of the recommended screening interval results in satisfactory diagnostic performance — especially as regards specificity. The expense and invasiveness of the study are important considerations not discussed here. The American Cancer Society's interval screening recommendations for the early detection of cancer are examples of screening schedules designed from theoretical considerations and validated by extensive clinical experience (American Cancer Society 1980).

Choosing Among Evidential Studies

When a diagnostic alternative is only moderately likely, it is often unrealistic to expect to confirm or exclude it by the performance of a single laboratory study. Studies with the requisite performance characteristics may not exist. Instead, one or more evidential laboratory studies must be obtained to appreciably alter the level of likelihood. If the likelihood is increased as a consequence of the test result, a confirming study is then appropriate; if it is decreased, an excluding study should be considered. The problem for the clinician is to select the most useful evidential study from among the abundant number available. The solution is to choose the study that is the best diagnostic classifier at the given level of likelihood. Thus the increment in diagnostic information is maximized.

In Chapter 4 it was stated that minimum misclassification is achieved when a study's critical value is set so that the corresponding point on the performance characteristic curve has a slope equal to

$$\frac{prevalence - 1}{prevalence} .$$

When choosing among diagnostic techniques, the minimum misclassification is similarly identified. Each study's performance characteristic curve will contain a point with slope equal to

$$\frac{prior\ likelihood - 1}{prior\ likelihood} .$$

From the set of target lines with the above slope, the one with the largest value for the sensitivity axis intercept marks the performance point and hence the study and its critical value, which minimizes misclassification.

ORDERING STUDIES

It may seem unnecessary to devote space to the topic of ordering laboratory studies. Surely clinicians simply order the studies they select as appropriate in the diagnostic work-up of patients. What further is there to discuss? The answer is: those real-life considerations that not infrequently cause clinicians to deviate from the simple pattern of test ordering. These considerations include:

1. the availability of studies, the scheduling of studies, and the time it takes to receive study results
2. anticipated diagnostic needs
3. the physical, psychological, and financial costs of laboratory testing.

Sequential Versus Concurrent Ordering

When planning the diagnostic approach to a patient, the clinician must keep in mind the capabilities of the clinical laboratories. In the example used earlier in this chapter, it was found that an americium scan is the preferred study for excluding malignancy in a patient with an asymptomatic thyroid nodule. But americium scans are not performed in every hospital. Clinicians at some hospitals must rely upon different studies. Fortunately, the standards of medical care in this country are so high that, usually, when a laboratory study is not available, either an adequate substitute study is or the patient can be transferred to a medical center that does offer the needed test. The availability of laboratory studies can also be limited because of problems in test scheduling. A study that cannot be performed for days because of a full schedule may be no more useful than a study that is not offered at all. Alternative studies that can be obtained quickly are then ordered instead.

Another and more frequent consideration in test ordering is the time that elapses between requesting a study and receiving the study result. If the wait is short, a study can be ordered and the result received and analyzed prior to requesting the next study, if additional testing is indicated. This is sequential test ordering. It is diagnostically efficient because each study ordered contributes to the diagnosis and is cost-effective because the number of studies ordered is minimized. If the turnaround time is long, however, the patient's care is compromised by the cumulative delay in diagnosis occasioned by sequential testing. In that case, most or all of the potentially useful laboratory studies are ordered together and the results are interpreted en masse. This is concurrent ordering. It is not efficient but, when properly used, is cost-effective since the cost of a delayed diagnosis is minimized.

Concurrent ordering must not be confused with the indiscriminant ordering of laboratory studies by those who have the misconception that the greater the number of studies ordered, the greater the amount of information that will be available for use in the care of the patient. Data is not always information! Informative study results contribute to the care of the patient. Superfluous study results, at best, contribute nothing to the patient's care, often obscure informative results, and sometimes, because of imperfect study performance, misinform.

Data-Base Ordering

Besides ordering indicated screening studies and pertinent diagnostic studies, clinicians often request studies that will provide useful information in the event that a patient develops certain future diagnostic needs, so-called data-base ordering. If interindividual variability in the measurement of an analyte exceeds its intraindividual variability, the availability of the patient's baseline value enhances the interpretation of subsequent determinations. Baseline studies should be ordered for such analytes but only when there is a reasonable expectation of a future diagnostic need.

Cost Containment

That there are costs to the patients who undergo laboratory testing was mentioned in the preceding chapter's discussion of identifying threshold diagnostic likelihoods. It was pointed out that when the confirming study is costly, the threshold likelihood for accepting a diagnosis is lowered, and when the excluding study is costly, the threshold likelihood for rejecting a diagnosis is raised. That means that the chances of a diagnostic misclassification are increased. To minimize this vitiation of the diagnostic process, laboratory studies should be selected to minimize the costs of testing. Although this is not always possible because of appreciable differences in study performance, when possible, it is an important consideration in study selection.

EXERCISES

The following table lists the performance characteristics of a number of tests for prostate cancer.

TEST	NO. OF PATIENTS	SENSITIVITY	SPECIFICITY	PREDICTIVE VALUE		EFFICIENCY
				POSITIVE TEST	NEGATIVE TEST	
Rectal examination	300	0.69	0.89	67	91	85
Acid phosphatase — enzyme	300	0.56	0.94	72	88	84
Acid phosphatase — RIA	100	0.20	0.85	29	78	70
Acid phosphatase — CIEP	100	0.20	0.95	56	80	78
Urine cytology before massage	202	0.17	0.98	67	80	79
Prostatic-secretion cytology after massage	211	0.29	0.98	78	82	81
Urine cytology after massage	209	0.22	0.98	71	81	80
Aspiration cytology	200	0.55	0.91	65	88	83
Lactic dehydrogenase V/I ratio	132	0.47	0.82	44	83	73
Leukocyte-adherence inhibition	113	0.50	0.79	43	83	72

(From Guinan, P., Bush, I., Ray, V., et al. The accuracy of the rectal examination in the diagnosis of prostate carcinoma. N. Engl. J. Med. 303:499, 1980 © New England Journal of Medicine, Boston.)

The prevalence of prostate cancer in patients over 50 years old with symptoms referable to the prostate is approximately 0.25. The prevalence in asymptomatic men over 50 years old is about 0.01. Assume that the threshold likelihood for rejecting the diagnosis of prostate cancer is 0.075 for both populations.

6-1. Which of these studies can be used to screen for prostate cancer among asymptomatic men?

6-2. The performance characteristics listed in the table were found in a population of symptomatic men. What can be inferred about the likely performance among asymptomatic men?

6-3. Which of these studies can be used to exclude the diagnosis of prostate cancer in symptomatic men?

6-4. If the threshold likelihood for electing to biopsy the prostate for a definitive pathologic diagnosis is 0.5, which of these studies can be used to confirm the diagnosis of prostate cancer in symptomatic men? Which would you recommend?

6-5. Suppose a screening program for prostate cancer is established using acid phosphatase-enzyme as the screening study. What study should be used to follow up a positive screening result?

Mind-Expanding Exercise

6-6. The American Cancer Society's recommendation for the early detection of asymptomatic cancer of the cervix is that women 20 to 65 years old have a Pap test (cervical scrape cytology) performed "at least every 3 years after 2 negative exams 1 year apart" (American Cancer Society 1980). Comment on this interval screening procedure.

REFERENCES

American Cancer Society. ACS report on the cancer-related health checkup. CA 30:193, 1980.

Ashcraft, M.W. Analysis of techniques to evaluate thyroid nodules. In van Herle, A.J. moderator. The thyroid nodule. Ann. Intern. Med. 96:221, 1982.

Feinstein, A.R. Clinical Judgment. Robert E. Krieger, Huntington, New York, p. 145, 1967.

PART III:

PHYSIOLOGIC PRINCIPLES

Chapter 7

ORGAN FUNCTION

1. Synthesis and Clearance

Est modus in rebus, sunt certi denique fines,
Quos ultra citraque nequit consistere rectum.

Horace

MEASUREMENT OF ORGAN FUNCTION

Organ function is assessed by measuring how well an organ is doing what it is supposed to be doing. For example, the pump function of the heart is studied by measuring the cardiac output and the blood pressure; the cognitive function of the brain is investigated using intelligence tests. The functional status of secretory organs, organs of cell generation (such as the marrow), and organs of elimination can also be evaluated. The laboratory studies used to make these measurements may assay the organ's functional state directly, such as analyzing semen to determine testicular function. More often, though, the studies measure function only indirectly: the plasma concentrations of the products secreted by the cells from an organ are used as markers for that organ's secretory or generative activity, and the plasma concentrations of the substances or cells cleared by an organ are used to monitor that organ's elimination process.

PHYSIOLOGIC MODELS: MARKER SUBSTANCES

(Groth 1982; Murphy 1978)

Very often in medicine one wishes to obtain information that is not available through direct observation. For example, when a physician wishes to learn if a patient has suffered an acute myocardial infarct, he or she does not examine the patient's cardiac myocytes directly in a search for recent cell death. Instead, the plasma concentrations of certain enzymes are determined. Although the measurements of the enzyme concentrations do not, by themselves, provide any information, they can be interpreted within a conceptual framework, or **model**, wherein the enzyme con-

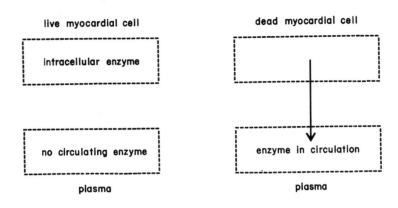

live myocardial cell

| intracellular enzyme |

no circulating enzyme

plasma

dead myocardial cell

enzyme in circulation

plasma

Fig 7-1   Model of Cardiac Enzyme Release

centrations relate in a predictable fashion to the physiologic
event "acute myocardial infarct." Hence, the measurements can be
used to make predictions about the presence or absence of an
acute myocardial infarct. Figure 7-1 depicts such a model. The
enzyme enters the plasma if, and only if, myocardial cells die
and liberate their intracellular stores of the enzyme. The appearance of the enzyme in the plasma, therefore, indicates the
death of myocardial cells.

This model is an example of the conceptualization of a **marker
substance**, a substance that marks or indicates a physiologic
process, even though it may be separated from the process by distance and time. Much of laboratory medicine is concerned with
the detection and measurement of marker substances, especially in
body fluids. Organ function can be evaluated by measuring the
plasma concentration of an organ's secretory product or the concentration of a plasma substance that is removed from the circulation by the organ. Cell injury and death is most often detected
by the appearance or the increased plasma concentration of an
intracellular substance present in the injured cells. The body
stores of an analyte can be quantified indirectly by measurement
of an intracellular substance released from or secreted by a cell
participating in the storage of the analyte. Hyperplastic and
neoplastic processes may be detected because of the release of
increased amounts of normal intracellular substances or secretory
products into the circulation. In addition, novel cellular
products may be secreted or released by neoplastic tissue. These
applications of marker substances are summarized in Table 7-1.

Table 7-1

Use of Marker Substances in Laboratory Medicine

	Marker substance		
	Intracellular substance	Secretory product	Eliminated substance
Organ function		+	+
Cell injury and death	+		
Body stores	+	+	
Hyperplasia/neoplasia	+	+	

SYNTHESIS AND CLEARANCE
(DiStefano 1976; Riggs 1976)

Organ function can be measured indirectly using the plasma concentration of a marker substance because in **steady state**, i.e., when the amount of substance in the system is constant over time, the plasma concentration of a substance is related to its production and removal according to the simple equation,

substance plasma concentration = synthetic rate/clearance rate.

The **synthetic rate** quantifies the entry of substance into the plasma. Its dimensions are substance per unit time (e.g., millimoles per hour). It appears in the numerator because the plasma concentration of a substance is directly related to its rate of entry; the more rapid the entry, the greater the concentration.

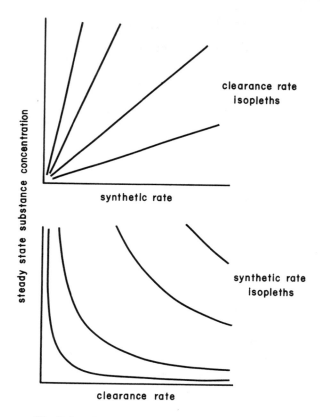

Fig 7-2   Steady-State Relationships
Among Concentration, Synthetic Rate, and Clearance Rate

The upper panel of Figure 7-2 shows the direct relationship between substance concentration and synthetic rate at various clearance rates.

The **clearance rate** quantifies the elimination of substance from the plasma. It has the dimensions volume per unit time (e.g., milliliters per minute) and can be thought of as the volume of plasma completely cleared of marker substance in a specified time interval. Substance concentration is <u>inversely related</u> to its rate of removal, so this term appears in the denominator. The lower panel of Figure 7-2 illustrates the hyperbolic relationship between substance concentration and clearance rate at different synthetic rates.

Although the synthetic rate is a familiar concept, the clearance rate is not. After all, most elimination processes do not completely clear plasma of marker substance during passage of the plasma through the organ. This leads to two questions: 1) Why does the clearance rate appear in the steady-state concentration expression rather than a more readily comprehensible term such as elimination rate? 2) If the clearance rate can be measured directly, how is it done?

The answer to the first question is that clearance rate appears in the concentration expression because it is the kinetic parameter that makes the equation work. Let the equation be rearranged thus:

plasma substance concentration · clearance rate = synthetic rate.

In this form, it is clear that the clearance rate is the constant of proportionality between concentration and synthetic rate. As such, it represents the volume of substance-free plasma that must be available per unit time so that substance entering the system is diluted to its steady-state concentration. Because in steady state an equal volume of substance-rich plasma must be cleared of that substance to serve as the source of substance-free plasma, this constant of proportionality also represents the volume of plasma that is completely cleared of substance per unit time.

It turns out that clearance rate and **volume of distribution**, the constant of proportionality between the concentration of substance in a fluid compartment and the amount of substance in the compartment, are the primary kinetic parameters. They determine the disposition and elimination of substance in a physiologic system. All of the derivative kinetic parameters, such as substance concentration and elimination rate, are determined by them.

The answer to the second question is that the clearance rate of a substance can be measured directly as the substance elimination rate divided by substance concentration. This equality is easily confirmed. Substitution of "elimination rate divided by substance concentration" into the steady state concentration equation in the place of "clearance rate" yields

plasma substance concentration = $\dfrac{synthetic\ rate}{(elimination\ rate/substance\ concentration)}$, which, on rearrangement, gives

elimination rate = synthetic rate.

This is certainly true for the steady state where the rate of entry of substance must be exactly balanced by the rate of loss of substance. Therefore,

clearance rate = elimination rate/plasma substance concentration.

When the substance elimination rate and plasma concentration can be measured directly, so can the clearance rate.

Volume of Distribution

The steady-state concentration equation indicates that the substance concentration does not depend upon the volume of distribution of the substance. To show that this is so, the following hydraulic analogy is offered.

Consider two fluid reservoirs, as pictured in Figure 7-3, one with a large horizontal surface area and one with a small surface

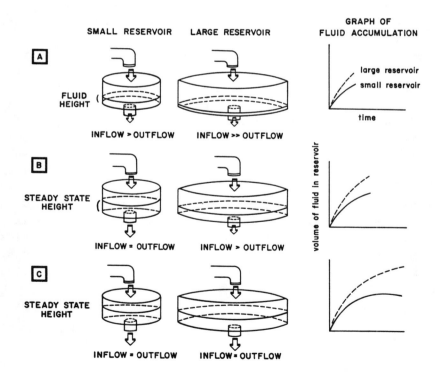

Fig 7-3   Hydraulic Analogy

- 134 -

area. Each reservoir is supplied from an overhanging spigot, and
fluid escapes each through equal-sized taps located at the container bottoms. At the start both reservoirs are empty. At some
point fluid begins to flow into the containers. Let the fluid
inflow be at a constant rate and equal for both reservoirs. At
the same time fluid begins to be lost from the containers through
the taps. The rate of fluid outflow depends upon the water pressure, which in turn varies directly with the height of fluid in
the container.

At first there is a large imbalance between the inflow and
the outflow. The rate of inflow is much greater, so fluid begins
to accumulate in the reservoirs. In the small reservoir, accumulation will result in a rapid elevation in the height of the
fluid and a brisk, steady increase in the outflow rate. In the
large reservoir, two competing effects operate. On the one hand,
a greater volume of fluid must accumulate to raise the fluid
level, thereby slowing the fluid rise in the container. On the
other hand, the lower fluid height causes a slower increase in
the outflow rate and, therefore, more rapid fluid accumulation.
The net result is that the fluid rises more slowly in the large
reservoir but a larger volume of fluid accumulates there (Figure
7-3, panel A). Continued fluid accumulation in the small reservoir will further raise the fluid height and therefore the rate
of fluid outflow. When the outflow is equal in magnitude to the
inflow, no further fluid accumulation will occur. At that time
the fluid in the small reservoir will have reached its steady
state height (Figure 7-3, panel B). Because of the less rapid
increase in the fluid level in the large reservoir, steady state
will be reached there later (Figure 7-3, panel C).

The steady-state height of fluid in the large reservoir will
be that which results in equivalence of fluid inflow and outflow.
Since the two reservoirs experience equal rates of fluid inflow,
the outflow rates from each must be equal in the steady state.
This means that the steady state fluid heights must, in addition,
be equal since the rate of fluid outflow depends solely upon
fluid height, given equal-sized taps. So in steady state, the
heights of the fluid in the reservoirs will be equal despite
differences in the (literal) volume of distribution of the fluid.

In contrast, the time needed to establish steady state does depend upon the volume of distribution. As a rule of thumb, steady state is achieved following five half-lives of the substance, where half-life equals

$$0.693 \cdot volume \ of \ distribution/clearance \ rate.$$

The time required to reach steady state is proportional to the volume of distribution.

The volume of distribution of a substance is a mathematical creation. It does not have a simple anatomic counterpart. It is common, for instance, to suppose that the compartment into which a substance distributes immediately following entry into the blood, called the central compartment, is the plasma and that the volume of distribution would be equal to the plasma volume. If a small, nonbinding solute enters, however, the calculated volume of distribution of the central compartment usually exceeds that of the plasma volume. This is so because, for most small solutes, diffusion into extravascular fluids is as rapid as within the plasma, making these fluids a part of the central compartment and adding to its apparent volume. If the substance additionally experiences significant rapid tissue binding or uptake, the central volume of distribution will be larger still. In such cases it can even exceed that of total body water (note that this central compartment is not homogeneous, but its apparent volume of distribution is calculated as though it were). Plasma protein binding and high molecular weight, on the other hand, will retard substance transfer into extravascular sites. For such substances the volume of distribution of the central compartment approaches that of the plasma volume. For substances that both diffuse rapidly and experience some protein binding, the volume of distribution of the central compartment will be intermediate between that of the plasma and that of the extravascular fluid.

ORGAN SYNTHETIC RATE

Direct measurement of the organ synthetic rate is possible only for a limited number of organs: the stomach, pancreas, and testes. The secretory products of all other organs are released in ways that disallow their collection. Consequently, the functional status of these organs must be assessed indirectly. The indirect measurement of organ synthetic rate is based upon the steady state relationship between the plasma concentration of a marker substance and its synthetic rate:

plasma substance concentration = synthetic rate/clearance rate.

Rearrangement yields

synthetic rate = clearance rate · plasma substance concentration.

If it is assumed that 1) the marker substance is secreted only by the organ of interest and 2) the clearance rate of the substance is a constant, then

organ synthetic rate = constant · plasma substance concentration.

Thus the organ synthetic rate can be estimated from the plasma concentration of the marker substance.

Because the relationship is not only linear but directly proportional, the magnitude of a change in synthetic function is exactly reflected in the proportional change in the concentration of the marker. A two-fold elevation in the marker substance levels, for instance, indicates a like, i.e., two-fold, increase in synthetic activity. A one-third reduction in the concentration of the marker reflects a one-third decrease in synthetic rate.

Similar reasoning is applied to the measurement of the generative rate of the bone marrow, such that

marrow generative rate = constant · cell concentration in blood.

ORGAN CLEARANCE RATE

The functional status of an organ of elimination is assessed by measuring the rate of removal of a substance eliminated by the organ. The organ clearance rate can be measured directly if the eliminated substance can be collected. The substance being removed is collected over time and its elimination rate is determined. During the collection a blood specimen is taken, and the concentration of substance in the plasma is assayed. The organ clearance rate is then calculated:

organ clearance rate = elimination rate/plasma substance concentration

For example, the renal clearance rate of creatinine can be measured directly:

$$\text{renal clearance rate for creatinine} = \frac{\left(\begin{array}{c}\text{concentration of creatinine}\\ \text{in time urine collection}\end{array}\right)\left(\begin{array}{c}\text{volume of}\\ \text{urine collection}\end{array}\right)}{\begin{array}{c}\text{concentration of creatinine}\\ \text{in plasma}\end{array}}$$

In routine practice the collection of eliminated substances is possible only for substances excreted into the urine. Direct measurement of organ clearance rate is thereby limited to the kidney.

Indirect Measurement

Indirect measurement of clearance function is required for such organs as the liver and lungs. The clearance function of the kidney can also be evaluated by indirect measurement, which is particularly useful when the collection of a timed urine specimen is impractical. Indirect measurements are based upon the steady-state relationship of the plasma concentration of a marker substance to the substance's clearance rate:

plasma substance concentration = synthetic rate/clearance rate.

Rearrangement yields

clearance rate = synthetic rate/plasma substance concentration.

If it is assumed that 1) the marker substance is eliminated solely from the organ of interest and 2) the rate of synthesis of the substance is a constant, then

organ clearance rate = constant/plasma substance concentration.

Therefore, the organ clearance rate can be estimated from the plasma concentration of the marker substance.

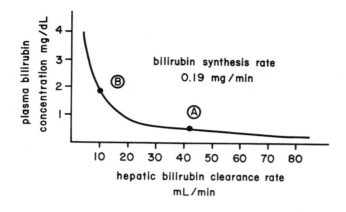

Fig 7-4   Steady-State Relationship of Plasma Bilirubin
Concentration to Hepatic Bilirubin Clearance Rate

Unlike the synthetic rate, however, this relationship is not linear but hyperbolic. Consequently, the magnitude of the change in the plasma concentration of a marker substance following an alteration in organ function will depend not only upon the magnitude of the alteration, but also upon the clearance rate present prior to the alteration. An example is given in Figure 7-4, which depicts the hyperbolic relationship between the hepatic bilirubin clearance rate and the plasma bilirubin concentration. In the presence of normal clearance rates (point A), a reduction in the clearance rate will result in no more than a modest elevation in the bilirubin concentration. When hepatic function is poor, however, and the bilirubin clearance rate is low (point B), even a slight additional reduction in the clearance rate will cause a marked increase in bilirubin level. Thus marker substances of organ clearance function show increasing sensitivity to changes in organ function as the organ's functional status deteriorates. Table 7-2 lists organ clearance studies that are commonly used clinically.

Table 7-2

Selected Organ Clearance Studies:
Endogenous Substances

Organ	Marker substance	Function measured
Lungs	Carbon dioxide	Alveolar ventilation
Liver	Bilirubin	(Hepatocyte) organic anion extraction
	Bile acids	(Hepatocyte) bile acid extraction
	Ammonia	(Hepatocyte) ammonia extraction
Kidneys	Creatinine	Glomerular filtration rate
	Urea nitrogen	Glomerular filtration rate
Spleen	Abnormal red cells	Red cell culling

Blood Flow as a Determinant of Organ Clearance Rate
(Cobby and Makoid 1980; Gibaldi and Perrier 1982; Wright 1982)

The rate of removal and hence the clearance rate of a substance by an organ depend not only upon the intrinsic capacity of the organ to clear the substance, but also upon the rate of plasma flow through the organ. At low rates of plasma flow, the elimination rate is low because, while the organ is able to remove much of the substance passing through it, the rate of delivery of substance is small. At high rates of plasma flow, the organ is able to remove only a small fraction of the substance in each passing volume of blood, but the elimination rate is high because the volume flux is great.

Figure 7-5 illustrates this phenomenon in a capillary. In the left panel, plasma enters the capillary at a flow rate designated Q. The plasma passes through the capillary in time t, during which the concentration of substance falls from C_{in} to C_{1out}. At twice the plasma flow rate, 2Q, as seen in the right panel, the substance concentration declines less, to C_{2out}, because the plasma resides in the capillary only half as long. It can be shown that the change in substance concentration at flow rate Q will be equal to or less than twice that at flow rate 2Q. Thus the elimination rate (which equals the product of the plasma flow rate times the change of the substance concentration) at 2Q is equal to or greater than that at Q.

- 140 -

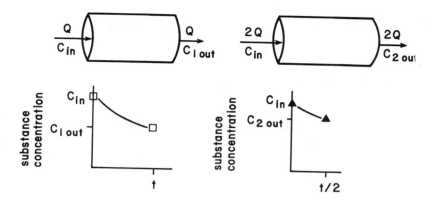

Fig 7-5   Elimination in a Capillary

An organ of elimination can be considered to be a large array
of capillaries arranged in parallel (the so-called "parallel
tube" model).   Then the results regarding the effect of blood
flow rate in a capillary can be extrapolated to the whole organ,
in particular:

1. The change in substance concentration across an organ of
    elimination decreases as the rate of plasma flow in-
    creases; however,

2. The elimination rate of the organ increases as the rate
    of plasma flow increases; and

3. Because the organ clearance rate equals the organ elimi-
    nation rate divided by the input concentration, the organ
    clearance rate increases as the rate of plasma flow in-
    creases.

    For the parallel tube model, the relationship of the organ
clearance rate to the rate of organ plasma flow (expressed as the
ratio of flow rate to the maximum organ clearance rate) is demonstrated in Figure 7-6.   At low relative flow rates, the organ
clearance rate is approximately equal to the plasma flow rate.
At high relative flow rates, the organ clearance rate asympto-
tically approaches the maximum substance clearance rate of which
the organ is capable, called the **intrinsic substance clearance
rate.**   The intrinsic substance clearance rate represents the
inherent functional capacity of the organ to clear substance.

    Also shown in the figure are the clearance characteristics of
two substances cleared by the liver.   Bile acids, typified by
chenodeoxycholic acid, have a large intrinsic hepatic clearance

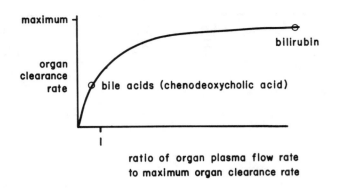

Fig 7-6   Relationship of Organ Clearance Rate
to Organ Plasma Flow

rate, somewhat greater than the hepatic plasma flow rate, so the ratio of the flow rate to the intrinsic clearance rate is less than one. That means that the hepatic clearance rate for bile acids roughly equals the hepatic plasma flow rate and, further-more, that changes in the plasma flow rate cause nearly equal changes in the organ clearance rate. The organ clearance rate is much less sensitive to changes in the intrinsic clearance rate. Bile acids, therefore, are good markers of liver plasma flow rate but not of liver functional capacity. The intrinsic substance clearance rate for bilirubin is small, about one-tenth that of the hepatic plasma flow rate, so the ratio of the flow rate to the intrinsic clearance rate is large. That means that the hepatic clearance rate for bilirubin is close to the intrinsic clearance rate. Changes in the intrinsic clearance rate cause equal changes in the organ clearance rate. The organ clearance rate is insensitive to changes in the plasma flow rate. Thus bilirubin is a good marker of liver functional capacity but not of liver plasma flow.

ORGAN CLEARANCE OF EXOGENOUS SUBSTANCES
(D'Argenio 1981; Dossing et al. 1983)

Exogenous substances can be used instead of endogenous sub-stances for the evaluation of clearance function. Renal clear-ance rates can be measured directly, but the clearance of exogenous substances by other organs must be measured indirectly. Of course, renal clearance can be measured indirectly also. As is true for endogenous substances, the exogenous marker substances must be eliminated solely from the organ of interest for the indirect measurements to be valid.

Indirect Measurement

If the exogenous substance is administered as a zero order, i.e., continuous, infusion its clearance rate can be calculated, once the steady state is achieved, by using the relationship

clearance rate = infusion rate/plasma substance concentration.

It is often impractical to administer a continuous infusion or to wait for steady state to be achieved, however. In such cases the substance can be given as a bolus (via intravenous injection) or by first order uptake (via gastrointestinal absorption). The plasma concentration of the substance is followed over time, and a **plasma clearance curve** is constructed, as shown in Figure 7-7.

The clearance rate can then be calculated using the formula

$$clearance\ rate = \frac{amount\ of\ substance\ administered}{area\ under\ the\ plasma\ clearance\ curve}$$

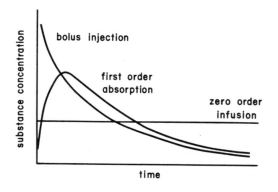

Fig 7-7   Plasma Clearance Curves

Table 7-3

Selected Organ Clearance Studies:
Exogenous Substances

Organ	Marker substance	Administration	Function measured
Liver	Indocyanine green	Bolus or zero order	(Hepatocyte) organic anion extraction
	Antipyrine/ aminopyrine	Bolus	(Hepatocyte) cytochrome P450 activity
	Galactose	Bolus	(Hepatocyte) galactose extraction
Kidney	Inulin	Zero order	Glomerular filtration rate
	^{51}CrEDTA	Bolus	Glomerular filtration rate
Spleen	Radiolabeled red cells	Bolus	Red cell culling

EDTA = ethylenediaminetetraacetic acid

This latter expression applies equally well to calculating the clearance rate during a zero-order infusion. Table 7-3 lists exogenous marker substances frequently used to measure organ clearance rate.

The number and timing of samples is of obvious practical importance when performing clearance studies. The sampling schedule should be designed to achieve minimum measurement variability in the estimation of the clearance rate while minimizing the discomfort and inconvenience to the study subject and the expense of analyzing the specimens. The following guidelines are based upon these considerations:

1. If the substance is administered by zero order infusion, two specimens should be taken after steady state is expected to have been achieved. Only one concentration determination is required to calculate the clearance rate, but a second is needed to confirm that the system is in steady state.

2. If the substance is administered as a bolus and has a monoexponential plasma clearance curve, two specimens should be taken, the first within minutes of the completion of the substance injection and the second at the

time equal to the anticipated turnover time of the substance, where turnover time equals the volume of distribution divided by the clearance rate.

3. If the substance is administered by a first-order process or has a multiexponential plasma clearance curve when administered as a bolus, multiple specimens will be needed. The number and timing of samples will vary considerably from substance to substance. The appropriate literature should be consulted as an aid in the design of the sampling schedule.

One-Sample Clearance Studies

In clinical practice, clearance studies usually rely upon a single concentration determination. This is because routine clearance studies do not include the actual estimation of the clearance rate but, rather, simply compare the extent of substance removal as indicated by the plasma concentration of the substance at a set time following the administration of that exogenous substance. Although this is a poor way to conduct a clearance study, its use is so widespread that a discussion of this approach is called for.

An important shortcoming of one-sample clearance studies is that the relationship between the substance concentration at the sampling time, t*, and the clearance rate is nonlinear. Consider the case of a bolus injection of marker substance as shown in Figure 7-8. The left panel of the figure shows the plasma

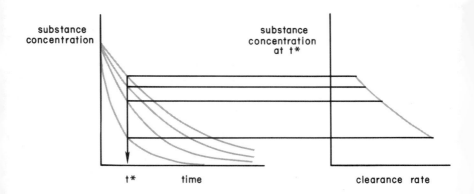

Fig 7-8   Relationship Between the Substance Concentration
at the Sampling Time and the Substance Clearance Rate
for a One-Sample Clearance Study
(t* = sampling time)

learance curves at four different clearance rates. The relationship between the substance concentration at the sampling
.me, t*, and the clearance rate is shown in the right panel. It
: convex. Therefore, as the clearance rate falls, the substance
ncentration at t* will increase, but not in proportion to the
ange in clearance rate.

Another difficulty in the use of one sample clearance studies
the variability in measurement that results from biologic
riability in the volume of distribution of the marker sub-
nce. This problem is illustrated for a bolus injection of
ker substance in Figure 7-9. Three plasma clearance curves
shown, representing studies in three individuals with dif-
ent volumes of distribution for the marker substance. The
arance rate for the substance is the same for all three.
ce that wide variability is present in the substance con-
ration and therefore in the estimate of the clearance rate
the study sample is taken soon after injection of the
er, e.g., at t_1*. Similarly, variability in the volume of
ribution of marker substance or in the rate of absorption of
ance will result in marked variability in the study result
wing first order absorption of the substance if the study
men is taken early. This is shown for the case of differing

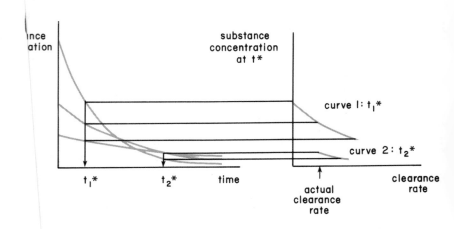

Fig 7-9   Effect of Different Volumes of Distribution
upon the Accuracy of a One-Sample Clearance Study
Following Bolus Injection of Marker Substance
(t* = sampling time)

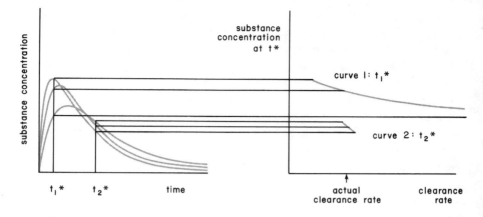

Fig 7-10   Effect of Different Volumes of Distribution
upon the Accuracy of a One-Sample Clearance Study
Following First-Order Absorption of Marker Substance
(t* = sampling time)

volumes of distribution in Figure 7-10.   Much less variability in
measurement is seen for both modes of administration when study
samples are taken later, e.g., at t_2*.

While the predetermined sampling time for a one sample clearance study may be set at a time that results in little measurement variability for a particular clearance rate, that time
cannot be well suited for measuring substance clearance in
patients with different clearance rates.   In particular, for
patients who have a clearance rate less than the one for which
the study performs well, the specified sampling time will fall
earlier in the plasma clearance of the substance, and thus the
effects of variability in the volume of distribution or in the
rate of substance absorption will be increased.   The greater the
reduction in clearance rate, the more profound will be the displacement of the sampling time.

MONITORING SYNTHETIC RATE AND CLEARANCE RATE

The purpose of monitoring a patient by using organ function
studies is to recognize a physiologic change before there is any
detectable clinical change. Such recognition allows early therapeutic intervention so that the consequences of a physiologic
insult can be minimized.   Alternatively, clinicians can monitor
for early signs of improved physiologic function that presage a
partial or complete return to health.   In either case it is

- 147 -

obvious that early indicators are to be preferred over late indicators. Thus for monitoring purposes, marker substances are
chosen on the basis of rapid changes in their plasma concentration following changes in organ function. These early indicators
are not always the same substances used to mark organ function in
steady state. For example, albumin, which is the standard marker
of hepatic protein synthetic function, has a low clearance rate
and, consequently, a very long half-life. Its plasma concentration changes very slowly following an alteration in synthetic
function. Even following nearly complete hepatic shutdown, as
occurs in fulminant hepatic necrosis, the plasma albumin concentration, corrected for changes in plasma volume, declines grad-
ually over a period of weeks. In contrast, prealbumin, which has
a very short plasma half-life, shows a marked reduction in its
plasma concentration in a matter of days following the onset of
hepatic failure.

Figure 7-11 depicts the plasma concentration of a synthesis
marker following a reduction in synthesis of the marker by the
organ of interest. Because there is unavoidable variability in
the laboratory measurement of the marker substance concentration,
the level of the substance must change by a certain amount before
the deviation can be attributed to an alteration in organ function rather than to chance. (This is discussed in detail in the
following subsection.) This amount is labeled "detectable
change" in the figure. The time required for the marker substance to fall to the concentration specified by the detectable

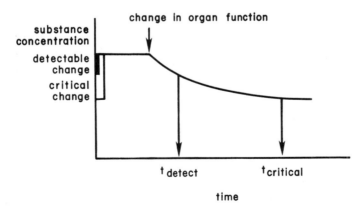

Fig 7-11   Monitoring Organ Function by Using
Marker Substance Concentration

change is labeled "t_{detect}." The larger the change in organ function, the earlier the change can be detected. "Critical change" and "$t_{critical}$" indicate, respectively, the magnitude of the change and time needed to achieve the change in concentration following a clinically significant alteration in organ function. Again, the greater the change in organ function, the earlier a significant change will be appreciated. Although "critical change" is drawn in Figure 7-11 as being larger than "detectable change," often it is not. It then follows that for those marker substances, one cannot detect small yet significant changes in organ function.

Two monitoring strategies for detecting a change in organ function arise from these considerations. If only small changes in organ function are expected, specimens should be obtained at intervals equal to $t_{critical}$ for the minimally significant, or t_{detect} for the minimally detectable, functional change. Here $t_{critical}$ approximately equals five times the plasma half-life of the marker substance. Using this interval, small changes in function will be appreciated no later than the second specimen after the onset of the function change. If large changes in organ function are likely, specimens should be drawn at intervals equal to t_{detect} for the minimum change expected. Then any reduction in function equal to or greater than that minimum change will be detected within two specimens. The general, but approximate, formula for t_{detect} given that the change in function will exceed K percent is

$$t_{detect} = -1.44 \left\{ \begin{array}{c} marker \\ half\ life \end{array} \right\} ln \left\{ 1 - (100/K) \ \frac{magnitude\ of\ detectable\ change}{initial\ concentration} \right\}.$$

Following a change in its synthetic rate, a plasma marker substance will require a period of time equal to five times its plasma half-life to achieve its new steady state concentration. After that its plasma concentration can be used to estimate the new level of organ function.

Magnitude of a Detectable Change
(Harris and Yasaka 1983; Winkel and Statland 1977)

Given that there is variability in laboratory measurement, how large a difference must exist between consecutive measurements in order to be confident that the difference is explained by a change in organ function, not by measurement imprecision?

Because Gaussian statistics can be used to describe the distribution of differences between consecutive measurements in a series of repeated analyte measurements, the following Gaussian formulas can be used:

$$significant\ deviation = 1.96 \left\{ \begin{array}{c} variance\ of\ differences \\ between\ measurements \end{array} \right\}^{1/2}$$

and

$$variance\ of\ differences = 2\ variance\ of\ the\ measurement$$
between measurements

where variance equals the standard deviation squared.

To use these formulas, an estimate of the variance of the measurement must be obtained. Ideally, the estimate is tailored to the individual patient and to the laboratory in which the study is being performed. This is called using the subject as his own referent. More frequently, the estimate is based upon typical values. The applicable formulas are listed in Table 7-4.

In the individual,

$$variance\ of\ the\ measurement = \begin{array}{c} variance\ of\ the \\ prior\ results \end{array} (1 + 1/number\ of\ results).$$

The term in parentheses corrects for inaccuracies in the estimation of the study variance due to a small sample size. Therefore,

$$detectable\ change = 1.96 \left\{ 2\ \begin{array}{c} [variance\ of\ the \\ prior\ results] \end{array} \quad [1 + 1/number\ of\ results] \right\}^{1/2}$$

The typical value for the variance of the measurement is calculated from typical variance values for the two sources of measurement variability, intraindividual biologic variability and analytic error. Because these sources of error are not correlated, the measurement variance equals the sum of the variances attributable to each of its components:

$$variance\ of\ the\ measurement = \begin{array}{c} typical\ intraindividual \\ variance \end{array} + \begin{array}{c} typical\ analytical \\ variance \end{array}$$

Therefore,

$$detectable\ change = 1.96 \left\{ 2\ \begin{array}{c} [typical\ intraindividual \\ variance \end{array} + \begin{array}{c} typical\ analytical \\ variance] \end{array} \right\}^{1/2}.$$

The formulas for the magnitude of a detectable change are valid only if the time interval between measurements is long. As

Table 7-4

Calculation of the Magnitude of a Detectable
Change in the Measurement of a Marker Substance
When the Interval Between Measurements is Long

Rule	Intraindividual variability	Analytic variability	Variability of difference in measurement	Magnitude of detectable change
Ideal	var_{intra} (actual patient value)	var_{anal} (actual laboratory value)	$2(var_{intra} + var_{anal})$	$1.96 \left[2(var_{intra} + var_{anal}) \right]^{1/2}$
Estimate using the subject as his own referent		Estimated from n prior study results	$2\,var_{prior\ results}\,(1 + 1/n)$	$1.96 \left[2(var_{prior\ results})(1 + 1/n) \right]^{1/2}$
Estimate using average value	var_{intra} (typical value)	var_{anal} (typical value)	$2(var_{intra} + var_{anal})$	$1.96 \left[2(var_{intra} + var_{anal}) \right]^{1/2}$

var_{intra} = intraindividual variance; var_{anal} = analytic variance the interval becomes shorter, the biologic component of the variability drops out because, for most analytes, only small changes in analyte quantity take place over a few hours. Consider, for example, the blood concentration of neutrophils. From day to day the concentration can vary as greatly as 3000 cells/μl around a mean level of 3500 cells/μl. Over a period of 2 to 3 hours, though, the variability is probably only one-third as great. Consequently, when measurements are taken at intervals of less than 3 hours, the differences in cell concentration between consecutive measurements will show much less variability than when measurements are made daily. The variability that is present will, in fact, be due largely to analytic variability.

The degree to which consecutive measurements are similar due to the sluggishness of biologic change is reflected in the Gaussian index, **serial correlation**. A serial correlation of one denotes absolute immobility of the quantity such that each measurement is identical to its predecessor. A value of zero indicates that the biologic change is rapid enough that, at the measurement interval specified, each measurement appears unrelated to the surrounding values. Incorporating the idea of serial correlation into the formula for the variability between consecutive measurements yields

variance of differences = 2 (1 - p[t]) variance of the measurement
between measurements   + 2 p[t] analytic variance

where p[t] is the serial correlation for the time interval, t.

For most purposes only the two extreme values for the serial correlation need to be considered. Either the measurement interval is assumed to be long relative to the time needed for biologic change, such that p[t] is equal to zero, or the interval is assumed to be short, with p[t] equal to one. The simplified formulas that result are

variance of differences = 2 variance of the measurement

if the interval is long and

variance of differences = 2 analytic variance

if the interval is short.

Table 7-5 lists typical magnitudes of detectable differences in measurement for short-term and long-term changes in selected organ function marker substances.

Table 7-5

Typical Magnitudes of Detectable Short Term and Long Term Measurement Change
for Selected Organ Function Marker Substances in Healthy Subjects

Analyte	Typical day-to-day intraindividual variability	Typical day-to-day analytic variability	Typical magnitude of detectable short term change	Typical magnitude of detectable long-term change
Albumin (g/dl)	0.11	0.14	0.4	0.5
Bilirubin (mg/dl)	0.22	0.10	0.3	0.7
Calcium (mg/dl)	0.20	0.20	0.6	0.8
Creatinine (mg/dl)	0.06	0.09	0.25	0.3
Glucose (mg/dl)	6.0	3.0	8	20
Hematocrit (%)	0.7	0.7	2	3
Hemoglobin (g/dl)	0.36	0.24	0.7	1.2
Immunoglobulins (mg/dl)	45	75	200	250
Lymphocytes (cells/μl)	200	60	165	575
Monocytes (cells/μl)	75	15	40	225
Neutrophils (cells/μl)	1125	135	375	3000
P_{CO2} (mmHg)	0.75	1.5	4	5
Phosphorus (mg/dl)	0.35	0.20	.6	1.1
Platelets (cells/μl)	10,000	12,500	35,000	45,000
Urea nitrogen (mg/dl)	5.2	1.6	5	15

Variability expressed as standard deviation.

Data from Ross and Fraser (1982) and Winkel and Statland (1977).

7-1. Plasma albumin concentrations decline in cirrhosis. Why?

7-2. The rate of carbon dioxide (CO_2) production in an average adult is 10.4 mmol/min. The pulmonary clearance of CO_2 averages 0.48 L/min. What is the steady-state blood concentration of CO_2?

7-3. The following figure depicts the steady-state relationship between the blood CO_2 concentration [expressed in terms of the partial pressure of CO_2 (P_{CO2})] and the pulmonary clearance rate of CO_2 (expressed as the pulmonary ventilation rate). Normally the P_{CO2} is 40 mmHg and the ventilation rate is 4 L/min, as indicated by the point on the curve.

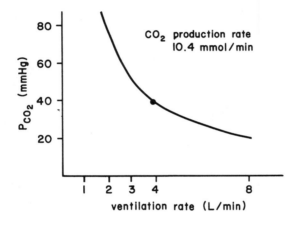

Compare this curve to the one for bilirubin on Figure 7-4. Here the normal set point is at the genu of the curve. What physiologic purpose is served by this location?

Your patient in a medical clinic has severe diabetic renal disease. She is 45 years old and weighs 60 kg. She had been told to collect a 24-hour urine specimen to bring to the clinic, but she started her collection late, so you have her wait in the clinic to complete the collection. Meanwhile a blood specimen is obtained, and a serum creatinine determination is performed. The result is 2 mg/dl.

7-4.   This patient is calculated to have a creatinine production rate of 1008 mg/24 hours. Assuming that she is in steady state, what is her plasma creatinine clearance rate (in ml/min)?

7-5.   She completes the urine collection and a renal creatinine clearance of 25 ml/min is calculated. What is her urinary creatinine excretion rate (in mg/24 hours)?

7-6.   Suggest an explanation for the difference between the clearance values obtained in this patient.

7-7.   For the four prior clinic visits, this patient's serum creatinine concentrations have been 1.4, 1.2, 1.6, and 1.7 mg/dl. Has there been a significant change in her renal function?

7-8.   The plasma concentration of bile acids is more sensitive than the plasma bilirubin concentration as a marker of early liver disease. Suggest possible mechanisms.

7-9.   The plasma concentration of bile acids 2 hours after a meal is also used as a marker of early liver disease. Explain the rationale of this laboratory study.

Mind-Expanding Exercise

7-10.   The blood clearance rate of radiolabeled, autologous, heat-damaged red cells is one measure of splenic fixed macrophage function. Peters et al. (1981) report that in patients with rheumatologic and hematologic disorders, the extraction fraction, that is the fraction of labeled cells cleared during a passage through the spleen, is directly related to splenic blood flow. This contrasts with the assertion in the text that the change in substance concentration across an organ of elimination decreases as the rate of plasma flow increases. Suggest an explanation for this disagreement.

REFERENCES

Cobby, J., Makoid, M.D. The use of marker drugs to measure organ function: A theoretical interpretation. Eur. J. Clin. Pharmacol. 18:511, 1980.

D'Argenio, D.Z. Optimal sampling times for pharmacokinetic experiments. J. Pharmacokinet. Biopharm. 9:739, 1981.

DiStefano, J.J. Concepts, properties, measurement, and computation of clearance rates of hormones and other substances in biologic systems. Ann. Biomed. Eng. 4:302, 1976.

Dossing, M., Volund, A., Poulsen, H.E. Optimal sampling times for minimum variance of clearance determination. Br. J. Clin. Pharmacol. 15:231, 1983.

Gibaldi, M., Perrier, D. Clearance concepts. In: Gibaldi, M., Perrier, D. Pharmacokinetics, ed. 2. Marcel Dekker, New York, pp 319-354, 1982.

Groth, T. Biodynamic models as pre-processors of clinical laboratory data. In: Heusghem, C., Albert, A., Benson, E.S. (eds.) Advanced Interpretation of Clinical L Marcel Dekker, New York, pp 151-170, 1982.

Harris, E.K., Yasaka, T. On the calculation of a "reference change" for comparing two consecutive measurements. Clin. Chem. 29:25, 1983.

Murphy, E.A. Some epistemological aspects of the model in medicine. J. Med. Philos. 3:273, 1978.

Peters, A.M., Ryan, P.F.J., Klonizakis, I. et al. Measurement of splenic function in humans using heat damaged autologous red blood cells. Scand. J. Haematol. 27:374, 1981.

Riggs, D.S. The Mathematical Approach to Physiologic Problems. MIT Press, Boston, 1976.

Ross, J.W., Fraser, M.D. Clinical laboratory precision. Am. J. Clin. Pathol. (suppl.) 78:578, 1982.

Winkel, P., Statland, B.E. Using the subject as his own referent in assessing day-to day changes of laboratory test results. Contemp. Top. Anal. Clin. Chem. 1:287, 1977.

Wright, F.S. Flow-dependent transport processes: Filtration, absorption, secretion. Am. J. Physiol. 24:F1, 1982.

Chapter 8

ORGAN FUNCTION

2. Homeostatic Systems

Concordia discors.

Horace

HOMEOSTASIS

(Riggs 1970)

One of the fundamental activities of physiologic systems is to maintain a constant internal environment despite perturbing stimuli. This is homeostasis (from the Greek <u>homoio-</u>, similar or like, and <u>sta-</u>, to stand). While homeostasis can be accomplished passively, such as the maintenance of a neutral blood pH by the plasma bicarbonate-carbon dioxide buffer system, most often it is accomplished actively. Figure 8-1 illustrates the essential components of active homeostatic regulation. The homeostatic setpoint of the target process is maintained by corrective responses of the regulator tissue to deviations of the process from the set-point state.

The regulator tissue controls the state of the target process through the magnitude of an effector signal. The effector signal

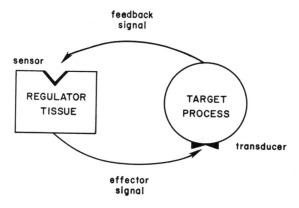

Fig 8-1   Basic Components of Active Homeostatic Regulation

is received by a biologic transducer, most often an effector tissue, the cells of which contain receptors for the effector signal. The regulator tissue maintains a vigilant surveillance of the target process. The magnitude of a feedback signal from the process is monitored by sensors in the regulator tissue. Alterations in the state of the process as reflected in alterations of the feedback signal initiate the corrective changes in the level of the effector signal. And the cycle is complete.

In higher animals systemic homeostasis is the responsibility of the endocrine glands. They are the regulators and their hormones are the effector signals. In contrast to the simplicity of the control model shown in Figure 8-1, however, hormone systems may produce multiple hormones, regulate multiple target processes, respond to diverse feedback signals and accessory influences, and in turn be regulated by other tissues. Additional complexity is found in the interdependent networks of endocrine regulation. Consider, for example, that the pituitary and adrenal glands produce hormones that act to counterbalance the regulatory effects of insulin on plasma glucose. And the pancreatic islets themselves are the source of the most important counterregulator hormone, glucagon. Still, the physiology of most endocrine glands is well represented by the comparatively simple model shown in Figure 8-2. The control tissue for an endocrine gland may be either another endocrine gland or an element of the central nervous tissue. In the first case, the control signal is the trophic hormone; in the second, the control signal is a hormone-releasing factor or a neurotransmitter.

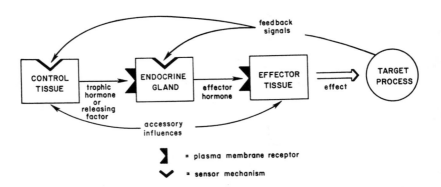

Fig 8-2   Simple Model of Endocrine Homeostatic Function

CLASSIFICATION OF ENDOCRINE DYSFUNCTION
(Blecher 1984; Pollet and Levey 1980; Verhoeven and Wilson 1979)
    Most classifications of endocrine dysfunction distinguish primary from secondary alteration in function. For primary disorders the dysfunction resides in the gland itself. The control or feedback signal becomes exaggerated in response to the inappropriate levels of circulating hormone, but, by definition, a return to normal glandular function is not achieved. Secondary dysfunction occurs when there is a disorder in the control tissue or the effector tissue, which leads to an abnormal level of stimulation or suppression of endocrine activity. As a result, the functional state of the gland is abnormal but appropriate. This classification scheme is summarized in Table 8-1.

Table 8-1

A Classification of Endocrine Dysfunction

State of control or feedback signal	Functional state of endocrine gland	
	Hypofunction	Hyperfunction
Stimulation	Primary hypofunction	Secondary hyperfunction
Suppression	Secondary hypofunction	Primary hyperfunction

    Primary endocrine dysfunction produces disease in which the clinical picture is consistent with the gland's functional state, but so does secondary endocrine dysfunction due to disordered control tissue. Consequently, the level of the control signal, i.e., the plasma concentration of the trophic hormone, must be measured to separate these two possibilities. In contrast, when secondary endocrine dysfunction is attributable to an abnormal effector tissue, the clinical findings referable to that effector tissue are inconsistent with the endocrine functional state. The diagnosis of secondary dysfunction is thereby readily made. Consistent findings can be expected, however, for other receptor tissues that are not abnormal.

EVALUATION OF ENDOCRINE GLAND FUNCTION
(Cryer 1979; Watts 1982)

The laboratory evaluation of endocrine gland function proceeds in two steps. First, the functional state of the gland, defined as the rate of secretion of its hormone product, is assessed using function markers, the most important of which is the steady-state plasma concentration of the hormone itself. For some disorders the measurement of function markers in the basal state does not yield adequate separation of the functional states. In these cases **stimulation** or **suppression** studies are required. Second, feedback markers or trophic hormones are measured to compare the gland's functional state to the level of physiologic stimulation of endocrine function. Such an analysis makes possible the segregation of primary from secondary dysfunction.

Function Markers

Because hormone clearance rates remain nearly constant in primary endocrine disease, the secretory rate of an endocrine gland, and hence its functional state, is directly proportional to the plasma concentration of the hormone:

$$synthetic\ rate = clearance\ rate \cdot plasma\ hormone\ concentration$$

where the clearance rate is a constant. For hormones that experience significant plasma protein binding, i.e., steroid and thyroid hormones, the concentration of physiologically available hormone must be measured rather than the concentration of total hormone. Similarly, it is the plasma clearance rate of the available hormone that remains constant in endocrine disease, not the clearance rate of total hormone. Therefore,

$$synthetic\ rate = \begin{matrix} clearance\ rate\ of \\ available\ hormone \end{matrix} \cdot \begin{matrix} concentration\ of \\ available\ hormone. \end{matrix}$$

The measurement of available hormone concentration is discussed in detail in Chapter 10.

When circulating hormone concentrations cannot be measured with adequate reliability, functional status is assessed by the measurement of some other function marker, the quantity of which is predictably related to the plasma concentration of available

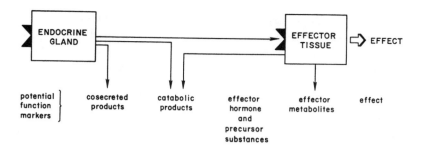

Fig 8-3   Model of Endocrine Homeostatic Axis
Showing Potential Function Markers

hormone. Figure 8-3 shows commonly used function markers. There
may be cosecreted products that are released from the endocrine
gland at rates proportional to the hormone secretion rate. Catabolic products arising from degradation of the hormone within the
gland itself and within peripheral tissues can be used. So can
effector metabolites, which are either intracellular messengers,
e.g., cyclic adenosine monophosphate, or products of intermediary
metabolism that are released from effector tissue in proportion
to the degree of hormone binding. These function markers may be
quantified by measurement of their plasma concentrations or by
measurement of their renal elimination rates. The hormone's
physiologic effect also may be assayed.

In diabetes mellitus, for instance, insulin secretory capacity is estimated from the plasma clearance rate of a glucose
load, insulin's physiologic effect. Insulin production by an
insulinoma is monitored by measurement of the plasma levels of
C-protein, a cosecreted product. The secretory activity of a
pheochromocytoma, in contrast, is estimated from the plasma
concentrations of catecholamines, catecholamine precursors, or
catecholamine catabolic products or from their urinary excretion
rates.

Feedback Markers and Trophic Hormones

Secondary forms of endocrine dysfunction, both hyper- and
hypofunction, are common. Measurement of the plasma concentration of the appropriate trophic hormone(s) is essential for
the identification of secondary dysfunction in the thyroid,
adrenals, ovaries, and testes. Confirmation of secondary
disorders of the posterior pituitary, parathyroids, or renin-
aldosterone system requires measurement of the magnitude of the
physiologic feedback signal or of a feedback marker substance.

Laboratory studies commonly used to evaluate secondary endocrine dysfunction are listed in Table 8-2. The classification of endocrine function based upon measurement of function and feedback markers is usually accomplished graphically, as shown in Figure 8-4.

Table 8-2

Common Laboratory Studies for
Secondary Endocrine Dysfunction

Endocrine gland	Hormone	Trophic hormone	Feedback marker
Posterior pituitary	Antidiuretic hormone		Plasma osmolality or sodium concentration
Thyroid	Thyroxine Triiodothyronine	Thyroid stimulating hormone	
Parathyroid	Parathormone		Plasma ionized calcium concentration
Adrenal	Cortisol	Adrenocorticotrophic hormone	
	Aldosterone	Renin	
Kidney	Renin		Urinary sodium excretion rate
Ovary	Estrogens	Follicle-stimulating hormone, luteinizing hormone	
Testes	Androgens	Follicle-stimulating hormone, luteinizing hormone	

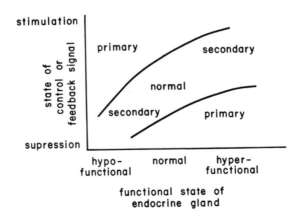

Fig 8-4   Laboratory Classification of Endocrine Function

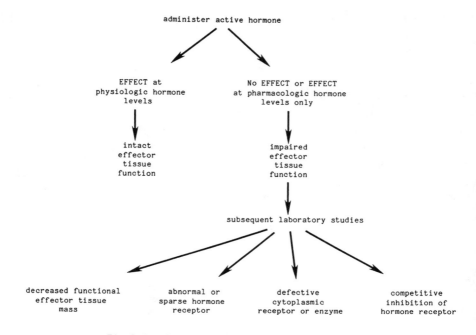

administer active hormone

EFFECT at
physiologic hormone
levels

No EFFECT or EFFECT
at pharmacologic hormone
levels only

intact
effector
tissue
function

impaired
effector
tissue
function

subsequent laboratory studies

decreased functional
effector tissue
mass

abnormal or
sparse hormone
receptor

defective
cytoplasmic
receptor or enzyme

competitive
inhibition of
hormone receptor

Fig 8-5   Evaluation of Effector Tissue Function

Testing Effector Tissue Function

When a patient suffers symptoms of endocrine hypofunction but has normal or elevated hormone levels, a defect in effector tissue function should be considered. Effector tissue function is tested directly by monitoring hormone effect following the administration of active hormone, as demonstrated in Figure 8-5. If physiologic doses of the active hormone produce a typical response, the effector tissue is functional. Some other explanation for the disparate clinical and laboratory findings must then be sought. If physiologic doses of hormone fail to evoke a response, the function of the effector tissue is impaired. Subsequent laboratory studies can be used to identify the cause of the dysfunction. Decreased functional mass of the effector tissue is the most common finding.

There are a few disorders of effector tissue function that occur frequently enough to warrant consideration during the evaluation of apparent endocrine hypofunction:

1. abnormal or sparse hormone receptors

    a. nephrogenic diabetes insipidus

    b. pseudohypoparathyroidism

    c. noninsulin dependent diabetes mellitus

2. decreased intracellular receptors or enzymes
   a. male pseudohermaphroditism
   b. pseudohypoaldosteronism
   c. vitamin D-dependent rickets.

STIMULATION AND SUPPRESSION STUDIES

The measurement of the quantity of an endocrine function marker rarely permits complete separation of patients according to functional status. Such ideal behavior is depicted in Figure 8-6. The empirical ranges of the marker quantity for each of the functional categories are indicated by the black bars. More typically, the functional categories overlap, sometimes extensively, when even the most reliable function marker available is assayed. This is illustrated in Figure 8-7.

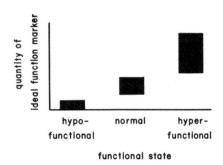

Fig 8-6   Classification of Endocrine Function
           by use of an Ideal Marker

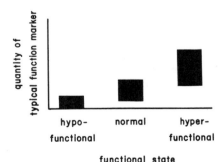

Fig 8-7   Classification of Endocrine Function
           by use of a Typical Marker

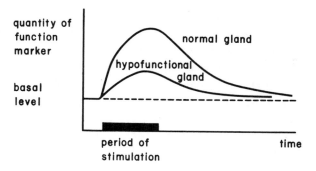

Fig 8-8   Time Course of an Endocrine Function
Marker During and Following Stimulation

To separate the functional categories more completely, an endocrine gland can be stimulated or suppressed. Stimulation of the gland by administration of its trophic hormone or by altering the feedback signal is especially useful in the separation of hypofunction from normal function. When transiently stimulated, a normal gland will, for a period of time, increase the rate of secretion of hormone. A hypofunctional gland will not respond to the stimulation with a comparable increase in secretion rate. Thus the two functional states can be differentiated.

Figure 8-8 depicts the time course of an endocrine function marker during and following stimulation of the gland. The area between the function marker curve and the line indicating the basal level of the function marker is proportional to the amount of hormone secreted in excess of the basal output:

area between the curves = amount of excess hormone secreted/clearance rate.

As the clearance rate for circulating hormone is usually the same in the setting of endocrine hypofunction as it is during normal function, the index "area between the curves" is a reliable marker of excess hormone secretion during stimulation. A hypofunctional gland will secrete less excess hormone and therefore will have a measurably smaller "area between the curves." In this way a hypofunctional gland can be distinguished from a normally functioning one.

Rather than following the full time course of the function marker, a single measurement, taken at a specified time (preferably at a time near the peak of a curve), can be used to quantify the amount of excess hormone released. The quantity of the function marker at the specified time will be linearly related to the amount of excess hormone secreted. Such a one-sample technique introduces measurement variability due to differences in the volume of distribution of the hormone, but experience has shown that satisfactory separation of functional categories is still often possible. The practical advantage of the one-sample technique over the multiple sample approach is obvious. The separation of hypofunction from normal function by using a one-sample stimulation study is illustrated in Figure 8-9. The empirical ranges of the marker quantity are indicated by the black bars.

The suppression of endocrine gland hormone secretion by alteration of the feedback signal can be used to improve the separation, of hyperfunction from normal function. During the period of suppression, a normal gland will markedly reduce its rate of hormone secretion. The reduction in the secretion rate will be less in a hyperfunctional gland. The extent of the reduction in the secretion rate, and hence the function state of the gland, can be evaluated using the multiple sample approach but most commonly is assessed using the one-sample technique. The results from a one-sample suppression study are shown in Figure 8-10. Table 8-3 lists stimulation and suppression tests in routine clinical use.

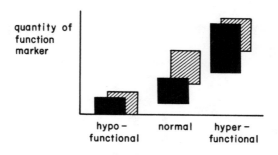

Fig 8-9   Classification of Endocrine Function
    by use of a One-Sample Stimulation Study

■   basal state
▨   following stimulation

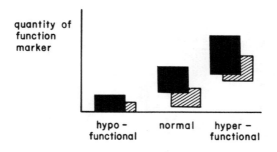

Fig 8-10   Classification of Endocrine Function
    by use of a One-Sample Suppression Study

■   basal state
▨   following suppression

Table 8-3

Common Stimulation and Suppression Tests

Hormone	Plasma function marker	Stimulation	Suppression	Diagnostic consideration
Antidiuretic hormone	(Urine) osmolality	Dehydration		Diabetes insipidus
Growth hormone	Growth hormone	Arginine, L-dopa, hypoglycemia		Pituitary failure
	Growth hormone		Hyperglycemia	Acromegaly, gigantism
Prolactin	Prolactin	Thyrotrophin-releasing hormone, phenothiazines, hypoglycemia		Pituitary failure
	Prolactin		L-dopa	Galactorrhea
Follicle-stimulating hormone, luteinizing hormone	Follicle-stimulating hormone, luteinizing hormone	Gonadotrophin releasing hormone, clomiphene		Pituitary failure
Thyroid-stimulating hormone	Thyroid-stimulating hormone	Thyrotrophin-releasing hormone		Pituitary failure
Adrenocorticotrophic hormone	11-Deoxycortisol	Hypocortisolemia (induced by metyrapone)		Pituitary failure
	Cortisol	Hypoglycemia		Pituitary failure
Cortisol	(Urine) cortisol		Dexamethasone (low dose)	Cushing's syndrome
			Dexamethasone (high dose)	Primary vs secondary Cushing's syndrome
	Cortisol	Adrenocorticotrophic hormone		Adrenal failure
Aldosterone	Renin, aldosterone	Dehydration		Hyperaldosteronism
	Aldosterone		Fluid loading, mineralocorticoids	Primary vs secondary hyperaldosteronism
Catecholamines	Catecholamines		Pentolinium	Pheochromocytoma
Insulin	Glucose	Hyperglycemia		Diabetes mellitus

EXERCISES

The synthetic and metabolic pathways for the catecholamines are

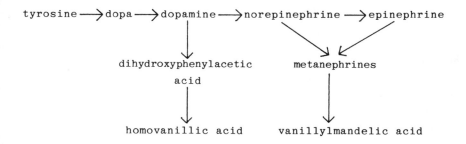

tyrosine ——>dopa ——>dopamine ——>norepinephrine ——>epinephrine

dihydroxyphenylacetic   metanephrines
acid

homovanillic acid   vanillylmandelic acid

Pheochromocytomas are catecholamine-secreting tumors of the adrenal medulla and extra-adrenal paraganglion system.

8-1. Suggest an explanation for the observation that small pheo-chromocytomas are detected most reliably by measurement of plasma epinephrine and norepinephrine concentrations, whereas large tumors are readily detected by measurement of the urinary secretion rate of metanephrines and vanillyl-mandelic acid.

8-2. What is indicated by the finding of an increased plasma concentration of norepinephrine but a normal or only slightly elevated epinephrine concentration?

8-3. List preanalytic factors that influence the measurement of plasma catecholamines and urinary catecholamine metabo-lites.

8-4. Draw a diagnostic graph similar to Figure 8-5 for use in the separation of primary and secondary hyperreninism.

8-5. The recently admitted patient you have been asked to see states that for the past week she has suffered from a ter-rible thirst and has been consuming very large amounts of water. Her response to your query about her urine output is that she urinates large volumes frequently. She is normoglycemic. Her urine has no detectable glucose and a very low osmolality. What two function studies should you perform?

8-6. Metyrapone inhibits the 11 β-hydroxylase enzyme in the adrenal cortex, thereby inhibiting the conversion of 11-deoxycortisol to cortisol. What will happen to plasma cortisol concentration? What will subsequently happen to the plasma adrenocorticotrophin (ACTH) and 11-deoxycortisol concentrations in patients with Cushing's disease (ACTHsecreting pituitary adenoma)? In patients with cortisol-secreting adrenal neoplasms? Why is this useful?

Mind-Expanding Exercise

8-7. Suggest a protocol for the evaluation of anterior pituitary function. Must every anterior pituitary hormone be evaluated?

REFERENCES

Blecher, M. Receptors, antibodies, and disease. Clin. Chem. 30:1137, 1984.

Cryer, P. Diagnostic Endocrinology, 2nd ed. Oxford University Press, New York, 1979.

Pollet, R.J., Levey, G.S. Principles of membrane receptor physiology and their application to clinical medicine. Ann. Intern. Med. 92:663, 1980.

Riggs, D.S. Control Theory and Physiological Feedback Mechanisms. Williams and Wilkins, Baltimore, 1970.

Verhoeven, G.F.M., Wilson, J.D. The syndromes of primary hormone resistance. Metabolism 28:253, 1979.

Watts, N.B., Keffer, J.H. Practical Endocrine Diagnosis, 3rd ed. Lea and Febiger, Philadelphia, 1982.

Chapter 9

METABOLISM

Dennis A. Noe, M.D. and J. David Bessman, M.D.

... it is not so deep as a well, nor so wide
as a church door, but 'tis enough, 'twill serve.

William Shakespeare

INTRODUCTION

The division of this chapter into discrete topics must not
mislead the reader into believing that the laboratory evaluation
of metabolic disorders can be accomplished in a similar dis-
jointed way. The body's metabolic pathways are complex and
extensively interconnected. Because of this, metabolic disorders
tend to have a multiplicity of systemic manifestations even when
the primary defect is localized anatomically. Similarly it is
usual for numerous laboratory abnormalities to develop with even
the simplest of metabolic disturbances. Necessarily, then, an
integrative approach is needed in the laboratory study of these
disorders.

WATER AND ABUNDANT METALS

(Beck 1981)

Figure 9-1 illustrates a simple scheme of water and abundant
metal dynamics. Water and metals absorbed from the diet enter
the plasma and are very rapidly dispersed in extracellular water.
Water distributes into the intracellular space and the metals

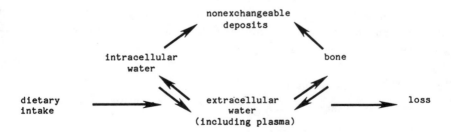

Fig 9-1   Simple Model of Water and
and Abundant Metal Dynamics

distribute into intracellular water and bone. Metal content in the intra- and extracellular water and in exchangeable deposits in bone together comprise the exchangeable pool for the metal. Metals subsequently may be irreversibly incorporated into cellular constituents or bone mineral. These are nonexchangeable body deposits. Body losses occur for the most part from the extracellular fluids. Metabolic balance is maintained by physiologic mechanisms that equalize body intake and losses.

Water equilibrates between the intra- and extracellular spaces in response to osmotic forces. The metals distribute between extra- and intracellular water so as to equalize diffusional transport and active ion transport at the cell membrane. Calcium and magnesium distribute between extracellular water and metabolically active bone under the influence of homeostatic processes that maintain a normal extracellular concentration of these cations. Sodium and potassium distribute between extracellular water and exchangeable deposits in bone, where they are constituents of the hydration shell that envelopes crystalline bone mineral. When there are changes in the content of body water or the abundant metals, they are first experienced in the extracellular space because it is the site of the external fluxes of substance. Secondary redistribution of substance leads to changes in content in the intracellular space and bone.

The anatomic distribution of water and the abundant metals in health is shown in Figure 9-2. The relative area of each circle represents the fraction of the exchangeable pool contained in the respective compartment. Sodium is mostly extracellular and potassium mostly intracellular. Each is the major determinant of the osmolarity in its water compartment. Because water freely diffuses between the intra- and extracellular compartments, so as to maintain equal osmolarity, its distribution between the compartments is determined largely by the cation content in each.

Cation concentration in its major compartment is determined by the content of the cation and the water content of the respective compartment:

$$[sodium]_{extracellular} = sodium\ content/extracellular\ water$$

$$[potassium]_{intracellular} = potassium\ content/intracellular\ water.$$

Substitution of the following relationships,

$$[sodium]_{extracellular} = [potassium]_{intracellular}$$

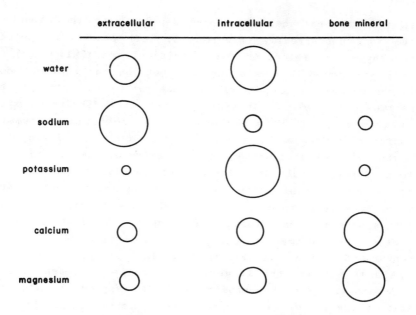

Fig 9-2   Distribution of Water and Exchangeable Pools
of Abundant Metals Among Anatomic Compartments

and

$$body\ water = extracellular\ water + intracellular\ water$$

into the cation concentration equations reveals that

$$[sodium]_{extracellular} = (sodium\ content + potassium\ content)/body\ water.$$

This equation indicates that the extracellular concentration of sodium and similarly the intracellular concentration of potassium depend upon body sodium content, body potassium content, and body water.

Pathophysiology

The clinical consequences of disordered water and abundant metal metabolism are due to

1. changes in extracellular water content
2. changes in intracellular water content
3. changes in the extracellular concentration of the metals.

Extracellular water content is reduced whenever body water content decreases. The fraction of the total water loss that comes from the extracellular space depends upon the amount of sodium lost concurrently (Figure 9-3, left panel). Hypotonic losses (hypotonic refers to the tonicity of the fluid lost) including pure water losses distribute between the anatomic compartments roughly in proportion to the prior water content of the compartments. Isotonic losses preferentially dehydrate extracellular water. This is so because that compartment remains isotonic; thus, there is no osmotic drive to redistribute water from the intracellular space into the extracellular space. Hypertonic losses result in extreme extracellular dehydration due to the combination of water loss and water redistribution into the intracellular space. Increases in extracellular water content always accompany total water excess. The distribution of the total excess between compartments is determined by the amount of concurrent sodium gain (Figure 9-3, right panel): the greater the gain in sodium, the larger the increase in extracellular water content. With hypertonic gains the expansion in extracellular water is due to water gain and water redistribution from the intracellular space.

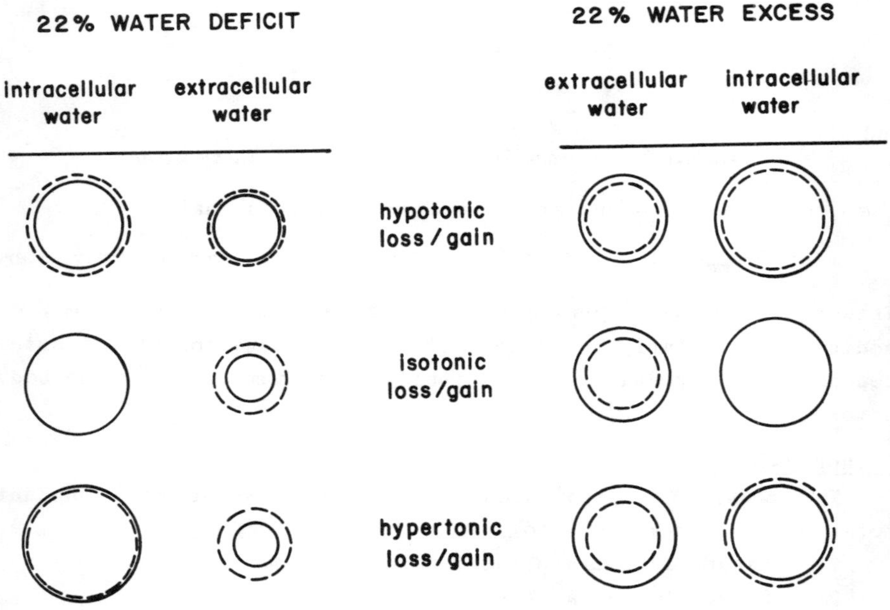

Fig 9-3   Distribution of Water Deficits and Excesses
Between Anatomic Compartments
Dashed circles: normal water content

Figure 9-3 also depicts how the content of intracellular water will increase, stay the same, or decrease with changes in total body water, depending upon the concurrent alterations in sodium content.

The extracellular concentration of the abundant metals is determined by the amount of the metal in the extracellular space and the water content of the space:

concentration of metal = amount of metal/content of water.

The concentration will increase if the amount of extracellular metal increases, if the extracellular content of water decreases, or if both increase or decrease but the amount of metal more so. The concentration will decrease if the amount of extracellular metal decreases, if the extracellular content of water increases, or if both increase or decrease but the amount of metal less so.

Changes in the extracellular concentrations of potassium, calcium, and magnesium are caused by changes in extracellular metal content due either to altered total body content or to redistribution of the metal from or to the intracellular space (potassium and magnesium) or bone (calcium). Changes in the extracellular concentration of sodium are caused by changes in extracellular water content due either to pure water deficits and excesses or to intercompartmental redistribution of water. In addition, the concentration is altered by combined changes in extracellular sodium and water content due to concurrent loss or gain of sodium and water. Hypotonic fluid losses and hypertonic fluid gains produce hypernatremia. Hypertonic fluid losses and hypotonic fluid gains lead to hyponatremia. Isotonic fluid imbalances do not change the sodium concentration.

Laboratory Measurement

The most reliable indicator of short-term changes in the content of body water is the basal body weight, which is defined as the body weight early in the morning before ingestion of food or fluid and after voiding and defecation. Daily changes in the basal body weight are due almost entirely to changes in body water content. Changes in the basal body weight occurring over days or weeks largely reflect water accumulation or loss and may be used to approximate the magnitude of water imbalance.

When the body content and distribution of osmolar substances is normal, changes in body fluid osmolarity, measured as plasma or serum sodium concentration, also reflect changes in body water

content.   An increase in the plasma sodium concentration indicates deficit of body water; a decrease indicates an excess. The
magnitude of the change can be calculated using the formula

$$\text{change in water content} = \frac{0.6 \left(\begin{array}{c}\text{initial body} \\ \text{weight in kg}\end{array}\right)\left(140 \text{ mmol/L} - \begin{array}{c}\text{current sodium} \\ \text{concentration}\end{array}\right)}{\begin{array}{c}\text{current sodium} \\ \text{concentration}\end{array}}.$$

If the body content of sodium is abnormal, an increase in the
plasma sodium concentration indicates a relative deficit of body
water; a decrease indicates a relative excess of body water.   The
absolute state of the body water <u>cannot</u> be derived from the
plasma sodium concentration when sodium stores are abnormal, however.   Absolute water deficit with relative water excess may be
seen, for instance, in adrenal insufficiency, and absolute water
excess with relative water deficit may appear, for instance,
after ingestion of large quantities of salt.

Body sodium content is not reliably indicated by the plasma
sodium concentration, which is determined by body water and
potassium content as well as by sodium content. Semiquantitative
assessments of sodium content can be made on the basis of clinical estimates of body water content, however.   If body water
content is increased, body sodium content is increased except in
the setting of a pure water excess.   If body water content is
decreased, body sodium content is decreased except when a pure
water deficit is present.

A rough estimate of the magnitude of the sodium deficit in
chronic sodium depletion can be calculated using the formula

$$\text{sodium deficit} = 0.6 \left(\begin{array}{c}\text{body weight} \\ \text{in kg}\end{array}\right)\left(140 \text{ mmol/L} - \begin{array}{c}\text{current sodium} \\ \text{concentration}\end{array}\right).$$

As this formula does not take into account the changes in body
water content that accompany sodium losses, it underestimates the
sodium deficit.   The formula cannot be used in acute sodium
depletion because during the acute phase of sodium depletion,
normonatremia is maintained at the expense of body water content.
Only in the chronic phase, when blood volume maintenance takes
precedence and body water is conserved despite continued sodium
depletion, is the degree of hyponatremia related to sodium
losses.

In the absence of intercompartmental redistribution, the body
contents of potassium, calcium, and magnesium are reflected in

the plasma concentrations of the respective cations. The hypercalcemia of pathologic bone resorption is an important exception.
Here body calcium content is reduced because of renal elimination
of the calcium liberated from the bone.

The changes in plasma concentrations of these metals are not
proportional to the alterations in their body content. Changes
in potassium concentration are exaggerated due to mechanisms that
minimize the fluxes of intracellular potassium at the expense of
extracellular potassium. Changes in the concentrations of calcium and magnesium are blunted owing to the operation of the
homeostatic processes, which serve to normalize their extracellular concentrations.

ACID-BASE BALANCE
(Stewart 1981)

The function of most of the body's metabolic activities is
influenced by the hydrogen ion concentration in the body fluids.
To maintain the concentration within the narrow limits that
permit optimal metabolic functioning, a balance must be achieved
among the factors that determine it. This is acid-base balance.

Acid-Base Physiology
(Stewart 1983)

At the level of refinement needed for clinical work, the body
fluids can be considered to be ionic solutions containing weak
acids, i.e., proteins, and carbon dioxide. In such systems the
equilibrium concentration of hydrogen ions is determined by three
factors: the partial pressure of carbon dioxide (P_{CO2}), the concentration of protein ([total protein species]), and the strong
ion difference ([SID]). Strong ions are those present only in
dissociated form under physiologic conditions. The major strong
ions in the body fluids are listed in Table 9-1. The strong ion
difference is the difference between the concentration of strong
cations and the concentration of strong anions.

The physical relationships governing the equilibrium state
are summarized in the following equations (concentrations are
expressed in electrochemical equivalents):

(1) water dissociation equilibrium

$$[H^+] \ [OH^-] = K_{water} \ [HOH]$$

K_{water} : *dissociation constant for water*

(2)   protein dissociation equilibrium

$$[H^+] \, [protein \, anion] = K_{protein} \, [protein]$$

$K_{protein}$: dissociation constant for protein

(3)   conservation of mass for protein

$$[protein] + [protein \, anion] = [total \, protein \, species]$$

(4)   carbon dioxide (CO_2) dissolution and ion formation equilibriums

$$[dissolved \, CO_2] = S_{CO2} \cdot P_{CO2}$$

S_{CO2} : CO_2 solubility coefficient

$$[H_2CO_3] = K_{carbonic \, acid} \, [dissolved \, CO_2][HOH]$$

$K_{carbonic \, acid}$: carbonic acid equilibrium constant

$$[H^+] \, [HCO_3^-] = K_{bicarbonate} \cdot P_{CO2}$$

$K_{bicarbonate}$: bicarbonate equilibrium constant

$$[H^+] \, [CO_3^{2-}] = K_{carbonate} \, [HCO_3^-]$$

$K_{carbonate}$: dissociation constant for bicarbonate

(5)   conservation of mass for carbon dioxide

$$[total \, CO_2] = [dissolved \, CO_2] + [H_2CO_3] + [HCO_3^-] + [CO_3^{2-}]$$

(6)   electrical neutrality

$$[H^+] + [SID] - [OH^-] - [protein \, anion] - [HCO_3^-] - [CO_3^{2-}] = 0.$$

All of these relationships must be satisfied simultaneously
for the equilibrium state to exist. That means that the equilib-

Table 9-1

The Strong Ions of the Body Fluids

Cations	Anions
Sodium	Chloride
Potassium	Sulfate
Calcium	Phosphate
Magnesium	Lactate
	Ketoanions

rium concentration of hydrogen ions can be calculated by combining and rearranging the equations into a single equation
relating the hydrogen ion concentration to the independent variables [SID], [total protein species], and P_{CO2}. The equation
that results is

$$[H^+]^4 + A[H^+]^3 + B[H^+]^2 - C[H^+] - D = 0$$

where

$$A = [SID] + K_{protein}$$

$$B = K_{protein} ([SID] - [total\ protein\ species])$$
$$- K_{water}[HOH] - K_{bicarbonate} \cdot P_{CO2}$$

$$C = K_{protein} (K_{water}[HOH] + K_{bicarbonate} \cdot P_{CO2})$$
$$- K_{carbonate} \cdot K_{bicarbonate} \cdot P_{CO2}$$

$$D = K_{protein} \cdot K_{carbonate} \cdot K_{bicarbonate} \cdot P_{CO2}.$$

The equation (a fourth-order polynomial) is formidable but
can be solved by the use of a computer. Its solution over a wide
range of values of P_{CO2} and [SID] is shown in Figure 9-4 (the
left panel expresses the hydrogen ion concentration in electrochemical equivalents; the right panel uses a pH scale). In this
figure [total protein species] is set equal to 19 meq/L. The
concentration of protein varies much less than that of the other
two determinants and only over a much greater period of time, so
in most cases it can be treated as a constant.

The figure illustrates that plasma hydrogen ion concentration
is directly proportional to P_{CO2}. Indeed, if [SID] is held constant, the two are very nearly linearly related. Note that this
is so when hydrogen ion concentration is expressed in electrochemical equivalents but not when it is expressed as pH. This is
why the concentration scale is much more appropriate than the pH
scale for clinical measurements of hydrogen ion concentration.

The plasma P_{CO2} is determined by the clearance of carbon
dioxide in the lungs, so disorders that alter effective ventilation and thereby carbon dioxide clearance cause alterations in
the plasma P_{CO2}. Disorders that decrease effective ventilation
and thus increase P_{CO2} produce a proportional increase in plasma
hydrogen ion concentration or acidemia. This kind of acid-base
imbalance is called respiratory acidosis. Disorders that increase effective ventilation result in a decrease in P_{CO2} and
cause a proportional decrease in plasma hydrogen ion concen-

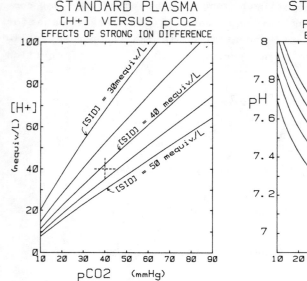
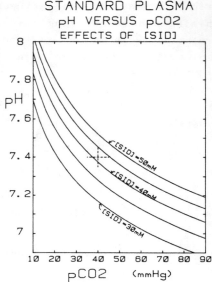

Fig 9-4   The Relationship Among the Concentration

of Hydrogen Ions in Plasma, the P_{CO_2}

and the Strong Ion Difference

(Concentration of Protein Held Constant)

(from Stewart, P.A.   Modern quantitative acid-base

chemistry.   Can. J. Physiol. Pharmacol. 61:1444,

1983 © The National Research Council of Canada, Ottawa)

To use the nomograms: Locate the P_{CO_2} in mmHg on the horizontal axis and the strong ion difference in meq/L among
the family of curves in the coordinate space.   Using a
straightedge, construct a line perpendicular to the horizontal axis passing through the stipulated P_{CO_2}.   Locate
the intersection of the line and the curve corresponding to
the strong ion difference.   Using a straightedge, construct
a horizontal line from the point of intersection to the
vertical axis.   The point on the vertical axis intersected
by the line is the hydrogen ion concentration; in the left
panel this is expressed as neq/L, and in the right panel as
pH.

tration, or alkalemia.   This imbalance is called respiratory
alkalosis.

Figure 9-4 also shows that plasma hydrogen concentration is
inversely related to [SID].   This means that metabolic disturb-

ances that lead to an unbalanced increase in strong anion concentration and thereby decrease [SID] produce acidemia. Those that generate an unbalanced decrease in strong anion concentration increase [SID] and cause alkalemia. These acid-base imbalances are called metabolic acidosis and metabolic alkalosis, respectively.

The changes in hydrogen ion concentration that are found in patients suffering from acid-base disorders are not as large as would be predicted, given the magnitude of the change in P_{CO2} or [SID]. This is because the homeostatic mechanisms that regulate the plasma hydrogen ion concentration in health also act to moderate alterations in the concentration in disease (Table 9-2). The effects of changes in [SID] are partially offset by compensatory changes in P_{CO2} brought about by alterations in respiratory rate. Alterations in P_{CO2} lead to compensatory changes in [SID] due to tissue buffering and renal mechanisms. Tissue buffering, including red cell buffering, occurs immediately, so it is operative in acute respiratory disorders. Renal compensation occurs over days, so its full effect is not seen except in chronic respiratory conditions.

Laboratory Measurement

The quantities that need to be determined when evaluating acid-base balance are the plasma hydrogen ion concentration and its determinants: P_{CO2}, [SID], and in certain cases, [total protein species].

Hydrogen ion concentration and P_{CO2} are measured in arterial blood by potentiometry using hydrogen and carbon dioxide ion-selective electrodes, respectively. Because of the multiplicity of assays that would need to be performed to derive [SID], it is not determined directly. Instead, the calculated concentration of bicarbonate ([HCO_3^-]) or the measured concentration of carbon dioxide ([total CO_2]) is used to estimate [SID].

To see why these estimates are valid, consider the equation describing the electrical neutrality of plasma:

$$[H^+] + [SID] - [OH^-] - [protein\ anion] - [HCO_3^-] - [CO_3^{2-}] = 0.$$

Rearrangement yields

$$[SID] = [HCO_3^-] + [CO_3^{2-}] + [protein\ anion] + [OH^-] - [H^+].$$

Under physiologic conditions, [HCO_3^-] is 10^2 times larger than [CO_3^{2-}], 10^4 times larger than [OH^-], and 10^5 times larger than

- 181 -

Table 9-2

Compensatory Mechanisms for Simple Acid-Base Disorders

Acid-base disorder	Primary effect	Compensatory mechanism	Compensatory effect	Net effect
Respiratory acidosis	Increase P_{CO2}			
Acute		Tissue buffering	Increase [SID]	$[H^+] = 0.75\ \Delta\ P_{CO2}$
Chronic		Increased HCO_3^- retention and Cl^- loss by kidney		$[H^+] = 0.3\ \Delta\ P_{CO2}$
Respiratory alkalosis	Decrease P_{CO2}			
Acute		Tissue buffering	Decrease [SID]	$[H^+] = 0.75\ \Delta\ P_{CO2}$
Chronic		Increased HCO_3^- loss by kidney		$[H^+] = 0.3\ \Delta\ P_{CO2}$
Metabolic acidosis	Decrease [SID]	Hyperventilation	Decrease P_{CO2}	$[H^+] = 1.5\ \Delta$ [SID] for Δ [SID] > -18 meq/L
Metabolic alkalosis	Increase [SID]	Hypoventilation	Increase P_{CO2}	$[H^+] = -0.5\ \Delta$ [SID] for Δ [SID] < 24 meq/L

[H^+], so the latter terms can be disregarded with no appreciable loss in accuracy. Thus,

$$[SID] = [HCO_3^-] + [protein\ anion].$$

As long as the protein concentration is nearly constant, [protein anion] will be too, so

$$[SID] = [HCO_3^-] + constant.$$

Therefore, [HCO_3^-] parallels [SID] and can be used clinically to estimate [SID].

The conservation of mass for carbon dioxide requires that

$$[total\ CO_2] = [dissolved\ CO_2] + [H_2CO_3] + [HCO_3^-] + [CO_3^{2-}].$$

Because under physiologic conditions [HCO_3^-] is 20 times larger than [dissolved CO_2], 10^2 times larger than [CO_3^{2-}], and 10^3 times larger than [H_2CO_3], these terms can be ignored, yielding

$$[total\ CO_2] = [HCO_3^-]\ .$$

Therefore, [total CO_2] is nearly equivalent to [HCO_3^-] and can be used in its stead to estimate [SID].

Total carbon dioxide concentration is measured by quantifying the amount of carbon dioxide released by acidification of venous plasma. Bicarbonate concentration is calculated from measurements of arterial hydrogen ion concentration and P_{CO2} by using the Henderson-Hasselbach equation:

or

$$[HCO_3^-] = K_{bicarbonate} \cdot P_{CO2}/[H^+]$$

$$log[HCO_3^-] = log(K_{bicarbonate}) + log(P_{CO2}) - pH\ .$$

Figure 9-5 shows the Siggaard-Andersen nomogram for this equation. Notice that this equation is listed in the preceding section as one of the physical relationships dictating the acid-base equilibrium state. It is often mistakenly asserted that this single relationship determines the equilibrium state. As has been discussed, it is in fact but one of many governing relationships.

Because the P_{CO2} of venous plasma is higher than that of arterial plasma, venous [total CO_2] can be expected to be greater than arterial [total CO_2] and therefore arterial [HCO_3^-], but

SIGGAARD-ANDERSEN ALIGNMENT NOMOGRAM

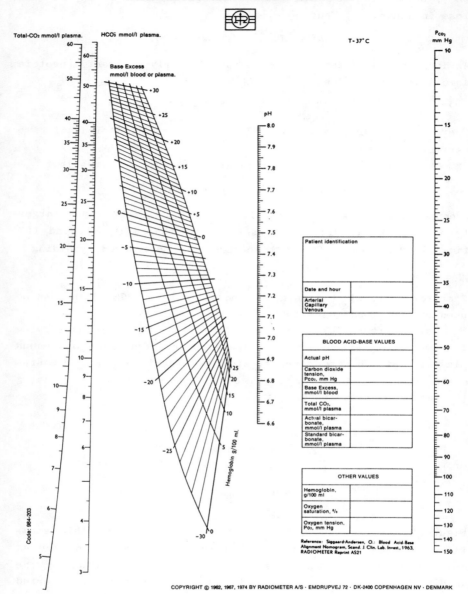

Fig 9-5   Siggaard-Andersen Alignment Nomogram
for the Henderson-Hasselbach Equation

To use the nomogram: Locate the P_{CO2} in mmHg on the right
axis and the pH on the center axis.   Connect the two points

only slightly. Empirically, venous [total CO_2] measurements are very close to arterial [HCO_3^-] calculations except at very abnormal levels of P_{CO2}. The relationship between the two, as reported by Brashear et al. (1979), is

$$venous~[total~CO_2] = 1.25~arterial~[HCO_3^-] - 6.25~meq/L$$

when both concentrations are expressed in milliequivalents per liter.

Information about the unmeasured components of the strong ion difference can be obtained by calculation of the anion gap. The anion gap is defined as the difference between the concentration of sodium and the summed concentrations of chloride and bicarbonate (or total CO_2):

$$anion~gap = [Na^+] - [Cl^-] - [HCO_3^-].$$

Sequential substitution of the formulas

$$[HCO_3^-] = [SID] - [protein~anions]$$

and

$$[SID] = [Na^+] + [other~strong~cations] - [Cl^-] - [other~strong~anions]$$

reveals that the anion gap indirectly measures the difference between the summed concentrations of protein and "other" strong anions and the concentration of "other" strong cations:

$$anion~gap = [protein~anions] + [other~strong~anions] - [other~strong~cations].$$

In most cases, the concentrations of protein anions and "other" strong cations are fairly constant, so changes in the anion gap reflect changes in the concentration of "other" strong anions. In this way the anion gap can be used to detect the retention of sulfate and phosphate in renal failure and the accumulation of

Fig 9-5, continued
with a straightedge. The point on the far left axis intersected by the straightedge is the carbon dioxide content in mmol/L; the point intersected on the center left axis is the bicarbonate concentration in meq/L. The near left axes are for the calculation of base excess or deficit (the difference between the titratable acids and bases of blood at a pH of 7.4, a P_{CO2} of 40 mm, and a temperature of 37° C).

organic acids in disorders such as lactic acidosis and ketoacidosis.

Clinical Evaluation
(Narins and Emmet 1980)

The questions to be answered in the evaluation of acid-base
balance prior to seeking an etiologic diagnosis are, in order,

1. Is an acid-base disorder present?
2. Is the disorder respiratory, metabolic, or both?

Acid-base disorders are usually screened for by measurement
of [total CO_2] in venous serum. Plasma hydrogen ion concentration and P_{CO2} are measured in arterial blood, which requires a
sampling procedure too invasive to be used solely for screening
purposes. The finding of an altered [total CO_2] indicates that
an acid-base disturbance is present. A normal or near-normal
value does not exclude this possibility, however. Normal
concentrations can be found in acute respiratory disorders and in
some mixed metabolic and respiratory disturbances. Because of
this, symptomatic patients and patients at risk for developing
acid-base problems should have their plasma hydrogen ion concentration and P_{CO2} measured. If a disorder is present, one or
both of these will be abnormal.

When an acid-base disorder is present, the concurrent measurement of plasma hydrogen ion concentration and P_{CO2} is used to
classify the disorder according to its pathophysiologic mechanism. The empirical ranges of the paired findings for the simple
acid-base disorders are mapped in Figure 9-6. Acidemia and an
increased P_{CO2} indicate respiratory acidosis; alkalemia and a
decreased P_{CO2}, respiratory alkalosis; acidemia and a compensatory decrease in P_{CO2}, metabolic acidosis; and alkalemia and a
compensatory increase in P_{CO2}, metabolic alkalosis. Patients
with respiratory disorders in whom a full compensatory response
has not yet developed will have result combinations in the
regions between the applicable acute and chronic respiratory
ranges. The result pairs for patients with mixed acid-base
disorders will be located in the regions between the applicable
metabolic and respiratory ranges.

The mechanism ascertained to underly a patient's acid-base
disorder will determine the direction of the subsequent clinical
search for the disorder's etiology. The finding of a respiratory
component indicates that there is a condition causing an alteration in effective ventilation. The finding of a metabolic com-

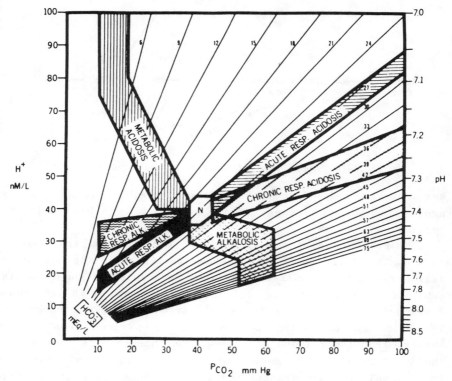

Fig 9-6   Diagnostic Classification of Acid-Base Disorders
[from Epstein, M., Oster, J.R. Acid-base disturbances: The
role of the kidney. In: Halsted, J.A., Halsted, C.H.
(eds.) The Laboratory in Clinical Medicine. 2nd ed.
1982, p. 305 © W.B. Saunders, Philadelphia]

ponent reveals the presence of disordered cellular metabolism or
a disturbance of the gastrointestinal tract or kidney.   In the
case of a metabolic acidosis, further classification of the
disorder in terms of normal versus high anion gap separates
diseases of the gastrointestinal tract and metabolic disturbances
of the kidney from renal failure and deranged cellular metabolism.

TRACE METALS AND VITAMINS

(Labbé 1981)

To protect against the development of shortages of trace
metals and vitamins during periods of dietary deprivation, they
are stored in the body, either as long-lived metabolically active
forms or as storage forms usually consisting of a complex of the

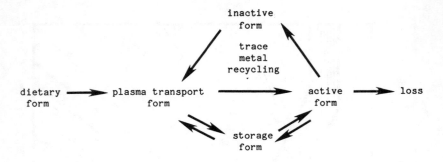

Fig 9-7   Simple Model of Trace Metal and Vitamin Dynamics

nutrient and a specific intracellular storage protein. Further
protection from shortages of trace metals is achieved by recycling.

A simple model of the dynamics of vitamins and trace metals
is shown in Figure 9-7. The tissues that produce the metabolically active form of a trace substance receive their supply of the
substance from the circulation, where it is present in its plasma
transport form, and from intracellular stores of the substance.
The trace substance transported in plasma arises from dietary
intake, from the release of stored substance, and in the case of
the trace metals, from recycling. Some of the vitamins and the
trace metal iron are transported in the plasma bound to specific
transport proteins. This facilitates the differential delivery
of these substances to the tissues utilizing them. Any trace
substance that is not removed from the plasma to produce the
active form of the substance is deposited in tissue stores in its
storage form. Trace substances are usually lost to the body in
their active form, such as by the catabolism of the enzyme co-
factor form of the vitamins, or in their storage form, such as by
the desquamation of epithelial cells containing trace metals.

The body stores of a trace substance are deficient when they
are not able to supply the body's needs for the production of the
active form of the substance. The accompanying clinical manifestations are due to the resultant reduction in the amount of the
active form of the substance.

A trace substance is present in excess, also called overload,
when the storage form of the substance is accumulated to the
point of damage to the storage tissue or when, because of increased body stores, there is sufficient deposition of the substance in nonstorage tissues to cause injury to them. Here the

clinical findings are attributable to the tissue injury and its sequela. The active form of the substance remains present in a normal amount unless one of the injured tissues is the site of synthesis of the active form.

Plasma Markers

Trace metals and vitamins circulate in the plasma not only in their transport forms but may also be present in their active and storage forms. Storage forms enter plasma as a result of leakage from dead storage cells. Active forms are secreted from their sites of synthesis into the plasma where they play their physiologic roles as plasma constituents.

The concentration of trace substance contained in its storage form can be used as a plasma marker of the body stores of the substance in deficiency and overload states. The plasma concentration of the storage form depends upon the rate at which the storage form enters the plasma. That entry rate is the product of the rate of death of storage cells and the amount of substance contained in each cell. In the absence of other perturbing influences, the rate of cell death among storage cells is constant. The plasma entry rate then depends only upon the amount of the storage form liberated per dead storage cell which is, in turn, determined by the overall body stores of the substance. Consequently, the concentration of the storage form is proportional to the body stores. When the cell death rate in the storage tissue is increased, however, as occurs with injury to the tissue and in neoplastic tissue, the release of the storage form is increased and its plasma levels will be elevated.

The plasma concentration of a trace substance contained in its transport form depends upon the rates of entry of the form into the plasma — from the diet, from body stores, and from recycling. If the major source of the transport form of the substance is the body stores, the concentration of the transport form will generally parallel those stores. If recycling supplies the transport form, its concentration will depend upon the rate of recycling, which may or may not correspond to the level of the body stores. If the transport form arises predominantly from dietary uptake, its plasma concentration will merely reflect the recent dietary intake of the substance regardless of the state of the body stores. The plasma concentration of the transport form also depends upon its rate of egress from the plasma into sites of synthesis of the active form and back into body stores.

Changes in clearance rate unrelated to the state of body stores will produce misleading alterations in marker concentration.

The circulating active form of a trace substance can be used as a marker of body stores in deficiency states. When stores are deficient, the reduced supply of the substance results in diminution in the rate of synthesis and secretion of the active form. Because the plasma concentration of the active form depends upon its rate of secretion, the magnitude of the deficiency in the substance stores will be reflected in the magnitude of the reduction in the circulating levels of the active form. Secretion of the active form will not be supranormal when body stores are increased, so the active form is not useful as a stores marker in overload states. Other influences upon the rate of secretion of the active form can cause alterations in its plasma concentration that can be confused with or can obscure changes due to abnormal body stores.

An additional plasma marker of the body stores of trace substances transported in the plasma bound to specific transport proteins is the transport protein itself. In deficiency states, the concentrations of specific transport proteins increase; in overload states, the concentrations decrease.

Table 9-3 lists plasma markers of the body stores of selected trace metals and vitamins. Iron and vitamin B12 (cobalamin) have circulating storage forms that are used as markers. Because the majority of the vitamin B12 in plasma is in the storage form, the total vitamin B12 plasma concentration (all circulating forms of the vitamin), which is more easily measured, is a reliable substitute marker. The trace metals copper and zinc have circulating active forms that can be used as stores markers in deficiency states. Overload states for these metals are indicated by an increased concentration of the transport form, as reflected in the increased total plasma metal concentration. Quantitative estimation of the excessive body stores is not possible using the plasma markers. The folic acid in plasma consists entirely of its transport form, most of which represents recent dietary intake. Consequently, there is no acceptable plasma marker of folate stores. Instead, tissue stores are assayed directly in circulating red cells.

Table 9-3

Plasma Markers of Body Stores of Selected Trace Metals and Vitamins

Trace substance	Major plasma form	Storage form released into plasma	Active form in plasma	Transport form in plasma	Assayable tissue storage site
Iron	Transport	Ferritin	(Red cell hemoglobin is the active form present in whole blood)	Iron-transferrin	Marrow macrophage
Copper	Active		Ceruloplasmin	Copper-albumin	
Zinc	Transport		Zinc metalloenzymes	Zinc-albumin	
Vitamin B12 (cobalamin)	Storage	Vitamin B12-transcobalamin I		Vitamin B12-transcobalamin II	Marrow blood cells
Folic acid	Transport			Free folic acid, folic acid-albumin	Red cells

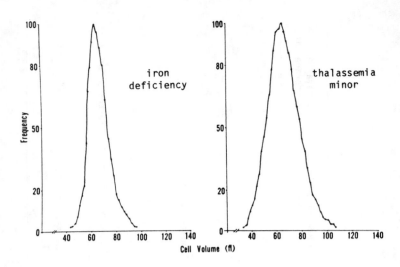

Fig 9-8   Normal and Abnormal Heterogeneity
of a Cytologic Characteristic
(from Bessman, J.D., Feinstein, D.I.   Quantitative anisocytosis as
a discriminant between iron deficiency and thalassemia minor.
Blood 53:288, 1979 © Grune and Stratton, Inc., Orlando)

Cellular Markers

(Bessman 1983)

Cells also can be used to detect and quantify physiologic processes.   There may be changes in the concentration of a particular type of cell, in the average amount of some cytologic characteristic per cell, or in the concentration of the characteristic (i.e., the product of the average amount of the characteristic per cell times the cell concentration).   In addition, laboratory techniques that measure a cytologic characteristic in large numbers of single cells can be used to identify changes in the distribution of the characteristic within the cell population.   In disease the variability, or heterogeneity, of a cytologic characteristic may be increased above its normal level.   No disorder has been found in which a characteristic's heterogeneity is decreased.   This suggests that heterogeneity, at least in part, represents the "quality control" of cell production, which may be expected to be optimal in normal individuals.   Figure 9-8 illustrates normal and abnormal heterogeneity graphically.

Disordered erythropoiesis due to deficient stores of iron, vitamin B12, or folic acid gives rise to a number of cellular markers:

1. decreased blood hemoglobin concentration and packed red
cell volume (anemia)

2. altered mean red cell hemoglobin content and volume (microcytosis or macrocytosis)
3. increased heterogeneity of red cell volume (anisocytosis).

Anemia develops late in the course of trace substance deficiency and therefore is not a sensitive marker of a deficiency state. Neither is it specific because there are numerous other conditions that can cause it. In contrast, when measured concurrently, mean red cell volume (or hemoglobin content) and cell volume heterogeneity are sensitive and moderately specific cellular markers. A decreased mean cell volume with an increased volume heterogeneity indicates iron deficiency. An increase in both markers implies vitamin B12 or folate deficiency. In both settings, the severity of the deficiency is reflected in the degree of the abnormality of the markers.

PLASMA PROTEINS AND BLOOD CELLS

The use of plasma proteins and blood cells as organ function markers has been considered previously. In that discussion it was stated that their role as markers depended, in part, upon constancy of the clearance rate. There are numerous disease states in which this condition is not met, in which, in fact, an increased protein or cell clearance rate may be the primary expression of the disorder. Hypoalbuminemia due to renal protein leakage (nephrosis), hypofibrinogenemia secondary to the intravascular coagulation/fibrinolysis syndrome, and anemia due to autoimmune hemolytic disease are important examples.

For these and similar disorders, the protein or cell concentrations are inversely related to the disease activity, as revealed by the steady state relationship

plasma concentration = synthetic rate/clearance rate.

Because the synthetic rate is usually not constant but increases in homeostatic response to depressed plasma concentrations, the relationship is not strictly hyperbolic. Disorders in which the capacity for synthesis of a protein or production of a cell type is compromised concurrent with an alteration in its clearance rate will demonstrate more nearly hyperbolic relationships. A reduction in the synthetic rate will exaggerate the decrease in plasma concentration. Chronic liver disease and megaloblastic anemia, for example, typically behave in this fashion.

In addition to decreased function of the synthesizing organ and increased plasma clearance rate, the concentration of a plasma protein may also be reduced due to a hereditary or acquired defect in the synthesis or secretion of the protein. Specific hereditary deficiencies represent a clinically important group of errors of inborn metabolism (Table 9-4).

Table 9-4

Plasma Proteins with Clinically
Important Hereditary Deficiency States

α_1-Antitrypsin

Ceruloplasmin

Antithrombin III

Complement components, especially

    C2, C1 esterase inhibitor

Clotting factors, especially

    Factor VIII, Factor IX

Immunoglobulins

CELLULAR METABOLISM
(Stanbury et al. 1983)

Nearly all of the inherited and most of the acquired metabolic disorders arise from a discrete defect in a metabolic pathway. The general model of metabolic fluxes illustrated in Figure 9-9 reveals the numerous locations at which such a defect can appear. There may be impaired transport of a precursor substance into the metabolic tissue (1), of end product out of the tissue (one mechanism of hereditary deficiency of a plasma protein), or of end product through its catabolic (5) and excretory (7 and 8) paths. Disordered metabolic transformations can occur in the metabolic tissue (2-4) or in the catabolic tissue (6).

As a rule, the presence of a metabolic defect results in the decreased appearance of substances in the metabolic pathway distal to the defect; the accumulation of substances proximal to the defect, especially of the substance immediately proximal; and, often, in the appearance of substances that are generated by

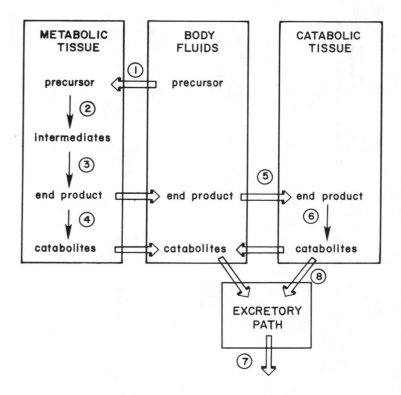

Fig 9-9   Simple Model of Metabolic Fluxes
with Clinically Important Sites of
Metabolic Defects Indicated

the shunting of the accumulated substances into alternative metabolic pathways.   The resulting pattern of substance deficiency,
accumulation, and appearance is highly specific for the underlying defect.

The diagnostic evaluation of a metabolic disorder may depend
upon the demonstration of the full pattern of metabolic abnormalities attendant upon it, but it can usually be accomplished by
the measurement of accumulated substances alone (the plasma protein deficiencies are important exceptions).   A diagnostic scheme
based upon accumulated substances is shown in Table 9-5.   Clinical examples from among the inborn errors of metabolism are indicated.   Note that the site of accumulation depends upon whether
there is cellular reflux of the substance.   When reflux does not

Table 9-5

Scheme of Substance Accumulation in Metabolic Disease

Tissue involved	Metabolic site and mechanism of defect[a]	Substance accumulated	Intracellular accumulation	Systemic accumulation	Clinical example
Metabolic tissue	1) Decreased uptake	Precursor		X	Familial hypercholesterolemia
	2) Decreased metabolism with reflux		X	X	Galactosemia
	3) Decreased production of endproduct	Intermediates			
	with reflux		X	X	Alkaptonuria
	without reflux		X		Glycogen storage disease
	with production of alternative end product	Intermediates and alternative end product		X	Congenital adrenal hyperplasia
	4) Decreased intracellular catabolism	End products			
	with reflux		X	X	Mucopolysaccharidosis
	without reflux		X		Lysosomal storage disease
Catabolic tissue	5) Decreased uptake	End products		X	Dysbetalipoproteinemia
	6) Decreased catabolism with reflux		X		Gilbert's syndrome (hereditary jaundice)
Excretory tissue	7) Decreased excretion	Catabolites		X	Renal tubular acidosis
	8) Decreased input into excretory path		X	X	Dubin-Johnson syndrome (hereditary jaundice)

[a] Numbering corresponds with sites shown on Figure 9-9.

occur to any appreciable degree, accumulation is intracellular. In such disorders cell contents must be submitted to laboratory study. When reflux does occur, accumulation is both intracellular and systemic. It then can be detected by measuring the appropriate substance concentration in body fluids.

EXERCISES

9-1. In which of the following disorders might the anion gap be increased? In which might it be decreased?
    hypocalcemia
    nephrotic syndrome
    multiple myeloma
    diabetes mellitus
While working in the emergency room you are brought a patient who is comatose. He is hyperventilating and he has a fruity breath odor. Because you suspect that he is comatose because of an acid-base disorder, you order a number of laboratory studies. The results include

plasma $[H^+]$	70 nmol/L
plasma P_{CO2}	20 mmHg
plasma anion gap	33 meq/L

(reference interval: 9-18 meq/L)

9-2. Is an acid-base disorder present? Is the disorder respiratory, metabolic, or both? Is there evidence of homeostatic compensation?
Further questioning of the family reveals that the patient weighs 4 kg less than usual and that he has had polydipsia and polyuria for the preceding few days. Other laboratory study results include

body weight	52 kg
plasma sodium concentration	131 meq/L
(reference interval: 135-145 meq/L)	
plasma potassium concentration	5.3 meq/L
(reference interval: 3.5-5.0 meq/L)	
plasma glucose concentration	27.5 mmol/L
(reference interval: 3.8-5.6 mmol/L)	

9-3. Because the patient has hyperglycemia he is experiencing an osmotic diuresis. What is the estimated magnitude of water loss? Assuming that the tonicity of the urinary losses is low, how much of the water loss is extracellular and how much is intracellular?

9-4. What is the state of body sodium content? What is the state of body potassium content?

9-5. You decide that the patient is suffering from hyperglycemia ketoacidosis due to diabetes mellitus. Indicate the site of the metabolic defect in diabetes mellitus in Figure 9-9. Explain why fasting hyperketonemia and hyperglycemia result from this defect.

Your next patient is an alcoholic who complains of weakness. He has a history of gastrointestinal bleeding, so you perform a stool guaiac test, which is positive for occult blood. You suspect that the patient is anemic due to blood loss. Laboratory study results include

hemoglobin concentration	12.0 g/dl
(reference interval: 13.2-17.4 g/dl)	
mean red cell volume	85.9 fl
(reference interval: 80.3-98.9 fl)	
red cell volume heterogeneity	17.6%
(reference interval: 12.2-14.6%)	
ferritin concentration	7.5 µg/ml
(reference interval: 10-200 µg/ml)	

9-6. Which laboratory findings suggest that the patient has iron deficiency secondary to chronic blood loss?

While the patient is in the hospital, his bleeding stops and oral iron therapy is begun. You see the patient 2 months after discharge to monitor his therapy. At that time laboratory study results include

hemoglobin concentration	13.0 g/dl
mean red cell volume	98.0 fl
red cell volume heterogeneity	15.5%
ferritin concentration	105 µg/ml.

9-7. Is the patient cured?

Mind-Expanding Exercise

9-8. The body stores of trace metals can be assessed by methods not mentioned in the text. Suggest how the administration of the trace metal of interest can be used to evaluate deficiency states.

Beck, L.H. (ed.) Body fluid and electrolyte disorders. Med. Clin. North Am. 65:247-452, 1981.

Bessman, J.D. Classification of anemia by MCV and RDW. Am. J. Clin. Pathol. 80:322, 1983.

Brashear, R.E., Oei, T.O., Rhodes, M.L., et al. Relationship between arterial and venous bicarbonate values. Arch. Intern. Med. 139:440, 1979.

Labbé, R.F. (ed.) Laboratory assessment of nutritional status. Clin. Lab. Med. 1:603-796, 1981.

Narins, R.G., Emmett, M. Simple and mixed acid-base disorders: A practical approach. Medicine 59:161, 1980.

Stanbury, J.B., Wyngaarden, J.B., Frederickson, D.S., et al. (eds.) The Metabolic Basis of Inherited Disease, 5th ed. McGraw-Hill, New York, 1983.

Stewart, P.A. How to Understand Acid-Base: A Quantitative Acid-Base Primer for Biology and Medicine. Elsevier-North Holland, New York, 1981.

Stewart, P.A. Modern quantitative acid-base chemistry. Can. J. Physiol. Pharmacol. 61:1444, 1983.

Chapter 10

PROTEIN BINDING IN PLASMA

When he killed the Mudjokivis,
Of the skin he made him mittens,
Made them with the fur side inside,
Made them with the skin side outside,
He, to get the warm side inside,
Put the inside skin side outside;
He, to get the cold side outside,
Put the warm side fur side inside,
That's why he put the fur side inside.
Why he put the skin side outside,
Why he turned them inside outside.

George A. Strong

PHYSIOLOGIC FUNCTIONS OF PROTEIN BINDING

(Kragh-Hansen 1981; Natelson and Natelson 1980; Ritzmann and Daniels 1975)

Many plasma constituents are partly or completely bound to plasma proteins. Four physiologic functions are served by this binding:

1. vehicle function
2. delivery function
3. storage function
4. buffer function.

Vehicle Function

Plasma constituents that have limited solubility in plasma achieve much greater plasma concentrations when transported bound to a protein.

Delivery Function

Certain plasma constituents are meant to be available to specific tissues and unavailable to others. One mechanism to accomplish this selective tissue delivery is for the plasma constituent to be bound to a protein for which the specific tissue has numerous high-affinity membrane receptors. Other tissues will have a lesser number of receptors or low affinity receptors and consequently will take up much less of the binding protein and its bound plasma constituent.

Storage Function

A plasma substance is stored when bound to a protein if the binding results in a decreased loss of that substance into the urine. This is one mechanism to reduce the dietary requirement for trace nutrients.

Buffer Function

For some plasma constituents, it is advantageous to have a circulating inactive species to serve as a ready source of the constituent when the active form is acutely depleted. Similarly, if the concentration of the active species is acutely increased, it is necessary to have a ready "sink" wherein the constituent is rendered inactive. This is the buffer function of protein binding: the protein bound form of the substance is physiologically inactive; only the unbound form is active. Plasma constituents that have binding proteins with a buffer function are characterized by homeostatic control of the concentration of the active, unbound form.

Table 10-1 lists the apparent physiologic functions of protein binding for a number of plasma constituents of clinical interest. The extent and distribution of protein binding for these analytes is presented in Table 10-2.

DELIVERY FUNCTION

(Steinman et al. 1983)

For binding proteins serving a delivery function, the rate of tissue uptake of the ligand depends upon the tissue density and affinity of cell surface receptors for the binding protein. Uptake is rapid when the tissue has either a high density of binding protein receptors or high-affinity receptors. Uptake is slow when the tissue has either a low density of binding protein receptors or low-affinity receptors.

After the binding protein-ligand complex is bound to the membrane receptor, the complex is internalized. This process is called receptor-mediated endocytosis. It proceeds by several steps. First, binding protein-ligand-receptor units aggregate over clathrin-coated domains of the plasma membrane. Then these regions invaginate and pinch off, forming clathrin-coated vesicles. Finally these vesicles migrate to lysosomes or to the Golgi organelle. The ligand is dissociated from its binding protein, and the surface receptors, now empty, return to the plasma membrane intact. The binding protein may be catabolized by the cell or it may reenter the circulation. The ligand, once freed of its plasma binding protein, is available either for immediate use or for cytoplasmic storage, which often is accomplished by the complexing of the ligand to a cytoplasmic binding protein.

Table 10-1

Physiologic Function(s) of Protein Binding for Selected Plasma Analytes

Analyte	Function			
	Vehicle	Delivery	Storage	Buffer
Bilirubin	Yes			
Free fatty acids	Yes			
Vitamin A (retinol)	Yes	Yes	Yes	
Vitamin D	Yes	Possible		
Vitamin B12	Yes			
Iron	Yes	Yes	Yes	
Hemoglobin		Yes	Yes	
Heme		Yes	Yes	
Copper			Probable	
Zinc			Probable	
Folic acid			Probable	
Calcium				Yes
Magnesium				Yes
Thyroxine				Yes
Triiodothyronine				Yes
Aldosterone				Yes
Cortisol				Yes
Testosterone				Yes
Estradiol				Yes
Progesterone				Yes

Table 10-2

Extent and Distribution of Protein Binding for Selected Plasma Analytes

Analyte	Typical % protein bound	Major specific binding protein	Distribution (%)		
			Binding protein	Albumin	Other globulins
Bilirubin	>99			100	
Free fatty acids	100			100	
Vitamin A (retinol)	100	Retinol-binding globulin	100		
Vitamin D	100	Vitamin D-binding globulin	95	5	
Vitamin B12	100	Transcobalamin II	20		80
Iron	100	Transferrin	100		
Hemoglobin	Varies	Haptoglobin	100		
Heme	100	Hemopexin	Varies	Varies	
Copper[a]	95			100	
Zinc[a]	90			60	40
Folic acid	Varies			100	
Calcium	45			90	10
Magnesium	25			100	
Thyroxine	>99	Thyroxine-binding globulin	70	10	20
Triiodothyronine	>99	Thyroxine-binding globulin	70	30	
Aldosterone	60	Cortisol-binding globulin	15	85	
Cortisol	90	Cortisol-binding globulin	75	25	
Testosterone Male	98	Testosterone-binding globulin	45	55	
Female	99	Testosterone-binding globulin	70	30	
Estradiol Male	98	Testosterone-binding globulin	40	60	
Female	98	Testosterone-binding globulin	20	80	
Progesterone: female	98	Cortisol-binding globulin	10	Varies	Varies

[a] Metals present in plasma enzymes are not included.

STORAGE FUNCTION

The rate of loss of a plasma substance into the urine is determined by the rate at which the substance is filtered at the renal glomerulus minus the rate at which it is recovered by renal tubular reabsorption. Therefore, trace nutrients in the circulation can be protected from wasteful renal loss by being unfilterable or by the presence of an efficient mechanism of tubular resorption.

Vitamin A (retinol) binds to the low-molecular-weight protein, retinol-binding globin (RBG). The pair then forms a complex with prealbumin, a minor thyroxine binding globulin. Unlike the vitamin A-RBG pair, the two ligand-two binding protein complex is too large to be filtered at the glomerulus. Thus the vitamin A is stored for tissue uptake. Copper, zinc, and folic acid circulate bound to unfilterable high-molecular-weight proteins, mostly albumin.

Iron storage is accomplished not only by the transport of plasma iron as transferrin but also by the protein binding of hemoglobin and heme following intravascular hemolysis. Urine loss of iron occurs only when the amount of hemoglobin released from a hemolytic episode exceeds the binding capacity of haptoglobin. Unbound hemoglobin then passes into the glomerular filtrate. Tubular resorption captures much of the filtered hemoglobin but some enters the urine. The reabsorbed iron, present in the tubular epithelial cells, reenters the circulation until the cells die and slough into the urine with their residual iron.

BUFFER FUNCTION

The protein binding of a physiologically active plasma substance serves to protect against sudden, large changes in the concentration of the substance. Given a change in the total plasma concentration of the substance, a lesser change will occur in the concentration of the active, that is, unbound, form. The difference between the two is accounted for by inactivation of added substance by protein binding or by release of active substance from the bound state when substance is removed. Figure 10-1 illustrates the protein buffering of an analyte when its concentration is changed from 8 to 16 units per volume. Of the 8 units added, 3 are bound to the protein carrier while only 5 remain unbound and active. Thus the protein binding has reduced by 37.5% the change in concentration of the active form that otherwise would have occurred.

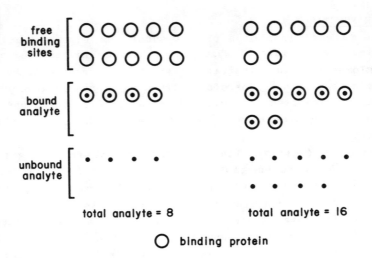

Fig 10-1   Buffering Effect of Protein Binding

The magnitude of the buffering effect of protein binding depends upon the **affinity** of the binding site for the plasma constituent and upon the plasma concentration of the binding sites, the **capacity** of the protein. This relationship is embodied in the equilibrium mass action equation:

$$\frac{[unbound\ analyte]}{[bound\ analyte]} = \frac{1}{K_a\ [free\ binding\ sites]}$$

where K_a is the association constant. The smaller the ratio of the unbound to bound analyte, the greater the buffer effect. The ratio is small if the association constant is large (high-affinity binding) or if the concentration of free binding sites is large (high-capacity binding). Conversely, the ratio is large and the buffer effect small if there is low-affinity or low-capacity binding.

Figure 10-2 shows the partition of a constant amount of ligand between bound and unbound forms for three binding proteins of equal capacity but unequal relative binding affinity. In this example, the association constants are 1.17, 0.21, and 0.06 for the high-, moderate-, and low-affinity binding, respectively. The concentration of unbound analyte is inversely related to the affinity of the binding protein.

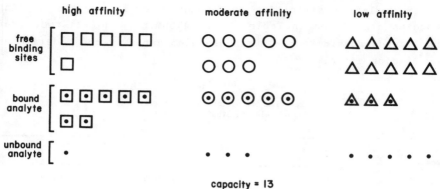

high affinity   moderate affinity   low affinity

free binding sites

bound analyte

unbound analyte

capacity = 13

total analyte = 8

Fig 10-2   Analyte Binding for Proteins of
Equal Capacity But Unequal Relative Affinity

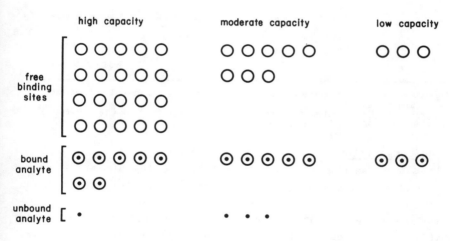

high capacity   moderate capacity   low capacity

free binding sites

bound analyte

unbound analyte

Fig 10-3   Analyte Binding for Proteins of
Equal Relative Affinity but Unequal Capacity

The effect of varying the capacity of a binding protein is depicted in Figure 10-3. The concentration of unbound analyte decreases as the capacity increases.

The relative affinities and capacities of selected binding proteins are listed in Table 10-3. Albumin is not listed. For the ligands considered, albumin has high capacity and moderate or low binding affinity.

Table 10-3

Relative Affinities and Capacities
of Selected Binding Proteins

Capacity	Affinity		
	High	Moderate	Low
High	TBG (triiodothyronine)	Prealbumin (thyroxine)	Prealbumin (triiodothyronine)
	CBG (testosterone, progesterone)	CBG (estradiol)	CBG (aldosterone)
	TeBG (estradiol)	α_1AG (testosterone, progesterone)	α_1AG (cortisol, estradiol)
Moderate	TBG (thyroxine)	CBG (cortisol)	TeBG (progesterone)
	TeBG (testosterone)		
Low			TeBG (cortisol)

The ligand binding to the protein with the stipulated affinity and capacity is indicated within the parentheses.
TBG = thyroxine-binding globulin; CBG = cortisol-binding globulin; TeBG = testosterone-binding globulin; α_1AG = alpha-1-acid glycoprotein

Binding Competition

It can be seen from Table 10-3 that the thyroid and steroid hormones distribute among multiple binding proteins, which leads to competition for binding sites on those proteins. This complexity makes the computation of the hormone binding partitioning prohibitively tedious. When certain simplifying assumptions are made, however, the equilibrium composition of these systems can be calculated using computers.

As an example, computer solutions for the steroid hormone system in the nonpregnant and pregnant female are presented in Figure 10-4. The differences in the binding distribution between the two conditions is attributable to the tenfold increase in the concentration of testosterone-binding globulin (TeBG) and the more modest 2.5-fold increase in the concentration of cortisol-binding globulin (CBG). The rise in TeBG concentration results in a greater percentage binding of estradiol and testosterone to

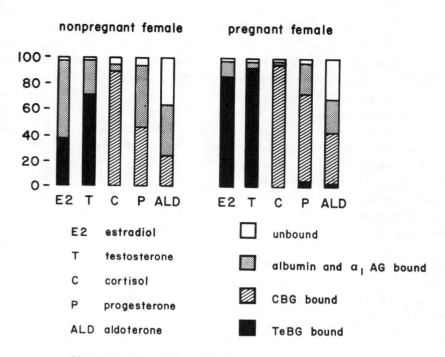

nonpregnant female   **pregnant female**

E2	estradiol
T	testosterone
C	cortisol
P	progesterone
ALD	aldoterone

☐ unbound

▨ albumin and α_1 AG bound

▨ CBG bound

■ TeBG bound

Fig 10-4   Plasma Distribution of Steroid Hormones
in Nonpregnant (Follicular Phase of Ovarian Cycle)
and Pregnant (Third Trimester) Females
[Adapted from Dunn et al. (1981)]

TeBG and a decreased percentage of estradiol and testosterone in available form. Because the estradiol concentration is increased 200-fold in pregnancy, the concentration of available estradiol is increased 40-fold. Similarly, the concentration of available progesterone increases markedly in pregnancy despite increased CBG concentrations because of the tremendous increase in progesterone concentration. The elevation in testosterone levels in pregnancy is small so the concentration of available testosterone is decreased twofold. These opposite effects upon the active fractions of the sex steroids are physiologically appropriate.

Homeostatic Regulation

The concentrations of protein-buffered plasma constituents are regulated by homeostatic systems. Because the concentration of the physiologically active unbound form is the one that is homeostatically controlled, changes in binding protein capacity or affinity will result in secondary alteration in the concentration of the total constituent. The concentration will be changed just enough to reestablish the set-point plasma concentration of the unbound species. In clinical practice, changes in binding protein capacity are common (see Table 10-4). Significant changes in binding protein affinity are uncommon.

An example of the physiologic response to an increase in binding protein capacity is shown in Figure 10-5. In this system the set-point concentration of unbound, active analyte is 3 units per volume. The system is perturbed by an increase in the concentration of binding protein, from 13 to 21 units per volume. As long as the concentration of analyte remains constant, this increase in binding capacity will lead to the conversion of unbound analyte to the bound form. This is labeled the intermediate state. The decrease in the concentration of unbound, active analyte will be detected by the homeostatic sensor, which will then activate mechanisms to increase the concentration of the analyte to 11 units per volume, so as to return the unbound analyte to its set-point concentration. This is shown as the final state.

Table 10-4

Common Causes of Altered Plasma Concentrations
of Selected Binding Proteins

Binding protein	Increased plasma concentration	Decreased plasma concentration
Albumin	Acute dehydration	Protein malnutrition, liver failure, nephrosis, protein-losing enteropathy, acute phase response
TBG	Hypothyroidism, pregnancy, hyperestrogenemia	Hyperthyroidism, protein malnutrition, liver failure, nephrosis, protein-losing enteropathy, acute phase reaction, hyperandrogenemia
CBG	Pregnancy, hyperestrogenemia	Liver failure, nephrosis, protein-losing enteropathy
TeBG	Pregnancy, hyperestrogenemia, hyperthyroidism, liver failure (in men)	Hyperandrogenemia, hypothyroidism (in women)

TBG = thyroxine-binding globulin; CBG = cortisol-binding globulin; TeBG = testosterone-binding globulin

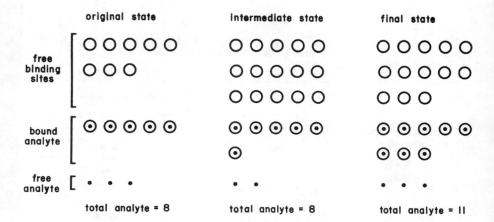

Fig 10-5   Homeostatic Control of a
Protein-Bound Plasma Substance

In Vivo Availability
(Jasen 1981; Pardridge 1981)

The availability of a protein-bound plasma substance for tissue interaction depends upon the distribution of the substance among its unbound, albumin-bound, and specific binding protein-bound forms. Unbound ligand is available. The unidirectional dissociation rate of albumin-substance complexes is much more rapid than the mean capillary transit times of the liver and most peripheral tissues. Therefore, substance release from albumin and subsequent tissue interaction can be accomplished during passage of the complex through the tissue capillary beds. Substance bound to its specific binding protein is available for tissue interaction only if the unidirectional dissociation rate of the complex is more rapid than the tissue's mean capillary transit time. If the unidirectional dissociation rate is slow compared to the tissue capillary transit time, the substance will not be released to the tissue. This scheme for in vivo availability is summarized in Table 10-5.

Because the mean capillary transit time is much longer in the liver, it is possible for a substance bound to its specific binding protein to be available there but not in the periphery. For example, triiodothyronine, estradiol, and cortisol behave this way.

Hormones that have a circulating fraction unavailable to the liver because of specific protein binding are partially protected from hepatic removal. The organ clearance rates that obtain at

Table 10-5

Tissue Availability of
Protein-Bound Plasma Substance

Circulating form of substance	Availability of substance	
	Periphery ($t_{cap} < 4$ seconds)	Liver ($t_{cap} > 5$ seconds)
Unbound	Available	Available
Bound to albumin	Available because $t_{dis} < t_{cap}$	Available because $t_{dis} < t_{cap}$
Bound to specific binding protein	Not available if $t_{dis} > t_{cap}$	Not available if $t_{dis} > t_{cap}$

t_{cap} = mean capillary transit time;
t_{dis} = unidirectional dissociation half-time

Table 10-6

Organ Clearance Rate of Protein-bound Plasma Substances

Unidirectional dissociation half-time for specific binding protein	Intrinsic substance clearance rate	
	High	Low
Rapid ($t_{dis} < 5$ seconds)	Organ plasma flow	f · intrinsic substance clearance rate
Slow	f · organ plasma flow	f · intrinsic substance clearance rate

t_{dis} = unidirectional dissociation half-time; f = fraction of substance in
unbound and albumin-bound forms

extremes of intrinsic organ clearance and unidirectional dissociation half-times are listed in Table 10-6.

LABORATORY MEASUREMENT

The extent of plasma protein binding must be considered when measuring the concentration of plasma constituents for which the protein binding has a buffer effect. The physiologic effects and homeostatic control of these constituents depend entirely upon the concentration of their available, active forms. Binding proteins that serve vehicle, delivery, or storage functions do not alter the physiologic activity of their ligands. The plasma concentration of the binding protein should be measured, however, whenever a congenital or acquired deficiency of the protein is a possible etiology for the decreased plasma concentration of an analyte.

The Active Fraction

Calcium and magnesium are physiologically active in their ionic form and exert their influence while in the extracellular fluids. Because of this, in vitro measurement of the concentration of the ionic species reliably indicates the in vivo concentration of the active species. The bound forms of these cations are made up of diffusable species (complexed calcium) and nondiffusable protein-, mostly albumin, bound complexes. For calcium, protein binding accounts for about 45% of the total calcium, and complexed calcium, for 10%. Total calcium levels are altered only very little by small changes in the plasma albumin concentration and small to moderate changes in the concentrations of the calcium-complexing anions (e.g., phosphate, carbonate, and citrate). The concentration of total plasma calcium then adequately reflects the ionic calcium concentration. Moderate changes in plasma albumin concentration and large changes in the concentrations of the calcium-complexing anions may alter the total calcium levels enough to obscure the true status of the homeostatic control of the ionic calcium concentration. In such settings the direct in vitro measurement of the concentration of ionic calcium is necessary.

Albumin-bound magnesium represents only 25% of the total magnesium, and complexed forms, about 15%. Only large alterations in the plasma concentration of albumin or the magnesium-complexing anions (e.g., phosphate, carbonate, and citrate) will change the total magnesium levels enough to disallow the use of the total magnesium level as the indicator of the ionic magnesium level.

Hormones are physiologically active in their available forms. The following rules can be used to identify hormones for which the extent of protein binding must be quantified because of a significant reduction in available hormone concentration in peripheral tissues due to the binding:

1. There is significant binding to the specific binding protein; in practice, this probably means greater than 50% protein binding.

2. The unidirectional hormone-binding protein dissociation rate is slow compared to expected mean capillary transit times in peripheral tissue; in practice, this probably means a dissociation half-time of 3 seconds or longer.

When applied, these rules yield:

Inclusions	Exclusions
thyroxine	aldosterone
triiodothyronine	estradiol
(marginal inclusion)	(marginal exclusion)
cortisol	progesterone
testosterone	

The hormones excluded by these rules show little influence of protein binding upon their in vivo availability. For these, measurement of the total hormone level is a reliable estimate of the in vivo concentration of available hormone.

Methods

Ideally the laboratory assay of an analyte showing significant protein binding should quantify the concentration of the in vivo physiologically active species. For calcium this is done by directly measuring the plasma concentration of ionic calcium by direct potentiometry using a calcium-selective electrode. Available hormone concentration can be determined by hormone-specific receptor radioassay or bioassay.

Typically, however, the in vitro concentration of unbound hormone is measured as an estimate of the concentration of available hormone. This concentration differs from that of the available fraction of the hormone because of the physiologic availability of the albumin-bound hormone.

Estimation of the concentration of unbound hormone can be accomplished by:

1. separation of the bound from the unbound species of the analyte and measurement of the concentration of analyte in the fraction containing the unbound form

2. calculation of the concentration of unbound analyte

3. calculation of an index proportional to the concentration of unbound analyte.

Methods used to separate bound from unbound hormone include equilibrium dialysis, ultrafiltration, kinetic radioimmunoassay, and chromatography. Equilibrium dialysis remains the reference technique for the measurement of unbound analyte concentrations for all protein bound analytes, but the technique is too tedious, time consuming, and imprecise for routine laboratory use. The separation techniques of ultrafiltration and kinetic radioimmuno-assay are practicable and are becoming increasingly popular for routine use. In vivo plasma ultrafiltration can be taken advantage of in the assay of cortisol. The renal glomerular filtration of unbound cortisol results in urine cortisol levels that can be readily and precisely measured. Empirically, the daily renal excretion of unbound cortisol correlates well with the mean daily circulating levels of unbound cortisol. The other hormones cannot be analyzed this way because their greater protein binding and lesser plasma concentrations result in urine hormone concentrations too small for accurate detection.

Calculation of the concentration of unbound hormone is accomplished by solving the following quadratic equation:

$$[unbound\ hormone]^2 + B\ [unbound\ hormone] - C = 0$$

where $B = [total\ binding\ sites] - [total\ hormone] + 1/K_a$ and $C = [total\ hormone]/K_a$. The hormone and binding site concentrations must be measured, and the hormone-binding protein constant of association must be known.

The solution to the equation can be derived by computation or by the use of nomograms. Two contrived nomogram representations are presented in Figure 10-6. The nomogram in the left panel is

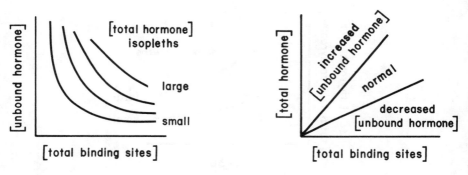

Fig 10-6   Nomograms for the Calculation of the
Concentration of Unbound Hormone

- 215 -

quantitative. The concentration of unbound hormone (vertical axis) can be calculated from the concentration of total binding sites (horizontal axis) and the concentration of total hormone (isopleths, i.e., lines of equal measure). The nomogram in the right panel is semiquantitative. The concentration of unbound hormone is expressed as increased, normal, or decreased.

The free thyroxine index (FTI) and free triiodothyronine index (FT3I) are indices that are related to the concentration of the unbound form of the hormones and have proven to be reliable indicators of thyroid function. The calculation of these indices is much easier than the calculation of the concentration of unbound hormone. Each is a simple product:

$$FTI = [total\ thyroxine]\cdot RT3U$$

$$FT3I = [total\ triiodothyronine]\cdot RT3U$$

where RT3U is the resin T3 uptake. The resin T3 uptake is a laboratory separation procedure that quantifies the extent of triiodothyronine protein binding. Because the hormones usually bind to the same sites, the RT3U is inversely related to the concentration of free protein-binding sites for both hormones. Thus the indices have the form of the equilibrium mass action expression:

$$[unbound\ hormone] = [bound\ hormone]\cdot \frac{1}{K_a\ [free\ binding\ sites]}\cdot$$

Total hormone concentrations substitute for bound hormone concentrations, which is reasonable because both hormones exhibit greater than 99% binding. In the graphic representation of these indices, values of the indices appear as hyperbolic isopleths in the hormone versus RT3U coordinate space (Figure 10-7).

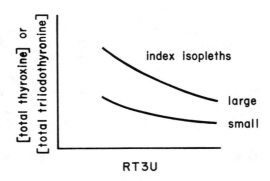

Fig 10-7   Thyroid Hormone Index Nomogram

EXERCISES

The effect of liver disease upon cortisol physiology is complex. This is so because the liver is the organ of clearance for cortisol as well as the organ of synthesis for the cortisol-binding proteins albumin and CBG. In liver disease the rate of clearance of cortisol is decreased, as are the rates of synthesis of albumin and CBG.

	Health	Liver disease
Concentration of total cortisol	10 µg/dl	
Concentration of CBG (binding capacity)	20 µg cortisol/dl	10 µg cortisol/dl
Binding of cortisol	see Table 10-2	

10-1. What is the concentration of cortisol available to peripheral tissue in health?

10-2. What is the concentration of cortisol available to the liver?

10-3. What is the association constant of CBG for cortisol? (Treat albumin-bound cortisol as though it were unbound.)

10-4. In liver disease, if the adrenal production of cortisol is unchanged but the hepatic clearance rate for cortisol is halved, what will the steady-state concentration of cortisol available to the liver be?

10-5. What will the steady-state concentration of cortisol available to peripheral tissues be? (Use the K_a calculated in Question 10-2.)

10-6. Will the adrenal production of cortisol remain unchanged in liver disease?

10-7. What will the steady-state level of total cortisol be then? (Again use the K_a calculated in Question 10-2.)

10-8. Following an exchange transfusion for hyperbilirubinemia, a neonate suffers a seizure. The house officer considers the possibility of hypocalcemia, but the plasma calcium concentration is normal. Has hypocalcemia been disproved?

10-9. Laboratory measurements of the plasma concentrations of unbound thyroxine correlate extremely well with the clinical assessments of the functional status of the thyroid gland. The concentration of available thyroxine includes that which is albumin bound, however. How can such excellent diagnostic accuracy be achieved while ignoring the albumin-bound species?

Mind-Expanding Exercise

10-10. Derive the quadratic equation for unbound analyte concentration presented in the text. (Hint: Start with the equilibrium mass action equation.)

REFERENCES

Dunn, J.F., Nisula, B.C., Rodbard, D. Transport of steroid hormones: Binding of 21 endogenous steroids to both testosterone-binding globulin and corticosteroid-binding globulin in human plasma. J. Clin. Endocrinol. Metab. 53:58, 1981.

Jasen, J.Aa. Influence of plasma protein binding kinetics on hepatic clearance assessed from a "tube" model and a "well-stirred" model. J. Pharmacokin. Biopharm. 9:1, 1981.

Kragh-Hansen, U. Molecular aspects of ligand binding to serum albumin. Pharmacol. Rev. 33:17, 1981.

Natelson, S., Natelson, E.A. Plasma Proteins in Nutrition and Transport. Plenum Press, New York, 1980.

Pardridge, W.M. Transport of protein-bound hormones into tissue in vivo. Endocrine. Rev. 2:103, 1981.

Ritzmann, S.E., Daniels, J.C. Serum Protein Abnormalities: Diagnostic and Clinical Aspects. Alan R. Liss, New York, 1975.

Steinman, R.M., Mellman, I.S., Muller, W.A., Cohn, Z.A. Endocytosis and the recycling of plasma membrane. J. Cell Biol. 96:1, 1983.

Chapter 11

TISSUE INJURY

> The young men of the world
> look into each other's eyes,
> And read there the same words:
> Not yet! Not yet!
> But soon perhaps, and perhaps certain.
>
> F.S. Flint

PLASMA MARKERS OF TISSUE INJURY
(Adolph and Lorenz 1982; Wilkinson 1976)

Injury to tissue causes a decrease in function or a diminution in the functional capacity of the tissue, the release of intracellular substances from damaged cells, and inflammation with its local and systemic effects. Those intracellular substances that enter the circulation after their release <u>and</u> are not otherwise present as plasma constituents can be used as plasma markers.of tissue injury. The overwhelming majority of plasma injury markers used clinically are enzymes.

A simplified model of the disposition of an intracellular substance following cellular injury is illustrated in Figure 11-1. Markedly increased cell membrane permeability permits the diffusion of intracellular material into the local extracellular

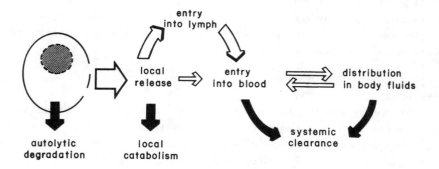

Fig 11-1   Distribution and Elimination
of Intracellular Substances

- 219 -

space. At the same time, autolytic degradation of the cellular contents results in substantial reductions in the amount of intracellular substance liberated, especially of those substances with high molecular weights. Once released the substance is either catabolized locally or is taken up in the lymphatic drainage, traverses the lymphatic circulation, and enters the blood. In tissues with permeable capillaries and venules, some of the substance enters the plasma directly. From the plasma the substance distributes in part into the other extracellular body fluids. Systemic catabolism and renal clearance of unchanged substance leads to elimination of the substance from the plasma and the body fluids.

When the rate of release of intracellular substance is constant over a prolonged period, the substance will achieve a steady-state concentration in the fluids into which it distributes. In particular, there will be a steady-state plasma concentration. Marker substances that are released from tissues with an appreciable rate of normal cell turnover will, therefore, be present in plasma at some constant concentration. Tissue injury that is persistent and relatively constant will also produce a nearly constant plasma concentration of marker substance, but one that is distinctly elevated. Episodic injury, on the other hand, will cause only a temporary increase in the plasma concentration of a marker. For a short period after the injury local release of the marker will overwhelm the local catabolic capacity of the tissue, and the marker will gain entry to the lymph and perhaps directly to the plasma. The marker will accumulate in the plasma, i.e., its concentration will increase, until the amount entering the plasma becomes less than the combined amount moving into the body fluids and undergoing systemic catabolism. When that happens, the plasma concentration will peak and then will fall.

Injury Versus Death
(Friedel et al. 1979)

An important question concerning the use of intracellular substances as plasma markers of tissue injury is whether release of the substances can occur when the damage to the cells is reversible or if marker release signifies cell death.

If marker release occurs while damage is still reversible, as seems to be true for hepatocytes, it is reasonable to expect that the amount of marker released per cell will depend upon the severity of the cellular injury. The amount of marker liberated as a result of injury to such a tissue is the product of the number of cells injured times the average severity of the injury. An extensive but mild process, such as uncomplicated viral hepatitis, can cause the release of as much marker substance as a severe but focal disorder, such as chronic active hepatitis. Another expectation is that the kind of markers released from an injured cell will vary according to the severity of the injury. Markers that reside in the cytosol, especially those of lower molecular weight, are released following slight injury. Higher molecular weight markers and those contained in membrane-bound organelles are released only if the injury is substantial. For example, only small amounts of the intramitochondrial enzyme glutamate dehydrogenase are released in the course of typical acute viral hepatitis, whereas abundant amounts are liberated in cases with fulminant hepatic necrosis.

When marker release occurs only with cell death, as seems to be true for cardiac myocytes, the amount of marker released from the tissue will depend only upon the number of cells lethally injured. For such tissues, estimates of the magnitude of injury based upon the measurement of marker release will correlate with the mass of the dead tissue.

Tissue Specificity

For a substance to serve as a specific plasma marker of tissue injury, it is necessary that the substance arise predominantly from the cells of the organ or tissue of interest. Otherwise, injury to other tissues containing the substance will cause its release into the circulation. This release will either be misinterpreted as resulting from injury to the tissue of interest when there is none or will interfere with the interpretation of plasma levels of the substance when there is concurrent injury.

Highly specific markers have been identified for a number of tissues (Table 11-1). A few are unique cell products, e.g., hemoglobin; some are enzymes found predominantly in the specialized tissue, e.g., lipase; and some are tissue-specific isozymes of widely distributed enzymes, e.g., the pancreatic isozyme of α-amylase. Isozymes are proteins that catalyze the same reaction but differ from one another in their structure. In the case of α-amylase, the isozymes arise from differences in posttranslational carbohydrate modifications of the enzyme.

Table 11-1

Tissue Sources of Selected Organ-injury Marker Substances

Analyte	Principle source(s) of plasma analyte	Minor source(s) of plasma analyte	Potential plasma contamination due to in vitro hemolysis
High-specificity markers			
Alanine aminotransferase	Liver	Skeletal muscle	Yes
α-Amylase, pancreatic isozyme	Pancreas		
Creatine kinase, MB isozyme	Heart	Skeletal muscle	
γ-Glutamyltransferase	Liver/biliary tract		
Lactate dehydrogenase, isozyme 1	Heart	Red cells, kidney	Yes
Hemoglobin	Red cells		Yes
Lipase	Pancreas	Pancreas	
Low-specificity markers			
Alkaline phosphatase	Liver/biliary tract, bone	Intestine, kidney	
α-Amylase	Pancreas, salivary glands	Intestine, female genital tract	
Aspartate aminotransferase	Liver, skeletal muscle, heart	Kidney	Yes
Creatine kinase	Skeletal muscle, heart		
Lactate dehydrogenase	Liver, skeletal muscle	Many	Yes

- 222 -

Table 11-1 lists a number of less specific tissue-injury markers that are frequently measured. Alkaline phosphatase and aspartate aminotransferase are useful as sensitive markers of mild liver injury. The total catalytic activity of α-amylase, creatine kinase, and lactate dehydrogenase can be assayed much more quickly and easily than the corresponding specific isozymes. This makes their measurement useful in emergent clinical situations where speed in obtaining a usable result is more important than obtaining a highly specific result. Because these markers are sensitive, they can also be used to identify those specimens that merit the performance of expensive and difficult isozyme determinations. Furthermore, in typical clinical situations, these three injury markers enjoy quite acceptable diagnostic specificity despite their inferior tissue specificity.

DETECTING TISSUE INJURY — THE DIAGNOSTIC WINDOW

The diagnostic window for a tissue-injury marker is that interval of time following an episode of injury during which measurement of the marker will demonstrate the occurrence of the injury. For highly specific marker substances, it is the interval during which the concentration of the marker exceeds the baseline concentration by an amount greater than that of a detectable change in the marker concentration. For less specific markers, it is the interval during which the marker concentration exceeds a critical value selected to yield a certain diagnostic performance for the marker. Marker substances that rapidly enter the circulation tend to have diagnostic windows that begin soon after the onset of the injury. These early indicators permit prompt detection of the injurious event and allow interventional therapy to be instituted. Those marker substances that are slowly cleared from the circulation generally have diagnostic windows that last long after the time of the injury. Such late indicators can be used to aid in establishing diagnoses' in those cases in which the patient has delayed coming to the physician. Figure 11-2 shows the plasma concentrations of two marker substances, one an early indicator and one a late indicator, following an episode of tissue injury. Diagnostic windows for the markers are also shown. Early indicators are usually cleared from the plasma rapidly, so the window for the early indicator is depicted as ending before the window for the late indicator.

The timing of an injury marker's diagnostic window is not constant but, rather, depends upon the magnitude of the injury

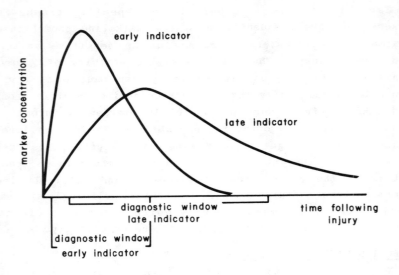

Fig 11-2   Marker Substance Concentrations
Following Tissue Injury

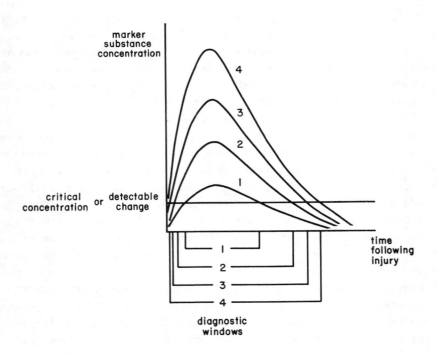

Fig 11-3   The Diagnostic Window as a
Function of Injury Severity

experienced. The more severe the injury, the earlier the window begins and the longer it lasts. Figure 11-3 depicts marker substance concentration versus time curves at four different levels of tissue injury (least severe: curve 1; most severe: curve 4). For each the corresponding diagnostic window is shown. Typically, differences in the magnitude of injury affect the time of termination of the diagnostic window much more than its time of appearance. Consequently, when monitoring a patient for the early detection of an episode of injury, little benefit is derived from adjusting the earliest time for sampling for differences in the anticipated degree of injury.

Magnitude of Detectable Change

Because of the presence of intraindividual and analytic variability in laboratory measurements, the concentration of a tissue-injury marker substance must change by a certain amount before that change can be ascribed to release of the marker substance rather than to measurement imprecision. Similarly, when a tissue-injury marker is being used to monitor the activity of a disease process characterized by persistent tissue injury, the plasma concentration of the marker must change by a certain amount before the change can be interpreted as indicating a change in the rate of release of marker substance. The same formula discussed in Chapter 7 (see Table 7-4) can be applied here to the calculation of a detectable change in marker concentration. In addition, the same qualification regarding the time interval between measurements applies. If the interval is long, both biologic and analytic variability contribute to the variability of measurement differences. If the time between measurements is short, the biologic component of the variability becomes negligible because of the short-term biologic inertia of most analytes. Table 11-2 lists typical magnitudes of detectable differences in measurement for short-term and long-term changes in selected tissue-injury marker substances.

Estimating the Magnitude of an Injury

If it is assumed that each cell in a tissue contains the same quantity of an injury marker, the magnitude of an injury to the tissue can be estimated from the amount of marker substance liberated. If in addition it is assumed that all or a constant fraction of the marker substance eventually enters the circulation, the magnitude of the injury can be estimated by measurement

Table 11-2

Typical Magnitudes of Detectable Short-Term and Long-Term Measurement Change
for Selected Tissue-injury Marker Substances in Healthy Subjects

Analyte	Typical day-to-day intraindividual variability	Typical day-to-day analytic variability	Typical magnitude of detectable short-term change	Typical magnitude of detectable long-term change[a]
Alanine aminotransferase (U/L)	1.3	1.1	3	5
Alkaline phosphatase (U/L)	1.2	1.8	5	6
Aspartate aminotransferase (U/L)	3.3	2.3	6	10
Creatine kinase (U/L)	10.3	4.0	10	30
γ-Glutamyltransferase (U/L)	0.8	1.1	3	4
Lactate dehydrogenase (U/L)	11.0	10.0	30	40

Variability expressed as standard deviations.
Data from Lohff et al. (1982) and Winkel and Statland (1977).
[a] See Table 7-4, rule 2.

of the amount of marker released into the plasma. Departures from the underlying assumptions lessen the reliability of such estimates. The cellular content of a marker may vary among individuals, as is true for those markers that are inducible enzymes. Also, an injury marker may not be uniformly distributed in a tissue, as is the case for the hepatic injury markers. Finally, the amount of marker released into the plasma may not be a constant fraction of that liberated, as is probably so for the cardiac injury markers.

The amount of marker substance that enters the circulation as a result of an episode of tissue injury can be calculated using the formula:

$$\begin{matrix} amount\ of\ marker \\ entering\ plasma \end{matrix} = \begin{pmatrix} plasma\ clearance \\ rate \end{pmatrix} \cdot \begin{pmatrix} area\ under\ the\ plasma\ clearance \\ curve\ for\ the\ marker \end{pmatrix}$$

If there is little biologic variability in the plasma clearance rate of the marker, the amount of marker entering the plasma can be estimated from the area under the clearance curve by using a typical value for the clearance rate. However, if the clearance rate displays appreciable biologic variability, the area under the clearance curve and the plasma clearance rate in the affected individual will need to be measured to accurately estimate the amount of marker substance entering the circulation. In practice, the measurement of marker clearance rates in individual patients can be accomplished only for those marker substances that show monoexponential kinetic behavior. Then the marker clearance rate equals the product of the exponential rate of decline in the marker's plasma concentration times the estimated volume of distribution of the marker in the patient.

A much less demanding but also less precise way to estimate the amount of injury marker released into the plasma is to measure the plasma concentration of the marker just once, at some specified time following the onset of tissue injury. If there is no variability in the kinetic behavior of the marker substance, the plasma concentration at any given time after the injury will be proportional to the amount of marker entering the plasma (Figure 11-3).

Of course, it is never true that the kinetic behavior of an injury marker shows no variability. Although the variability may be little enough that the one sample method of estimating marker substance release is clinically reliable, usually appreciable kinetic variability is present. Figure 11-4 illustrates the effects that such variability has upon the performance of the one sample technique. The upper left panel depicts the plasma clearance curves for a marker substance in three individuals who have different rates of clearance of the marker. The amount of marker substance released into the plasma is the same in each case. If the sample is taken at the average time of peak marker concentration, t_{peak}^*, there are substantial differences in marker concentration among the individuals despite equivalent amounts of marker release. At later times, for example t_2^*, the differences

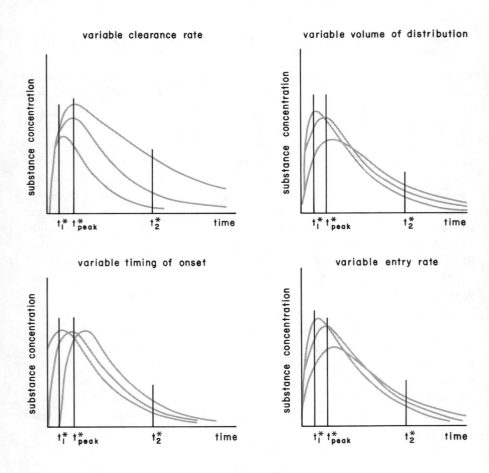

Fig 11-4   Effects of Variability in the Kinetic
Behavior of an Injury Marker Substance upon
the Performance of One Sample Estimation
of the Magnitude of Tissue Injury

in marker concentration are even greater. Sampling at an earlier time, for example t_1^*, results in less variability in marker concentration. The upper right and lower right panels show plasma marker clearance curves for individuals with different volumes of distribution for the marker and different rates of entry of marker into the circulation, respectively. In both cases, there is moderate variability in the plasma concentrations early on, at both t_1^* and t_{peak}^*. Much less variability is seen for both when samples are taken later, for example at t_2^*. The effect of variability in the timing of the onset of tissue injury, a very real problem in clinical practice, is shown in the lower left panel. Only small differences in plasma concentration are seen at t_2^* and even at t_{peak}^*, but marked differences are found at earlier sampling times, for example t_1^*.

The selection of the sampling time for a one-sample estimation of injury marker release should be made with due consideration for the kinetic variability of the marker. If there is only slight variability in the marker clearance rate, the sample should be taken at a time following the average time to peak marker concentration. A time 1.44 plasma half-lives of the marker after the average time to peak is suggested. If there is appreciable variability in clearance rate of the marker, the sample should be taken at a time prior to the average time to peak marker concentration. This sampling time should be selected so as to balance the measurement imprecision attributable to the variability in clearance rate with that arising from variability in timing the onset of injury.

SYSTEMIC RESPONSE TO TISSUE INJURY
(Dinarello 1984)

Tissue injury elicits an acute inflammatory reaction. Its local manifestations constitute many of the symptoms and signs associated with injury. The systemic effects contribute to the clinical presentation and can be useful, albeit nonspecific, markers of the presence and severity of tissue injury.

Acute inflammation produces a characteristic triad of systemic effects: fever, neutrophilia, and alterations in the concentrations of a number of plasma proteins. This triad is referred to as the acute phase response. Each of the effects appears to be mediated by the monokine Interleukin-1 (also called leukocytic pyrogen), which is a low-molecular-weight protein secreted by activated monocytes. Fever, which may have a suppressive effect upon microorganisms and a stimulatory effect upon host defense mechanisms, results from the Interleukin-1-induced resetting of the hypothalamic set point for the body's core temperature. Neutrophilia results from the Interleukin-1-stimulated discharge of neutrophils from marrow reserves. This provides cells for participation in the inflammatory reaction. Interleukin-1 also activates neutrophils, causing partial degranulation of the cells while they are in circulation. The lactoferrin thereby liberated binds plasma iron and is then rapidly cleared from the plasma. The resulting hypoferremia probably has an antimicrobial effect.

Those plasma proteins that are present in increased concentration during acute inflammation are called acute phase proteins. They include:

1. concentrations increased 1.5-to threefold:
   a. α_1-antitrypsin
   b. ceruloplasmin
   c. haptoglobin
   d. fibrinogen
   e. α_1-acid glycoprotein
2. concentrations increased up to 1000-fold:
   a. C-reactive protein
   b. serum amyloid A protein.

The first four appear to have functional roles at the site of inflammation, which may explain the biologic utility of their increased plasma concentrations during the acute phase. α_1-Antitrypsin inhibits, and thereby limits, the activity of proteases liberated by phagocytes; ceruloplasmin inactivates superoxide ions generated by phagocytes; haptoglobin binds hemoglobin released by red cell lysis, which may reduce the local iron concentrations; and fibrinogen is the substrate for plasma clotting and the scaffold for tissue repair. The apparent biologic effect of the increased concentration of α_1-acid glycoprotein is to bind plasma cortisol, thereby lowering the concentration of free cortisol in circulation. C-reactive protein and serum amyloid A protein appear to dampen any concurrent immune response.

The increased plasma concentrations of the acute phase proteins result from Interleukin-1-induced increases in the rates of hepatic synthesis of the proteins. The synthetic rates of the other plasma proteins secreted by the liver are decreased. The reductions in the concentrations of a number of plasma proteins with long half-lives, notably albumin and transferrin, are not caused by their reduced rates of synthesis, however. These proteins, which are sometimes called "negative acute phase proteins," are simply diluted by the increase in plasma water that occurs in the acute phase.

The magnitude of the systemic effects of tissue injury is determined by the extent of the injury and the cause of the injury, as indicated in Table 11-3.

Table 11-3

Variability in the Expression of the Acute Phase Response
According to the Cause of Tissue Injury

Systemic response	Cause of tissue injury			
	Bacterial infection	Viral infection	Rheumatologic disease (chronic)	Sterile infarct (acute)
Body temperature	+++	+++	+	±
Neutrophil concentration	+++	±	+	+
Acute phase protein concentration	++	±	++	+

+++, marked elevation; ++, moderate elevation; +, mild elevation; ±, mild or no elevation

Laboratory Measurement

Although the acute phase response is nonspecific, it can be used to detect the presence of otherwise clinically silent injury, to confirm the presence of injury, and to monitor the severity of persistent injury. Depending upon the clinical situation (refer to Table 11-3), the acute phase response may be detected and monitored by the measurement of body temperature, blood neutrophil concentration, or plasma concentration of acute phase proteins. Often these measurements are used in combination.

The temperature of peripheral tissue depends upon the body's core temperature, local tissue factors, and the environmental temperature. Therefore, measurement of body temperature at peripheral sites serves only as an estimate of the core temperature. Those peripheral sites that approximate core temperature in a warm environment are the mouth, the rectum, and the axilla. The temperature recorded at the mouth is $0.5°$ to $1°$ C lower than that of the rectum and approximately $0.5°$ C higher than that of the axilla. The temperature of the skin of the forehead, the measurement site recommended for liquid crystal thermometry, is not reliably related to the core temperature.

The neutrophil concentration in blood is calculated as the product of two measurements: the blood concentration of nucleated cells and the fraction of nucleated cells that are neutrophils, i.e., the cell differential. Both of these measurements have also been used individually as markers of the acute phase response, but they are less informative than the neutrophil concentration. Increases in the concentrations of circulating hyposegmented neutrophils (band neutrophils) and immature neutrophils (metamyelocytes and myelocytes) are specific but not sensitive markers of the acute phase. Regrettably, when measured manually, the quantification of band neutrophils is subject to considerable interobserver measurement variability, which makes this otherwise useful marker unreliable.

Of the acute phase proteins, only C-reactive protein is routinely measured directly as a marker of the acute phase response. Fibrinogen is an excellent marker, but it is not measured for this purpose directly. The presence of an increased plasma concentration of fibrinogen produces two rheologic effects that have been used as the bases of laboratory studies

Effect	Study
elevated plasma viscosity	plasma viscosity
elevated red cell aggregability	erythrocyte sedimentation rate (ESR).

Viscosity is an indirect measure of plasma protein concentration. It depends most upon the concentration of fibrinogen, less upon the immunoglobulins, and not at all upon albumin and the other globulins within the physiologic ranges for these proteins. The ESR is an indirect measure of plasma protein concentration — primarily of fibrinogen and much less so of the immunoglobulins — and also of the red cell concentration. The measurement of plasma viscosity has been demonstrated to be superior to the ESR for all of the clinical situations for which measurement of the acute phase response is indicated.

MEDIATORS OF TISSUE INJURY

As well as establishing the presence of tissue injury in a patient, a clinician must also uncover the cause of the injury so that appropriate therapy can be instituted. Sometimes this can be accomplished without the aid of laboratory studies, but more often laboratory identification of the mediator of the injury is necessary. The major categories of injury mediators detected using laboratory studies are listed in Table 11-4.

Etiologic category	Clinical examples	
	Mediator	Disease
Microbiologic	Klebsiella pneumoniae Coxsackie B virus	Klebsiella pneumonia Viral myocarditis
Immunologic		
Autoantibodies	Antibody to gastric parietal cells Anti-red cell antibodies	Pernicious anemia Autoimmune hemolytic anemia
Immune complexes	Anti-gamma globulin antibodies (rheumatoid factor) Antinuclear antibodies	Rheumatoid arthritis Systemic lupus erythematosus
Gammopathies	Monoclonal immunoglobulin	Multiple myeloma
Toxic (endogenous)		
Inborn errors of metabolism	Uric acid α_1-Antitrypsin (deficiency)	Gout Panlobular emphysema
Trace substance overload	Copper	Wilson's disease
Autodigestion	Gastric acid	Peptic ulcer disease
Toxic (exogenous)	Mercury Paraquat	Renal tubular necrosis Pulmonary fibrosis

The following figure illustrates the typical chronologic behavior of two cardiac enzymes released following an acute myocardial infarct.

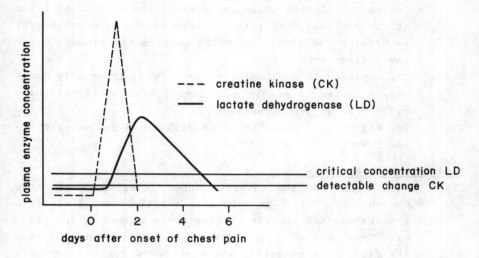

11-1.   What is the diagnostic window for creatine kinase?
11-2.   What is the diagnostic window for lactate dehydrogenase?
11-3.   Suggest two reasons for the later timing of the diagnostic window for lactate dehydrogenase.
11-4.   List disorders other than myocardial infarction in which creatine kinase or lactate dehydrogenase may be elevated.
11-5.   A 50-year-old man presents to your emergency room on Monday saying that he experienced an episode of severe chest and left arm pain on Friday afternoon. He has been on a fishing trip over the weekend (one he didn't want to miss). Today he feels tired and has noticed a few "twinges" of chest pain, so he has come to the hospital. You order plasma creatine kinase and lactate dehydrogenase determinations. To your surprise the creatine kinase is moderately elevated. After a moment's thought, you realize why this may be so. Why?
11-6.   The isozymes of creatine kinase are composed of two subunits. Each subunit is either an H (heart) type or an M (muscle) type. How many isozymes of creatine kinase are there and what are their subunit structures?

11-7.   The isozymes of lactate dehydrogenase are composed of
         four subunits. Each subunit is either an H (heavy) or an
         L (light) type. How many isozymes of lactate dehydroge-
         nase are there and what are their subunit structures?

11-8.   Patients with acute viral hepatitis show marked eleva-
         tions in the two aminotransferases, aspartate aminotrans-
         ferase and alanine aminotransferase. Sometimes the ratio
         of their plasma activities is less than one; sometimes it
         is greater than one. In which case is the prognosis for
         the patient worse?

11-9.   The erythrocyte sedimentation rate (ESR) is usually mark-
         edly elevated in multiple myeloma (plasma cell malignan-
         cy). What is the mechanism?

11-10.   The ESR may be normal in immunoglobulin M-producing myel-
         oma. Why?

Mind-Expanding Exercise

11-11.   When injury to the liver includes intrahepatic biliary
         obstruction, very high molecular weight forms of alkaline
         phosphatase and γ-glutamyltransferase appear in the plas-
         ma. Treatment with detergents releases the enzymes from
         the lipid-rich material, which accounts for the increase
         in molecular weight. What might the high-molecularweight
         form be? A unique plasma lipoprotein, lipoprotein X, is
         also found. How might it arise?

REFERENCES

Adolph, L., Lorenz, R. Enzyme Diagnosis in Diseases of the Heart, Liver, and Pancreas. S. Karger, New York, 1982.

Dinarello, C.A. Interleukin-1. Rev. Infect. Dis. 6:51, 1984.

Friedel, R., Diederichs, F., Lindena, J. Release and extracellular turnover of cellular enzymes. Adv. Clin. Enzymol. 1:70, 1979.

Lohff, M.R., DiSilvio, T.V., Ross, J.W., et al. Analytic clinical laboratory precision. Am. J. Clin. Pathol. (suppl.) 78:634, 1982.

Wilkinson, J.H. The Principles and Practice of Diagnostic Enzymology. Year Book, Chicago, 1976.

Winkel, P., Statland, B.E. Using the subject as his own referent in assessing day-to-day changes of laboratory test results. Contemp. Top. Anal. Clin. Chem. 1:287, 1977.

Chapter 12

NEOPLASIA

Daniel F. Cowan, M.D., C.M.

All knowledge resolves itself into probability.

David Hume

INTRODUCTION

Neoplasia is the process of abnormal new cell growth. The neoplastic cell is a modified cell, i.e., one that, while having many normal processes, expresses certain metabolic defects such as abnormal cell growth, abnormal consumption or metabolism of nutrients, and abnormal synthesis of cell products. Although the anatomic distortions related to new growth are obvious and evident in every case and indeed define the concept of neoplasia, expression of biochemical defects is quite variable. In one instance a patient with a relatively modest physical burden of tumor tissue may die of a severe metabolic derangement resulting in cachexia; another patient may remain surprisingly well until organ failure results from destructive growth of his cancer.

This chapter deals with the diagnosis and monitoring of neoplasia, based on recognition of anatomic and metabolic changes. Recognition of impairment of organ function, whether caused by neoplasia or another disease process, is discussed elsewhere and is not repeated here, although of very great importance. Here those morphologic and chemical methods that relate more or less specifically to neoplasia are considered. Most of the morphologic methods are well established, and their validity is universally accepted. The chemical (including immunologic) methods are relatively new, and their roles are not firmly established. There are as yet no certain human tumor-specific chemical tests. Although periodically new procedures generate interest and enthusiasm, they seldom live up to initial expectations. This is not the case with some tumor-associated antigens, which have a definite place in the laboratory study of people with tumors.

LABORATORY IN DIAGNOSIS

Laboratory examinations may 1) detect the presence of a neoplasm or risk factors relating to neoplasia, 2) establish the diagnosis of neoplasm, 3) determine the extent of the neoplasm, and 4) suggest the recurrence of a neoplasm after treatment.

The applicability of diagnostic measures is determined mainly by the site of the suspected lesion and its character, i.e., whether it is on a surface or exposed site or in the deep tissues. Neoplasms may be so situated as to be either apparent or inapparent to physical examination. Tumors of the skin, mouth, tongue, breast, and cervix uteri, for example, may be diagnosed with a degree of accuracy that can occasionally approach 100% on visual inspection alone. Laboratory examination may be merely to confirm the nature of the disease. Tumors of inapparent sites, such as the brain, stomach, and lungs, among others, are diagnosed only with the aid of laboratory studies.

Some laboratory methods are conceptually merely an extension of the physican examination and are designed to display changes in gross or microscopic anatomy. Others are designed to detect functional, physiologic, or chemical changes produced by neoplastic tissue or in organs damaged by tumor growth.

Selection of the appropriate laboratory study requires clear formulation of a clinical question, i.e., screening versus diagnosis, a knowledge of the behavior of tumors in general, and of the particular type suspected in any given patient. Interpretation and application of results demand, in addition, knowledge of the accuracy (sensitivity and specificity) and precision of the laboratory method and of the sources of measurement error.

DETECTION OF NEOPLASIA IN ASYMPTOMATIC PEOPLE
(American Cancer Society 1980)

Screening is the search for disease or its risk factors in asymptomatic people. Screening procedures address the questions "Who in this population has cancer?" and "Who in this population is prone to develop cancer in the future?" Screening has generally been a disappointment and is of limited value for three main reasons: 1) the prevalence of cancer is generally low in the population, 2) the sensitivity of screening tests is generally low, and 3) the specificity of tests is less than 100%. Two notable exceptions have proven to be of great value, however. The first and foremost has been cytopathologic study to detect cervical cancer and its major risk factor, epithelial dysplasia.

Cytopathology is the study of pathologic processes by means of desquamated (exfoliated) or aspirated cells. In its classic application, exfoliative cytology emphasizes the study of cells shed or scraped from mucous surfaces, especially the uterine cervix and vagina. The technique applies equally well to cells scraped from the lining of the mouth, brushed from the gastric mucosa, and aspirated in fluid from a body cavity or from a solid organ. Careful comparison of collected cells with the tissue from which they are derived has established criteria that allow very refined diagnosis based on cell features alone. Indeed, conclusions regarding invasion, an architectural change, may be drawn from isolated cells. Owing to the success of a continuing public education program and the routine cytopathologic examination of the cervix, the incidence of invasive cervical carcinoma has fallen greatly. Once a very common disease, it is now a rather uncommon one.

Examination of the stool for blood to detect colorectal cancer is a second important exception to the general rule about the low value of screening tests for neoplasia.

DETECTION OF NEOPLASIA IN SYMPTOMATIC PATIENTS

The limited value of screening contrasts sharply with the effectiveness of laboratory studies when applied to a particular patient, when the questions now become "Does this person have cancer?" and "Is the likelihood of this symptomatic person having cancer sufficiently high to justify an invasive procedure to establish a diagnosis?" In this situation the screening has been accomplished by the patient who presents himself to a physician with a suspicion of disease based on an observed physical change or suggestive symptom. The presence of symptoms justifies the use of techniques that are an extension of the physical examination: a way of visualizing internal anatomy.

Diagnostic Imaging

Physical examination is very effective in finding superficial tumors, but this direct approach cannot reveal internal ones. Access to these is gained indirectly, by the use of diagnostic imaging. Imaging is useful in the detection and localization of tumors. The major imaging techniques are radiographic studies, with or without dye contrast or computer enhancement; scanning using radioisotopes; ultrasonic imaging; and nuclear magnetic resonance scanning.

Radiographic Studies

Radiographic studies may reveal the presence, location, and to a degree, the extent of tumors. Radiographic methods depend on the differential density of tissues; that is, the ease of penetrance of x-ray beams through the tissue. For example, erosion of a bone by a neoplasm (or any other process) produces a focus of decreased density, whereas stimulation of bone may produce a focus of increased density. Only relatively large changes in bone density may be detected by radiographs. Somewhere in the order of a 30-50% change is necessary.

Subtle differences in radiodensity of a focus of tissue, especially if numerous readings of the same spot from different angles are made, may be detected and enhanced by computer analyzers integrated into the radiographic equipment. This is the basis for computed tomography scanners. The machines produce a computer-generated image representing sectional "slices" through the part of the body being studied.

In soft tissues, density differences may be greatly enhanced by the use of radiodense dye contrast media, or of very lucent air as a contrast medium. Infusion of a contrast medium into hollow organs (e.g., colon, stomach) may show displacement of the medium or filling defects caused by tumor growth. Injection of radiopaque dyes into vessels may show displacement of normal vessels by tumor growth or formation of new, abnormal vessels supplying the tumor. Dyes may be concentrated and excreted by particular organs, notably the liver and the kidney, imaging the excretory duct systems that may be distorted by new growth.

Isotopic Scanning

Isotopic scanning reflects the propensity of neoplastic tissue to be more or less able to take up certain metabolites than the normal tissue from which it orginates. This characteristic has allowed development of test procedures using metabolites with radioactive labels as indicators. External scanning detection devices register and record the intensity of radiation at points over the surface of the organ being tested. As an example, some but not all adenomas of the thyroid have a greater than normal avidity for iodine. Administered ^{131}I is taken up and concentrated more in the adenoma than in the surrounding thyroid, producing a focus of increased radioactivity known colloquially as a "hot nodule." Carcinomas of the thyroid have a less than normal avidity for iodine and with ^{131}I produce a focus of below normal radioactivity or a "cold nodule" relative to the surrounding thyroid. A carcinoma of the thyroid metastatic to bone may produce a radioactive focus relative to the surrounding bone on dosing with ^{131}I. Many isotopic scanning procedures relying on a combination of functional and morphologic characteristics of tumor growth are now available. Scanning studies using a variety of carrier molecules for investigation of the liver, spleen, and brain for primary or metastatic tumor growth are in common use. The use of radiolabeled antibodies against specific tumor antigens is a current focus of active research.

Ultrasound Imaging

Ultrasound imaging uses penetrating high-frequency sound waves as a detection medium. It depends on differential absorption and reflection of the sound waves by tissues of various densities. The echoes are detected and recorded, producing an interpretable visual image. Apparently safer than x-ray beams, sound waves lack the resolving power of that form of radiation. Ultrasonic imaging has its greatest application in the study of masses of soft tissue, i.e., the abdomen.

Nuclear Magnetic Resonance

Nuclear magnetic resonance (NMR) is an imaging technique that does not rely on tissue attenuation of x-ray beams or external detection of concentrations of internally administered radiolabeled antibodies or metabolites. For this reason, and because it has a high potential for very detailed resolution of internal structures, NMR imaging has a great potential for the detection of tumors. The technique depends on ascertaining the behavior of elemental nuclei in a uniform applied magnetic field when exposed to brief bursts of alternating magnetic fields. Energy absorbed and released by these nuclei is measurable as a small electric voltage. Computer analysis and processing of the electric signals generated in tissue produces the image. The great power of this technique rests on its apparent ability to produce a kind of map of biochemical activity in groups of cells and to image tissue structure with great fidelity. If it proves to be safe, there seems little doubt that it will become an extremely important imaging modality.

Tumor Markers

(Imura 1980; Kyle 1982; Pearse 1980; Statland and Winkel 1982; von Kleist and Breuer 1981; Waldenström 1978)

Tumors may produce abnormal chemical substances or normal ones in abnormal amounts. While these are probably metabolized or excreted by normal mechanisms, they may reach blood and urine concentrations that can be detected in the laboratory as tumor markers. In addition, physiologically active substances may occur in concentrations sufficient to produce signs and symptoms, i.e., clinically distinctive paraneoplastic syndromes. Laboratory measurements of some tumor markers are widely accepted as diagnostic aids, while measurements of others are still being evaluated. In this section, five classes of substances are discussed: oncofetal antigens, polyamines, enzymes, hormones, and immunoglobulins. Certain other general phenomena, such as the frequent elevation of the erythrocyte sedimentation rate in cancer patients and changes in calcium metabolism, will not be considered. A discussion of organ system failure caused by neoplastic disease, such as diabetes insipidus, is beyond the scope of this chapter.

Oncofetal Antigens

In some tumors substances normally present only in the fetus or embryo may reappear in the tumor tissue and may circulate in the blood, to be excreted in urine or feces or to disappear in the normal metabolic channels. These substances, recognizable through their antigenicity, are called fetal antigens or oncofetal antigens. Many are known compared to the few that are of clinical utility.

Carcinoembryonic antigen (CEA) is a normal cell surface glycoprotein with a molecular weight of about 200,000. It was characterized in tissue extracts of the fetal gastrointestinal tract. Since normal cells secrete CEA mostly into the lumen of the gut, in healthy people the serum concentration is low. In tumors of the gastrointestinal epithelium, CEA is absorbed into the body fluids, and elevated levels can be found in the blood of a high proportion of people with colon cancer. Originally thought of as a tumor-specific antigen, it is now known to occur in some cancers not of gastrointestinal origin and may be found in the serum of tobacco smokers and in persons with inflammatory disease of the bowel, lung, and pancreas, among other organs. It is therefore of no value as a diagnostic study. It can be of considerable value in following cases of known intestinal cancer, however, and in formulating prognoses.

Alpha-fetoprotein (AFP) is a glycoprotein with a molecular weight of about 70,000. It is normally present in fetal liver and is a normal component in fetal serum and in maternal serum during gestation. Shortly after birth, the serum AFP concentration falls to a very low level and remains there throughout life. In cases of rapid liver cell growth, as in regeneration after a severe case of hepatitis, and in many cases of hepatocellular carcinoma, a protein immunologically identical to AFP appears in the serum. Low but elevated levels suggest benign disease, whereas high levels suggest liver cancer. In hepatocellular carcinoma, levels 10,000 times normal are common. AFP is by no means a specific liver protein, any more than it is specific to hepatic malignancy. Teratoid tumors of ovary and testis, especially those with yolk sac differentiation, may also produce AFP.

Other oncofetal antigens are under investigation. Among the more promising of these are the Tennessee antigen, the pancreatic oncofetal antigen, and the fetal sulfoglycoprotein antigen.

Polyamines

Polyamines (putrescine, spermine, spermidine) are low-molecular-weight compounds formed as breakdown products in the metabolism of ornithine. They are present in every cell, and because they are involved in cell growth, their accumulation parallels the cell proliferation rate. Considerable interest has been shown in the use of polyamines as possible tumor markers. However, they have a very short half-life in serum, the sensitivity of measurements used in screening is low, and they lack specificity, i.e., they occur in increased amounts in many non-neoplastic diseases. It is unlikely, therefore, that the polyamines will find wide application in laboratory diagnosis of neoplasia or in the evaluation of treatment effectiveness.

Enzymes

Certain enzymes or isozymes may be produced in great excess by a neoplasm. The particular enzyme is coherent with the tissue of origin of the neoplasm; that is, it is an enzyme normally found in that tissue. Usefulness in diagnosis depends on tissue specificity. Some enzymes may rise but be so nonspecific as to be of little practical value as a clue to tissue of origin (e.g., lactate dehydrogenase). Conversely, some neoplasms lose normal enzyme activity characteristic of the differentiated cell. For example, leukocyte alkaline phosphatase may be diagnostically low in chronic granulocytic leukemia.

Acid phosphatase is an enzyme found in a number of tissues but in greatest concentration in the prostate as the prostatic isozyme, which may be identified either chemically or immunologically. Serum levels are commonly elevated in patients with metastatic carcinoma from the prostate. It is seldom necessary to use enzyme levels to make an initial diagnosis of prostatic cancer. Biopsy methods are quite reliable. However, in the occasional case in which the presenting signs relate to metastatic disease, serum levels of prostatic acid phosphatase may be useful in disclosing the prostate as the primary site.

Alkaline phosphatase is very useful in the evaluation of tumors of bone, but it is not very specific. Elevated serum levels may be produced either by increased production in bone disease or by impaired elimination of normal bone production by diseases of the hepatobiliary tract. Biliary tract disease may cause elevation of serum levels by increased release of the enzyme from biliary epithelium. Levels may be elevated into the five times the normal range by diseases as disparate as osteosarcoma, Paget's disease of bone, parathyroid adenoma, carcinoma metastatic to bone, certain benign bone diseases, and biliary tract obstruction. The higher the serum level of alkaline phosphatase, the more likely it is to be caused by a proliferative lesion of bone. Levels hundreds of times greater than normal are common in osteosarcoma.

The "Regan isoenzyme" is a heat-stable isozyme of alkaline phosphatase initially described in a patient (Regan) with lung carcinoma but also found in 10-15% of patients with ovarian or uterine carcinoma, and in cases of breast carcinoma.

Hormones

Hormones may be secreted by neoplasms, either benign or malignant. The secreted hormone may be appropriate to the tissue involved, or it may be inappropriate or ectopic, that is, not normally associated with that tissue. Most are normally continually present at low levels but may be greatly increased by tumor production. Chorionic gonadotrophin (hCG), on the other hand, is normally absent from the serum except during pregnancy but may be detected when elaborated by gonadal germ cell neoplasms that contain a trophoblastic element.

It should be no surprise that a tumor of an endocrine tissue can produce the hormone of that tissue. It is usual for the hormonal effects of an endocrine neoplasm to be the presenting disorder and for the tumor to be discovered in the course of the diagnostic work-up. Laboratory investigation will be directed toward demonstration of elevated serum levels of the hormone likely to produce the clinical syndrome or of metabolites of the hormone in the urine.

The more obvious syndromes produced by endocrine neoplasms are gigantism, feminization and virilization, hyper- and hypoglycemia, hypercalcemia, and Cushing's syndrome. Less obvious ones include disturbed maintenance of blood pressure by oversecretion of pressor hormones.

In the instances cited, the hormones secreted are biologically active, i.e., they produce hormonal effects, and are immunlogically active in that they are detectable using antibodies directed against them. Elaboration of complex molecules by neoplastic tissue may be defective, so that in the case of hormones, the molecule may be biologically inactive but retain immunologic activity. Thus two patients may have similar serum levels of tumor-derived hormone as detected by antibody methods, while only one might have physiologic hormonal effects.

In addition to the production of excess amounts of biologically active hormone produced by endocrine glands, hormones may be produced ectopically, by tissues not normally associated with their production. Extensive study of tissues and tumors by sensitive immunologic and histochemical methods has led to the concept of a diffuse endocrine system or "organ." It consists of cells that have in common derivation from the neural crest, cytoplasmic neurosecretory granules, and the retained facility of producing both polypeptide and amine hormones. The cells of this system have been named the amine precursor uptake and decarboxylation (APUD) cells. Although the concept of the system has evolved beyond the original description, the idea of a diffuse system remains valid. Neoplasms of this system may produce many if not all of the hormones of the system. The clinically important syndromes produced by APUD cell tumors involve mainly five hormones: adrenocorticotrophic hormone (ACTH), calcitonin, enteroglucagon, serotonin, and histamine, although other peptide hormones including glucagon, insulin, parathormone, antidiuretic horomone, and somatostatin have been described. Steroid hormones are never produced by APUD tumors, although hyperadrenocorticism due to excess adrenal steroid production is a well recognized consequence of APUD tumors, owing to the production of ACTH by the tumor.

Oat cell carcinoma of the lung is probably the most versatile producer of ectopic hormones, often producing several simultaneously. Conversely, specific hormones, especially ACTH, may be produced by a variety of APUD tumors. Carcinoids, as APUD derivatives, are active producers of biogenic amines, which are the direct cause of the syndromes associated with these tumors. Serotonin (5-hydroxytryptamine) is the dominant carcinoid hormone.

Laboratory detection of these tumors depends upon demonstrating excessive amounts of the hormones or their metabolites in blood or urine. Of course, excess hormone production does not of itself distinguish appropriate from ectopic production or the kind or location of the hormone-producing neoplasm.

Immunoglobulins

Lymphoreticular cell proliferation and immunoglobulin production are normal responses to antigenic stimulation. Immunoglobulins thus formed are typically directed specifically against the provoking antigens. Neoplastic proliferation of lymphoreticular cells may be accompanied by excess production of immunoglobulins. These are not responding to or directed against a challenging antigen and indeed may be blank, having no useful or detectable antibody activity.

In contrast to the peptide hormones that appear to be coded for by single genes, immunoglobulins are the product of the coherent activities of several genes. The complete immunoglobulin molecule is composed of two pairs of polypeptide chains, one "heavy" (molecular weight, 55,000) and one "light" (molecular weight, 25,000). Two varieties of light chain, kappa and lambda, and five varieties of heavy chain are recognized. Each variety of chain is coded for by a single gene. It is believed that individual lymphoreticular cells produce only one type of heavy and one type of light chain. A clone derived from a single lymphoreticular cell would be expected to produce a single pair of chains and a characteristic, monoclonal immunoglobulin molecule.

Immunoprotein secretion responding physiologically to antigenic challenge is typically polyclonal, due to the production of immunoglobulin from many normal clones of lymphoreticular cells. Neoplastic secretion resulting from proliferation of a defective clone is typically monoclonal. The demonstration of monoclonicity is the goal of most laboratory techniques directed toward the detection of neoplastic immunoglobulin secretion.

The early response of the lymphoreticular system to antigenic challenge is the proliferation of lymphocytes with the production of a high-molecular-weight antibody of low specificity. With persistent challenge, proliferation of plasma cells is associated with the production of a lighter, more specific antibody. Abnormal proliferation of lymphocytes with persistent production of high molecular weight immunoprotein (immunoglobulin M) produces macroglobulinemia (Waldenström's macroglobulinemia). Neoplastic proliferation of plasma cells (myeloma) typically results in production of excess globulins of lower molecular weight (immunoglobulin G) and molecules similar or identical to kappa or lambda chains. The light chains may be lost in the urine in large amounts, where they may be recognized as Bence-Jones proteins (proteins that precipitate at $60^{O}C$, disappear at $100^{O}C$, and reappear on cooling to $60^{O}-80^{O}$ C). Excessive production of light chains is believed to be a manifestation of disordered synthesis of globulins in which production of heavy and light chains is not appropriately synchronized. Although excess light chain production is more commonly encountered, the rare excess heavy chain production, or heavy chain disease, is also recognized.

Cryoglobulins are abnormal serum proteins arising either from polymerization of excess monoclonal proteins or from immune complexing of abnormal globulins and antibodies against them. As the name implies, cryoglobulins are cold-precipitable proteins. Cooling of the blood from the $37^{O}C$ of deep tissue to $25^{O}C$ (room temperature) in superficial vessels may allow precipitation of cryoglobulins, leading to vascular thrombosis, Reynaud's phenomenon, or renal damage.

HISTOPATHOLOGIC DIAGNOSIS

Tumors are recognized by morphologic features, e.g., cytohistologic appearance, shape, and relation to surrounding structures. These characteristics have acquired definition and meaning because they have prognostic value; that is, long experience has taught that a given set of morphologic features in a given tissue or locale correlate with a reasonably well defined course of events. Indeed, histologic diagnosis remains the reference test against which all other approaches to tumor diagnosis are evaluated. A diagnosis based on biopsy is taken as a proven diagnosis. All other approaches are suggestive, and if results conflict with those of the biopsy, the biopsy determines the diagnosis. This is the state of the art today. It may change in the future as analytical methods become more specific and precise.

Biopsy

Biopsy is the fundamental or reference procedure. It consists of taking a piece of the lesion for microscopic examination. Several methods of biopsy are available, and selection among them is based upon the size and location of the lesion. Excisional biopsy is preferable when the size and location of the lesion permit it. In one operation the lesion is both diagnosed and removed. If removal is complete, then the diagnostic procedure is curative as well.

A lesion may be so large, of a kind, or so situated that attempts at complete excision for diagnosis are unwise, unnecessary, or undesirable. For instance, surgical excision may be too destructive or hazardous, some treatment other than surgery (e.g., radiation, chemotherapy) may be more appropriate, or planning of therapy may require time after diagnosis. Such lesions may be sampled by incisional biopsy. A piece of tissue is removed for study, and on the basis of the findings, a plan of treatment of the remainder is developed. Incisional biopsy may be done with a knife, or if the lesion is internal, e.g., in the stomach, colon, or bladder, an instrument using a modified knife blade, a curette, or a hot wire may be used to remove tissue. In all of these the piece of tissue is removed under visual direction, either by the unaided eye or by use of an endoscope.

Needle biopsy is a form of incisional biopsy used mainly to sample internal organs, such as liver and kidney, and increasingly, more superficial organs (e.g., thyroid and breast) when incision is deemed unnecessary or undesirable. A special hollow needle with a sharp cutting edge is inserted into the organ, occasionally under fluoroscopic direction, but most commonly by the use of anatomic landmarks as guides. A core of tissue is obtained for histologic evaluation. While this method has the advantage of sparing the patient exploratory surgery, its value may be limited by focal distribution of disease in the organ being biopsied. Thus a normal examination may represent a sampling error rather than an absence of disease.

Cytopathology may be used to establish a diagnosis. Scrapings or brushings from surface lesions or aspiration of cells from deep-sited lesions through fine needles may provide samples fully adequate for diagnosis. Fine needle aspiration is simply a form of needle biopsy, the main difference being that the biopsy produces a core of more or less intact tissue, whereas the aspirate produces clusters of cells and single cells. Aspiration cytology is less traumatic than core biopsy and is less likely to be complicated by bleeding. Almost every organ in the body is accessible to the aspiration needle. Although a very powerful tool, cytopathology has certain drawbacks: sampling error may fail to reveal disease; the lesion must be present at the surface sampled in order for its cells to be included in scrapings or brushings; and desquamated cells in urine or effusions may deteriorate past the point of usefulness.

Microscopy

Histologic study of tissues and cells with the light microscope is the keystone of morphologic diagnosis of neoplasia. Appropriate use of histochemical methods may reveal specific structural or chemical features of a tissue, as well as more general nuclear and cytoplasmic characteristics. The binding of the most widely used dyes, hematoxylin and eosin (H&E) is to structures that are, respectively, basic or acidic in reaction. As a rule, diagnosis of a neoplasm and classification of it as benign or malignant can be made using only these two dyes. In the great majority of cases, further classification as to tissue of origin can readily be made based on the cytologic or architectural features revealed by them. Special stains of a higher degree of chemical specificity may be used to identify the cell line of origin of the neoplasm when it is not readily apparent on H&E staining. They may be used to demonstrate cell products such as keratin, bile, melanin, mucin, and others, inside or outside the cell. Enzymes (e.g., acid phosphatase) and numerous other substances may be stained directly by histochemical or cytochemical methods.

Immunohistologic methods rely on the affinity of specific antibodies for antigenic sites on the cell surface or within the cell. A very large array of antibodies against cell membrane and cytoplasmic constituents has been developed. Labeled with ultraviolet-reactive fluorochromes or pigment-producing substances such as peroxidase, these are exquisitely sensitive methods of demonstrating specific antigens. Important applications of these methods include the identification of specific hormone-associated granules in the pituitary gland, pancreatic islets, APUD cells, and other endocrine tissues; classification of the subtype of the cells in lymphoproliferative disorders; and classification of soft tissue tumors according to intermediate filament type.

Unfortunately, in many instances neoplastic dedifferentiation of a degree sufficient to cause specific morphologic features to be lost may also cause functional biochemical characteristics to be lost, and application of special stains is not helpful. In such cases electron microscopy (EM) may be useful. EM almost never contributes to the resolution of the problem of benign versus malignant. If that judgment cannot be made by light microscopy, it is highly unlikely that it will be made by EM. EM in tumor diagnosis is used in a way analogous to a special stain. It may reveal cytoplasmic structures specific to or suggestive of a particular cell line when these are too small to be resolved by the light microscope or are found only in a fragmentary or grotesque form. EM is prone to sampling error, as only extremely minute bits of tissue may be studied using current methods.

Morphologic study of tumors, then, is based on the use of chemical dyes of various degrees of specificity, with or without the mediation of antibodies to reveal specific or suggestive structural or functional characteristics of the cells of origin. Identification and classification of the tumor allow it to be related to past experience with similar lesions and enables predictive and therapeutic judgments to be made. Only the rare tumor cannot ultimately be identified as to line of origin, and these undifferentiated neoplasms themselves constitute a diagnostic and prognostic category.

DETERMINING THE EXTENT OF A NEOPLASM

It is usually insufficient merely to establish that a neoplasm is present in the body, especially if the neoplasm is malignant. If prognosis is to be accurate and treatment rationally planned, the extent of the lesion must be determined. Whether the tumor is treated by local excision, radiation, or chemotherapy all depends on knowing not only that a neoplasm is present, and what kind it is, but also its local destructive effect and its spread throughout the body.

By their nature benign neoplasms are entirely local, that is, they do not extend by metastasis from their place of origin.

Once the diagnosis is established, treatment is based on the size of the lesion, its relation to vital structures, and its size.

If a diagnosis of malignancy is established, two crucial questions must be anwered: "Is this malignant focus the primary lesion, or is it a metastasis?" and "If it is a primary lesion, has this malignancy metastasized?" The decision about the primary or metastatic nature of a malignant neoplasm may range from easy to near impossible. With some cancers the general configuration, the relation to adjacent structures, and the histologic type may make the decision easy. With tumors in unusual locations, or with atypical or highly undifferentiated histologic features, the decision may be very difficult and may depend on the use of histochemical, immunochemical, or ultra-structural features. If the first appearance of the malignancy is unquestionably a metastasis, for example, a focus of carcinoma in bone, then the primary site must be determined to plan appropriate treatment.

The search for inapparent or occult metastases may involve all of the imaging techniques described earlier. A combination of chemical studies to reveal the existence of metastatic disease somewhere in the body and imaging to localize the metastases to a particular organ or place is commonly used.

The local extent of neoplasms on superficial surfaces may be judged by eye, with confirmation of total excision based upon microscopic examination of resection margins by the surgical pathologist. This is adequate for benign lesions and for basal cell carcinomas of the skin. Certain malignant lesions arising on surfaces or in superficial structures are approached surgically by removal of the lesion and surrounding tissue, and by sampling or excision of tissues with an anatomically defined relationship to the site of the primary, for example, sampling of regional lymph nodes. The principle of block excision of anatomically defined, related structures such as lymphatic drainage fields is widely followed for internal malignancies as well. All removed tissues are examined grossly and microscopically by the surgical pathologist, and certain critical information is recorded. This includes a definition and description of the neoplasm and its degree of departure from normal differentiation (histologic grading), the size of the lesion and its relation to resection margins and anatomic landmarks, and the presence or absence of metastatic tumor in adjacent tissues and lymph nodes (staging). All of these have been found by long experience to have prognostic significance.

A number of specific and general systems have been developed to record and unambiguously communicate this descriptive anatomic information. The TNM system has gained currency. In this sytem, the primary lesion is noted as T1 through T4, with increasing size. NO indicates no nodal metastasis, N1 and N2 few or many nodes involved; and MO indicates no distant metastases, M1 and M2 few or many distant metastases. Details of the system vary with the organ concerned.

RECURRENCE AFTER TREATMENT

The aim of treatment of neoplastic disease is its total eradication from the body. In the case of benign tumors, this is commonly accomplished by surgery. Malignant tumors, if they have not metastasized and are resectable on anatomic grounds, may also be eradicated by surgery. Some cases of malignancy may be cured by removal of the primary lesion and local node metastases. Still others are not eradicable by surgery, although surgery may be needed to reduce tumor bulk, establish or reestablish physiologic continuity in organs, control bleeding, or attain other limited therapeutic objectives.

Very often it cannot be ascertained at the time of initial surgical treatment whether metastases exist or not, and so the patient enters a period of watchful waiting. During this period the judicious use of tumor marker assays may be helpful. If it is known that the tumor in question is associated with a particular marker, then the continued absence of the marker after treatment suggests that treatment is successful, whereas the reappearance of the marker indicates that the disease has spread beyond the field of treatment. For example, in cases of colon cancer with elevated serum CEA levels, the CEA may decline to normal after removal of the primary lesion. Failure to return to normal may reflect the presence of metastatic disease at the time of surgery. Fall to normal with subsequent rise may indicate recurrence of the tumor — actually, growth of tiny metastatic deposits present at surgery to a size able to produce detectable serum levels of CEA. Maintenance of normal CEA levels after treatment is a very hopeful sign but may also mean that any metastasis present simply does not produce CEA. Similarly, persistent or recurrent elevations of hCG or alpha-fetoprotein after removal of the primary germ cell neoplasm indicate metastasis containing trophoblastic or yolk sac elements.

For malignancies not amenable to surgery, eradication may be attempted with radiation or chemotherapeutic agents. Tumor markers may then be used to monitor the efficacy of treatment. Monitoring tumor markers following trials of treatment also allows selection of the most efficacious drugs. These may change over time in the course of established metastatic malignant disease.

CONCLUSION

The great importance of approaching the laboratory in a thoughtful, analytic way has been stressed throughout this book. The laboratory is a source of information about organ structure and function, disease process and causes of disease. Requests for laboratory data are in fact questions posed to test hypotheses about the structure, physiology, or chemistry of a patient, based on careful prior study of historical data and the physical status of the patient as assessed by hand and eye. Nowhere is this approach more important or more amply rewarded than in the use of the laboratory in the study of neoplasia.

EXERCISES

A 55-year-old man complains that the color of his urine has changed. It used to be "normal urine color" but now it frequently is pink or reddish. He has no pain. He has been otherwise well and has noticed no change in his sense of well-being or in his weight.

12-1. Which laboratory procedure will be of most use in defining this man's problem in medical terms?

12-2. This man's complaint has been found to be caused by a papillary tumor of the bladder. What is the most important bit of information to be gained from biopsy?

12-3. What test (if any) done on serum will be helpful in defining the nature of this man's disease?

A 23-year-old man complains of a slightly tender enlargement of the left testis. He can recollect no injury to the area. Palpation reveals a mass in the testis. The right testis is normal. The remainder of the physical examination is normal.

12-4. What is the differential diagnosis of this lesion?

12-5. What test (if any) done on serum will be helpful in defining the disease and managing the case?

A 55-year-old man has a long history of hepatic cirrhosis. He is slightly jaundiced and also has a small amount of blood in the stool. An important finding on physical examination is a mass in the liver. Owing to mild obesity, this finding is difficult to substantiate.

12-6. Outline a series of studies to elucidate the case.

Mind-Expanding Exercise

12-7. By a critical examination of the recent medical litera-ture, determine the clinical usefulness of a tumor marker measured in the clinical laboratories you use. Consider its application in screening, detection, and monitoring.

REFERENCES

American Cancer Society. Report on the cancer-related health checkup. Ca. 30:194, 1980.

Imura, H. Ectopic hormone syndromes. Clin. Endocrinol. Metab. 9:235, 1980.

Kyle, R.A. The laboratory evaluation of immunosecretory states. Clin. Pathol. Ann. 1:383, 1982.

Pearse, A.G.E. APUD concept and hormone production. Clin. Endo-crinol. Metab. 9:211, 1980.

Statland, B.E., Winkel, P. (eds.). Laboratory measurements in malignant disease. Clin. Lab. Med. 2:429-681, 1982.

von Kleist, S., Breuer, H. (eds.). Contributions to Oncology. Vol. 7: Critical Evaluation of Tumor Markers. Karger, Basel, 1981.

Waldenström, J.G. Paraneoplasia: Biological Signs in the Diag-nosis of Cancer. John Wiley and Sons, New York, 1978.

Chapter 13

THERAPEUTIC DRUG MONITORING

Karen M. Kumor, M.D.

The truth is rarely pure, and never simple.

Oscar Wilde

PHILOSOPHY

Drugs are administered for the purpose of achieving a particular goal. This is the most important fact in all of drug therapeutics, yet it is very often overlooked. The tendency of the inexperienced physician is to look up the recommended dose of a drug, write an order or hand the patient a prescription, and expect a "good result." Thus it is not unusual to encounter a young house officer who is uncomfortable because the medication he prescribed has not yielded a "good result." It is also not unusual to come upon patients who have developed a relative overdose of a medication because the prescribing physician failed to notice that the disease process has significantly altered the patient's disposition of the drug. And it is common to find individuals who are being treated ineffectively with many drugs meant to ameliorate one problem.

The goal of the therapy must be kept clearly in mind. Without an explicit therapeutic objective, there is no clear definition of failure of the therapy and thus there exists inertia to modifying it. In addition, we physicians dislike having to recognize the failure of a therapeutic maneuver. We tend to rationalize failures and tell our patients and ourselves that we can do no better. Sometimes it may be that we must settle for less than we would wish, but this should be an uneasy peace.

The practice of writing <u>concrete</u> goals for therapy in the patient's chart is a valuable one with practical benefits. The best place to note this information is in the plan of therapy. It is then easy to find later. This practice helps to prevent us from lessening our expectations when we reevaluate the patient's course. It also conveys the intended therapeutic goals to subsequent care-givers. In this way the responsibility to accomplish these goals is less easily shrugged off.

Therapeutic Monitoring
(Tognoni et al. 1980)

Once an objective is set, there must be a way to evaluate or measure whether it is achieved. The process by which one evaluates the effectiveness and safety of therapy is called **therapeutic monitoring**. A good physician frequently monitors the response of his patients. This practice, diagrammed in Figure 13-1, necessitates a reconsideration of the therapeutic plan based on the current state of information and prevents stagnation of the physician's planning.

Often it is best to monitor the patient's progress directly by history and physical examination. The response of the disease to therapy and improvement in the subjective feelings of the patient are the primary objectives of therapy. However there are circumstances in which it is warranted to substitute an indirect goal for a direct goal. When would it be impossible to assess the disease of the patient directly? When would it be dangerous?

If we treat someone prophylactically to prevent disease, as we do when we give immunizations or when we treat the family of the patient with meningococcal meningitis, we cannot perform therapeutic monitoring in the usual sense because the goal is to prevent disease entirely. Therefore, an indirect goal is substituted. It is to replicate the drug regimen determined to be the optimum prophylaxis. We use the particular dose or method of administering the drug that has been shown to be most effective in avoiding disease in the population at risk.

In other cases it may be dangerous to attempt direct monitoring of certain disease states. This occurs in two circumstances: when the toxicity of the therapeutic agents is severe or irreversible and when the disease process is a serious threat to life or causes permanent damage. If there are no clinical findings that can herald impending harm to the patient in time to allow the physician to respond effectively, a substitute goal, such as achieving a certain plasma concentration of the drug, must be used. This is called indirect monitoring. It is this kind of monitoring that usually comes to mind upon hearing the term therapeutic monitoring. In fact, though, indirect monitoring is only one small aspect of therapeutic monitoring. Sometimes this is forgotten or misplaced and there are indi-

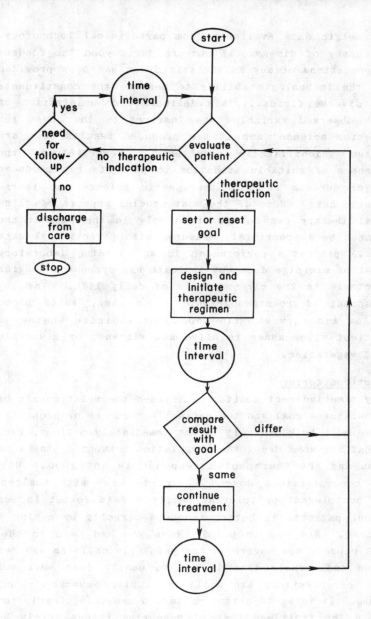

Fig 13-1   Therapeutic Monitoring Flowchart

viduals who become carried away by the "hard science" part of indirect therapeutic monitoring. What follows is a warning for those likely to be enraptured by such ideas (Feinstein 1971):

Rather than confronting and solving the problems of clinical data, clinicians have substituted the plethora of metric data available from paraclinical technology. An assay of dimensional numbers far beyond the fondest expectations of any Kelvinistic dream has been provided by the technologic ability to measure the constituents of diverse fluids....This deliberate dehumanization of the observed variables was inspired by the quest for "better science" and it has produced results that are often scientifically excellent. Nevertheless, the absence of suitable attention to patients has produced major defects in both therapeutic science and therapeutic care. Some of the most crucial aspects of clinical therapy can be discerned only in the patient and cannot be appropriately measured with paraclinical data ....A patient's performance in an isolated laboratory test of exercise does not indicate his dyspnea or angina pectoris in the circumstances of daily life. The assessment of roentgenographic tumor size, white blood count and survival time does not indicate whether a patient with cancer is alive and vibrant, or miserable and vegetating.

Indirect Monitoring

Any time indirect monitoring is used the relationship between the substituted goal and the patient's response or probability of response must be known. It is not immediately obvious, for example, that for some drugs the correlation between a plasma concentration and the therapeutic response is not good. Morphine plasma concentrations do not correlate well with analgesia in either nontolerant or tolerant people. Pain relief in mentally competent patients is better assessed directly by asking simple questions. Are you in pain? Have you had pain in the last several hours? How severe is the pain? In children and mentally impaired individuals this is not so easily done, but morphine plasma concentrations are still meaningless numbers — uninterpretable. It is an important matter to see this clearly in order to avoid the fruitless task of measuring things merely because they can be measured and might correlate with disease activity. This is inappropriate in the practice of clinical medicine, although posing questions about the possibility of a relationship is a perfectly legitimate and honorable activity for the medical scientist.

The Plasma Concentration-Response Curve: the Therapeutic Window

The relationship between the concentration of a drug in plasma and the therapeutic response in a population of patients is determined in research trials. If the variation in the drug concentration accounts for a large fraction of the variation in the patients' responses, monitoring the drug concentration may be clinically helpful.

A graph of the cumulative percent of patient subjects experiencing a therapeutic benefit versus the drug concentration can be prepared and a curve can be fit to the data points. Similarly, such a graph can be prepared for adverse effects. The resultant graphs can be used to determine the therapeutic window, also called the therapeutic range. The therapeutic window defines the range of drug concentrations that maximizes the percent of the patient population deriving a therapeutic effect while minimizing the percentage having adverse effects. This is the optimal concentration range for a population. In Figure 13-2 the limits of the therapeutic window for a hypothetical drug are defined by the vertical dashed lines. When the concentration of the drug is 1 U, approximately 20% of the patient population experience benefits from the drug. This is defined here as the lower limit of the therapeutic range. The upper limit is 3 U.

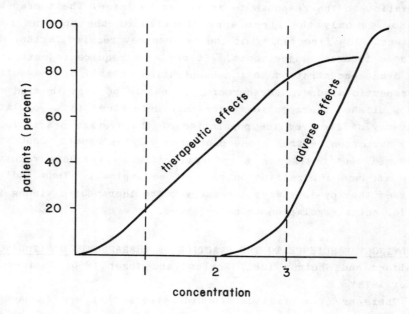

Fig 13-2   Therapeutic Window

At that concentration 15% of the patient population have an adverse reaction. Notice that at 3 U of the drug, approximately 20% of the patients are still not receiving any benefit from the medication.

The therapeutic window is defined individually for each drug. In Figure 13-2 the therapeutic benefit and adverse effects are not stated. If, for example, the adverse effects were death or blindness and the benefit, improvement of a chronic lung disease, then the therapeutic range should be shifted, perhaps to an upper limit of 2 U of the drug. On the other hand, if the adverse effect were tremor, then it might be reasonable for the upper range of the therapeutic window to be greater than 3 U of the drug concentration.

In practice the physician begins drug therapy with a dose of medication that has been shown to achieve concentrations within the therapeutic window for most people. Then the blood concentration of the drug is measured at the appropriate time, and the dose of the drug is adjusted as needed to achieve a plasma concentration within the desired range. This is a good strategy. However, it is important to remember that the therapeutic window refers to the frequency of effects in a population. It does not define an optimal result in an individual. Indeed, interpatient variation in the response to drugs can be large. The therapeutic window is only the first approximation of the optimum for a patient. The fine tuning of the regimen may require further dose or dose interval adjustments. It may even require adjustment of the drug concentration to a concentration outside of the defined therapeutic window. Furthermore, it should be kept in mind that the published therapeutic windows are determined in a population that may differ from the population of the average practitioner. This may often be true since published work is usually done at an academic center that is a referral center. Patients receiving care at such an institution may not be typical. Thus individualized therapy is always necessary. The therapeutic window is a guide, not a regulation to be enforced.

APPLYING THE SCIENCE TO THE PRACTICE OF THERAPEUTIC MONITORING

(Holford and Sheiner 1981; Rowland and Tozer 1980; Sheiner and Tozer 1978)

There are two practical considerations that are fundamental to the interpretation of drug concentrations. Both are related to the choice of when to collect the sample: 1) How long should one wait after the initiation of the therapy to sample fluid for monitoring?   2). When during the dosing interval is it best to sample?

Steady State

In pharmacology, steady state means a state in which the amount of drug taken into the body per dosing interval equals the amount removed per dosing interval. This state results in constant plasma concentrations with continuous infusions and periodic concentrations with intermittent dosing regimens. With intermittent dosing a drug has repeated, identical concentration curves with equally spaced peaks and troughs.

Steady state is achieved as a result of the plasma concentration of a drug rising to a level such that its elimination rate equals the administration rate of the drug. Initially, as doses of drugs are given, the administration rate exceeds the elimination rate. Consequently, the drug accumulates in the body, which leads to increasing plasma concentrations. The elimination rate of the drug increases as a result of the increased drug concentrations. Eventually enough drug accumulates so that the elimination rate exactly balances the administration rate.

It takes time for the accumulation of the drug to achieve steady-state equilibrium. This presents a difficulty in the interpretation of the plasma concentration. If the physician orders a drug concentration before steady state is achieved, he may be able to interpret the likely effect of the drug at the time the blood sample was drawn but may be unable to determine what eventual blood concentration will be achieved by the drug. Therefore, it is often best to draw blood samples during steady state. Occasionally, though, it is important to draw blood samples before steady state is achieved for the purpose of avoiding a dangerous, unpleasant, or permanent toxic side effect. And sometimes it is important to achieve a minimal therapeutic level early in therapy. For example, as is shown by the plasma accumulation curves in Figure 13-3, sampling after the second dose for the C dosing regimen demonstrates a toxic concentration well before steady state is achieved. In this situation it is clear that the dose must be decreased. However, sampling after the second dose for regimen B yields a concentration that is below the therapeutic window; yet in this case the drug will continue to accumulate to a steady-state concentration that is

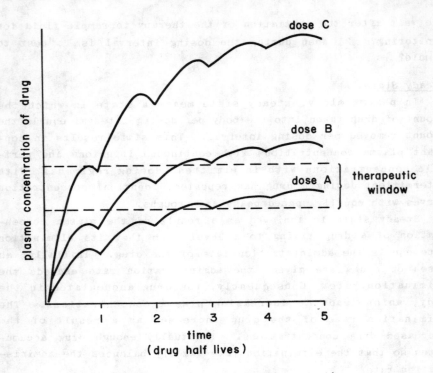

Fig 13-3   Time Course of Drug Concentration
Resulting from Three Different Doses

above the therapeutic window. Here the clinician needs to
decrease the dose, but this is not apparent from the early
results. For regimen A, sampling after two doses reveals a
concentration below the therapeutic window; yet the steady-state
concentrations will be within the window. The correct course is
to continue the regimen unless there is an urgent need to achieve
the target concentration immediately, in which case a loading
dose would be advisable.

For some drugs there are published nomograms and. equations
for the calculation of the probable concentration of the drug in
steady state given a concentration of the drug at some particular
time after the first dose. Such nomograms generally describe
drugs with long half-lives, such as the antidepressants, and they
are useful, although they should be checked, confirming the
estimate by measuring the concentration at steady state. These
equations have not come into general use, and it remains to be
seen whether there will be enough advantage to patient care to
justify having the average clinician attempt to keep up with the
various methods for calculations.

An often quoted rule is that it takes about four half-lives to achieve steady state. This is a result of the fact that the usual routes of elimination for drugs, hepatic metabolism and renal filtration, are first-order processes. First-order processes are described by the equation

$$-dC/dt = KC$$

where C is the concentration of drug, t is time, and K is the first-order rate constant. The rate constant expresses the fraction of the drug eliminated per unit time. An elimination constant of 0.01 per hour, for instance, means that one hundredth of the drug is removed per hour.

Solving the differential equation gives rise to the familiar equation

$$C = C_o e^{-Kt}$$

where C_o is the initial concentration of drug. The half-life of the drug can be derived from this equation by setting C equal to $C_o/2$ and substituting $t_{1/2}$ (half-life) for t:

$$t_{1/2} = 0.693/K.$$

Therefore half-life is a time constant inversely proportional to the rate constant. The half-life of the drug eliminated with a rate constant of 0.01 per hour is 69.3 hours.

Since steady state by definition requires that the administration rate of the drug is equal to the elimination rate of the drug, the length of time to steady state is dependent on the elimination rate constant, which can be expressed conveniently as the half-life. After one half-life has passed, the concentration of the drug (and the amount of drug in the body) is one-half of the steady-state accumulation. After two half-lives, the concentration will be 75% of that in steady state, and so on. The formula for the plasma concentration of the drug as a percentage of the steady-state value is

$$\% \ steady \ state = 100 \ (1 - 0.5^N)$$

where N is the number of half-lives elapsed. Thus after four half-lives the drug is about 94% of the maximum steady-state concentration. The equation implies that steady state is never actually attained but is approached exponentially. The small changes in the concentration after five or more half-lives are clinically unimportant.

It is important to realize that steady state requires four or five half-lives, whether one is accumulating drug to a plateau or discontinuing the drug. When the drug is discontinued, a concentration of zero is the steady-state concentration. It also takes four half-lives to reach a new steady state if the dose of drug is changed or if the elimination rate is changed by disease of the liver or kidneys. The absolute differences in the concentration of the drug from the new steady state will be less than when approaching steady state from a zero concentration and may even be inapparent after two to three half-lives (see Figure 13-4).

Some patients may never reach steady state because the capacity to eliminate the drug is constantly changing. For example, a patient with acute tubular necrosis experiences a precipitous decline of renal function that over several days may improve back to normal. Caring for such individuals requires that the serum concentrations of the drugs of interest be measured periodically while frequently monitoring signs and symptoms of disease that may reflect a change in the elimination capacity of the patient.

When using the monoexponential equation

$$C = Coe^{-Kt}$$

it is implicitly assumed that the drug is given as a bolus and

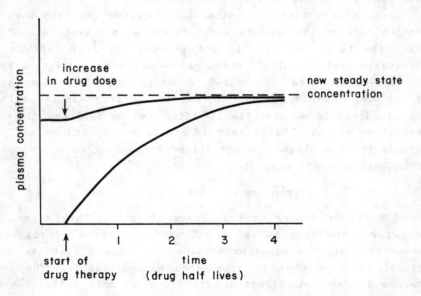

Fig 13-4   The Approach to the Steady-State Plasma Concentration

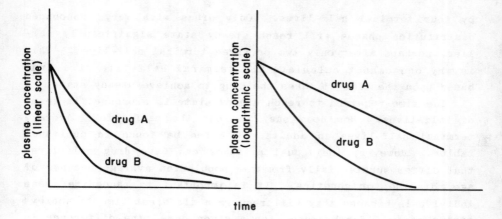

Fig 13-5   Plasma Clearance Curves for Two Drugs
with the Same Terminal Rate Constants but
Different Elimination Rate Constants
(Note: each is graphed on linear and log-linear scales.)

Drug A: Monoexponential clearance curve
$$C = e^{-K_n t}$$
Drug B: Biexponential clearance curve
$$C = 0.8e^{-3.125K_n t} + 0.2e^{-K_n t}$$

instantly mixes with all body tissues.   This is the one-compartment model.   However, many drugs are not well described by this
model.   Instead they have multicompartmental characteristics in
that multiple exponential functions are needed to describe their
serum concentration versus time curves.   That is,

$$C = C_o e^{-K_o t} + C_1 e^{-K_1 t} + C_2 e^{-K_2 t} + \ldots C_n e^{-K_n t}$$

where K_n is the terminal rate constant of the drug.   The elimination rate constant, called K_{el}, does not equal K_n.   Instead,

$$K_{el} = (C_o/K_o + C_1/K_1 + C_2/K_2 + \ldots C_n/K_n)^{-1}.$$

In Figure 13-5 the two drugs A and B have identical terminal rate
constants, but K_{el} is not the same.

As with the one-compartment model, the time needed to achieve
steady state in the multicompartment model is approximately four
times the half-life of the elimination rate.   However, neither
K_{el} nor the elimination half-life can be routinely calculated for
individual patients.   Fortunately, it can be shown that the
elimination rate half-life is always shorter than the terminal
half-life.   Therefore, steady state will be reached no later than

by four terminal half-lives. Only drugs with very pronounced distribution phases will reach steady state significantly earlier, perhaps after only two or three terminal half-lives. This is why one cannot calculate the terminal half-life of a drug based upon the time it takes the drug to achieve steady state.

The time required to reach steady state is expressed in terms of half-lives. How does one find out the half-life? Average terminal half-lives in adults can often be found in published tables. However, individual patients can have drug half-lives that differ substantially from the population average because of age, disease, or genetics. It is important to recognize these individuals because they will require a different time to achieve steady state. Furthermore, for a given dose, the difference in the elimination rate will result in a different steady-state drug concentration.

Sampling with Respect to Time Elapsed Since Previous Dose

Drugs exert their effects at sites that lie in some body tissue. Consequently, the relationship between a pharmacologic response and the plasma concentration must be defined with due consideration for the time course of distribution of the drug to the target tissue. For some drugs the distribution is nearly instantaneous so that throughout the dosing interval the plasma concentrations parallel the drug response. This applies, for example, to heparin. Heparin given intravenously is extremely rapidly bound to antithrombin III in the blood, thereby producing a conformational change in the antithrombin III and making the complex a potent inhibitor of the clotting process. As a result the anticoagulant effect of the drug is immediately and directly related to its plasma concentration. Most drugs, however, are not conveniently injected into, mixed, and confined to their effector organ. Most are transported via the blood to the target tissues.

The absorption of drug from the body site of administration into the blood, the circulation time, and the distribution or uptake of drug into the target organ cause a delay in the response. During distribution the plasma concentration and the physiologic response are often inversely related. The relationship is inverse because the target organ uptake is much slower than the absorption and the circulation time. This is shown for digoxin in Figure 13-6. It takes a relatively long time for the drug to distribute from the blood into the heart and

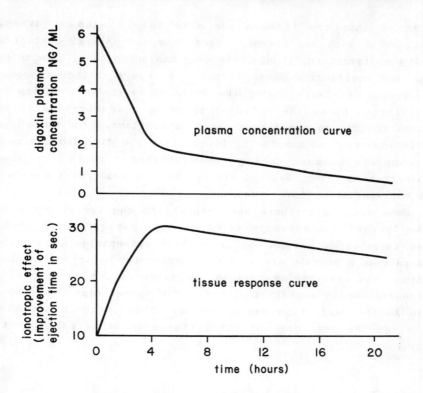

Fig 13-6   Time Course of Digoxin Plasma
Concentrations and Ionotropic Effect

other tissues. The digoxin concentration in heart tissue is
directly correlated with the ionotropic effect, as measured by
the ejection time.   Shortly after an intravenous injection of
digoxin, the concentration in the plasma is high relative to
later plasma concentrations.   Yet at this time the ionotropic
response is nearly baseline. For the next few hours there is an
inverse relationship between the plasma concentration and the
ionotropic effect.   At approximately 4 hours the relationship
changes and the plasma concentration and tissue response curves
become parallel to each other. This parallel portion of the
curve is sometimes called the pseudoequilibrium phase or simply
the equilibrium phase.   During this portion of the curve, the
plasma concentration of digoxin conveys information about the
ionotropic effect on the heart (therapeutic response) and the
risk of toxicity (adverse response). This is because during this
part of the curve, the plasma concentration bears a constant
relationship with the ionotropic effect.   The drug has dis-

tributed into the tissues and come into a kind of dynamic equilibrium with the plasma. Even from the initial instant of drug administration, though, the drug has begun to be eliminated. Thus the equilibrium phase is never a true equilibrium because the system is always losing the drug. Nevertheless, during the equilibrium phase the ratio of the drug concentration in the plasma to that in the target organ is constant. For most drugs it is important to sample the blood after the distribution phase is complete because during the equilibrium phase the blood concentration often, but not always, has a linear relationship to the therapeutic or toxic response.

Some drugs distribute very rapidly to the target organ but take longer to distribute to other body parts (Figure 13-7). Thus intravenous boluses of drugs like epinephrine, lidocaine, and calcium gluconate are dangerous during the distribution phase because the equilibrium between the target organ and the blood concentration is rapidly achieved. The target organ is responsive to the early high concentrations of the drug in the blood although the drug has not yet diffused to other parts of the body.

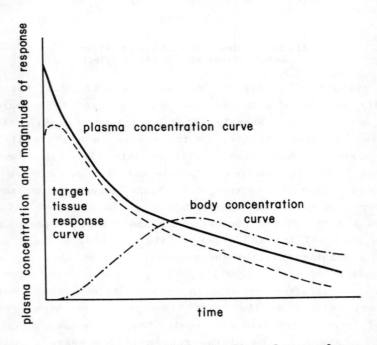

Fig 13-7   Plasma Concentration and Tissue Response Curves
for a Drug with Rapid Distribution to the Target Tissue

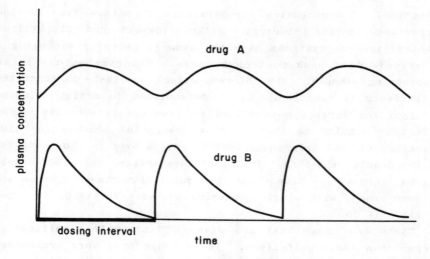

Fig 13-8   Plasma Concentrations of Two Drugs
(A and B) Given by Intermittent Dosing

Drug A: Long absorption and elimination half-lives
Drug B: Short absorption and elimination half-lives

To safely give such drugs intravenously, they should be administered at a rate that roughly equals the rate of distribution. The dosing schedule of these drugs as found in clinical manuals accomplishes this, thereby allowing a slow accumulation of the drug in the blood and avoiding toxic concentrations at the target organ. Therapeutic monitoring is performed using clinical signs and symptoms or bedside laboratory studies. For epinephrine, lidocaine, and calcium gluconate the electrocardiogram is monitored.

Drugs that have a long half-life compared to the dose interval (perhaps a ratio of 3 to 1) do not have large changes in the serum concentration during a dose interval. The resultant curve of the drug concentration is similar to a flat plateau, with the concentration varying only a little from the beginning of the equilibrium phase to the trough. Phenobarbital, which has an average terminal half-life of 85 hours, has these characteristics. For these drugs one gains similar information from taking a blood sample immediately after entering the equilibrium phase or at the trough because the concentrations differ little.

As shown in Figure 13-8 (drug A), drugs that have slow or prolonged absorption relative to the half-life also show only small changes of drug concentration from peak to trough. Phenytoin has a long half-life and is absorbed slowly from the small intestine. Pharmaceutical preparations that have time-release properties slowing absorption like Slow-bid and Slophylline theophylline preparations have the same property of producing a relatively flat peak-to-trough curve. Chloramphenicol is an interesting example. The chloramphenicol succinate administered to patients is inactive. It is metabolized to active chloramphenicol and further metabolized to inactive metabolites. The effect is similar to that of slow absorption because the biotransformation of chloramphenicol to active drug is slow compared to the drug's half-life. In all of these cases, the blood sample can be taken at any time after the equilibrium phase is begun and in some drugs, with single-compartment characteristics, any time at all will do.

There are drugs that are given at intervals significantly longer than their half-lives. These drugs have very pronounced differences between the plasma concentrations at the beginning of the equilibrium phase, hereafter called the peak, and at the trough (drug B in Figure 13-8). For example, if a drug has a half-life of 3 hours and is given every 6 hours, its plasma concentration will have dropped to 25% of the concentration attained at the time of administration by the time of the next dose. For this reason, the time lapsed since the drug was given is an important consideration in therapeutic monitoring.

For drugs administered at intervals that are as long or longer than the terminal half-life of the drug, the therapeutic window is defined not only by a range of plasma concentrations but also by a time after drug administration. Gentamicin levels, for instance, are often measured 1 hour after the completion of the drug infusion. They are measured at this time because there exists a body of research that demonstrates the relationship between gentamicin's therapeutic efficacy and toxicity and its plasma concentration based upon blood sampling 1 hour after drug administration.

In order to obtain an ideal specimen for the therapeutic monitoring of drugs given intravenously, both the duration of the drug infusion and the interval from termination of the infusion to blood sampling must be timed accurately. In the example of gentamicin, a blood sample should be taken 1 hour after the completion of a 30-minute infusion. If the infusion lasts 1 hour instead of 30 minutes, the 1-hour postinfusion level will be lower. This is so because the clearance rate is constant for drugs eliminated by first-order processes, such as gentamicin.

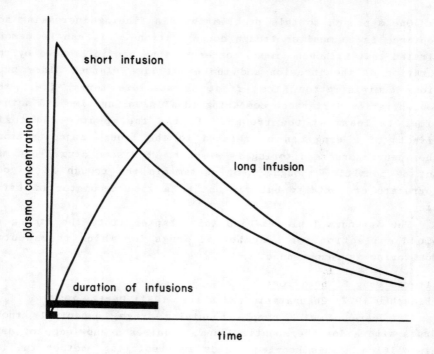

Fig 13-9 Influence of Infusion Time on the
Plasma Clearance Curve of a Drug
(The total doses and AUCs are equal)

Because the clearance rate equals the dose divided by the area
under the plasma clearance curve, if clearance is a constant and
if the dose is constant, then it follows that the area under the
plasma clearance curve (AUC) must also be constant. As illustrated in Figure 13-9, if the duration of an infusion is ex-
tended, the concentrations must be lower so that the AUC will be
equal to that during the shorter infusion. Whatever the duration
of the infusion, if the dose is equal, the AUC is equal. The
duration of the drug infusion influences the concentration of the
drug during and after infusion.

Sampling at the stipulated time following drug administration
is also problematic. Nurses often have great difficulty drawing
blood samples at a precise time. They are busy with other tasks.
House officers have the same problem, only worse. Blood-drawing
teams are unable to render this service unless they are affili-
ated with the pharmacy or a clinical pharmacology or clinical
pathology group. So while proper sample timing is a desirable
goal, it is seldom achieved.

One approach to this problem that is finding increasing acceptance is to monitor trough concentrations. It can be demonstrated that although trough concentrations are influenced by the duration of the infusion and the exact time elapsed since previous administration, the effect in absolute terms, i.e., the concentration difference comparing ideal sampling time and actual time, is least at the trough. If the therapeutic and toxic effects of a drug can be related to the trough concentration, therapeutic drug monitoring is simpler. For some drugs this may not be possible, though. For gentamicin the trough is a good correlate of toxicity but may not be a good predictor of efficacy.

The Appendix Table 13-1 to this chapter lists the timing of blood collection for a number of drugs for which therapeutic monitoring is recommended.

Altered Drug Disposition

(Blaschke 1977; Chennarasin and Brater 1981; Dettli 1977)

The care of sick people receiving drugs, especially those drugs with a low therapeutic index, requires a knowledge of drug disposition. This knowledge aids in predicting whether the individual patient is likely to have altered drug kinetics. The question arises, what is the best method for therapeutic drug monitoring in an individual suspected to have altered drug disposition? One approach would be to treat the patient initially with a lower than usual dose of drug. Then measure the drug concentration after four times the upper limit of the normal range of half-lives for the drug and again one or two half-lives later. If the concentration increases by more than about 20% (depending upon the analytic variability of the assay), it may be concluded that the patient has a reduced clearance of the drug. In such an individual repeated determinations at similar intervals may be justified until steady state is attained. When the drug is very dangerous, careful direct monitoring of the patient's status is important. A sample taken after one half-life can be useful in this situation. After one half-life has elapsed, the drug concentration should be half of the steady-state level. If the drug concentration in the patient is greater than half the maximum therapeutic concentration, it is very probable that the steady-state concentration will be outside the therapeutic window. In such an individual the drug dose should be decreased and drug concentrations should be measured regularly.

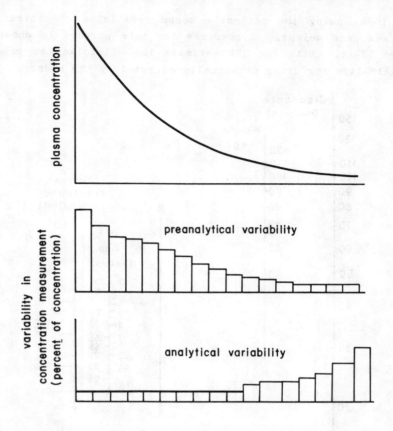

Fig 13-10   Analytic Variability as a Function
of Drug Plasma Concentration

When monitoring drug levels after one half-life, the peak
concentration is not optimal because this early concentration is
not greatly influenced by the terminal elimination rate.   These
early concentrations are more influenced by distribution.   Therefore, one should use a trough level for this type of monitoring
because the trough level is influenced by all drug disposition
factors.   The only difficulty with using the trough is that if
the usual trough levels are quite low, the analytic variability
of the drug assay may be high (Figure 13-10).   Knowing the magnitude of the variability of the assay at the trough concentration allows for more confident comparisons of the drug concentrations.

For patients in whom renal function alone is impaired, there
are methods for calculating the patient's glomerular filtration

rate (GFR) using the patient's serum creatinine concentration, age, sex, and weight. A nomogram for this purpose is shown in Figure 13-11. With the GFR estimate the clinician can predict the half-life for drugs principally excreted by the kidney. This

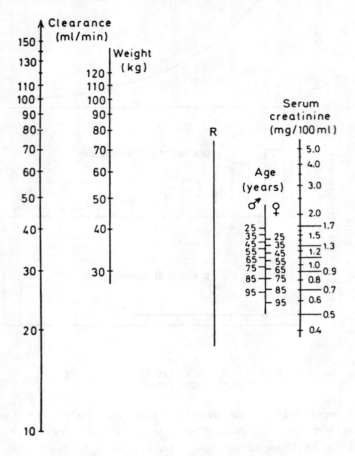

Fig 13-11   Nomogram for the Calculation of GFR
(From Siersbaek-Nielsen, K., Hansen, J.M., Kampmann, J., Kristensen, M. Rapid evaluation of creatinine clearance. Lancet i:1133, 1971 © The Lancet Ltd., London, England)

To use the nomogram: Locate the patient's weight on the near left axis and the patient's age on the near right axis.   Use a straightedge to connect these two points.   Note the point of intersection with the middle axis (labeled R). Locate the patient's serum creatinine concentration on the far right axis. Use a straightedge to connect the indicated point on the center axis and the point on the serum creatinine concentration axis. The point of intersection with the far left axis is the patient's creatinine clearance rate.

allows the steady-state concentration of drugs with the characteristics of a one-compartment model, such as the aminoglycosides, to be predicted with reasonable accuracy. Despite this, such nomograms are seldom used by persons who are not specialists in drug therapy, although the principles are not difficult. One particular advantage of these methods is the fact that they can be used to adjust dosing regimens for patients who have rapidly changing renal function.

Liver dysfunction is another matter. Impairment of the liver's ability to metabolize drugs is not quantifiable using any laboratory study. This is because hepatocytes are specialized according to their placement in the sinusoid. Each drug has an individual topographic pattern of drug metabolism, so each disease process has a different pattern of impaired drug metabolism, depending upon the location of the key enzyme systems within the sinusoids. For example, the cells near the central vein have more cytochrome P-450 than those close to the portal area. They also are more susceptible to ischemic damage because the oxygen concentrations at the terminal portion of the sinusoid are lower than in the surrounding tissue.

The traditional markers of liver injury and function, hepatic enzymes, albumin, and bilirubin concentrations, and the prothrombin time do not share the enzymatic pathways most important in drug metabolism. It is probable that this explains their failure to reflect alterations in drug metabolism. Therefore, for drugs largely dependent on liver metabolism, the best procedure is the empirical approach of repeated measurements.

OTHER CONSIDERATIONS
(Rowland and Tozer 1980)
Protein Binding

Drug concentrations are usually measured as total drug per unit volume of plasma. However, it is the concentration of drug unbound to protein that is more closely related to drug efficacy and toxicity. Unbound drug in the plasma is in dynamic equilibrium with unbound drug in the tissues, and the unbound drug in the tissues is usually the active species at the drug effector site. The unbound drug in the plasma is also the drug species filtered by the kidney, extracted by the liver, or removed by the lungs.

In plasma, basic drugs usually bind to alpha-1-acid glycoprotein and acidic drugs to albumin. The extent to which a drug binds to serum proteins can be altered in disease states and by the administration of other drugs. This in turn will cause changes in the plasma concentration of the drug. For the most part these changes have a small magnitude and are short lived. As such they are seldom clinically important. They do not disrupt the concentration-versus-response relationship that lies at the heart of therapeutic drug monitoring. However, drugs that are highly protein bound in the plasma are susceptible to protein-binding changes that can change their plasma concentration substantially without appreciably altering their concentration at the effector site.

Figure 13-12 depicts the effects of a reduction in binding capacity upon the plasma concentrations of a drug that is normally 90% protein bound in plasma. The upper panel of the figure shows the steady-state distribution of the drug in a person with a normal binding protein concentration. The amount of drug in the various compartments is indicated. The middle panel shows the redistribution of drug that accompanies a 50% reduction in the drug binding due to a disease-induced reduction in binding protein levels. The drug displaced from the binding protein distributes into the other compartments so as to maintain equal unbound drug concentrations in plasma and tissue and a constant ratio of unbound to bound drug in tissue. As a result the amounts (and concentrations) of unbound drug in plasma and tissue are slightly increased whereas the total amount (and concentration) of drug in the plasma is markedly decreased. Because the plasma concentration of unbound drug is increased, its elimination rate is increased. That means that there will be a net loss of drug from the body. As this happens the drug will redistribute. In the new steady state, when drug elimination again equals drug intake, the amount (and concentration) of unbound drug in plasma and tissue will have returned to normal, as will the amount of bound drug in the tissue (lower panel). The total amount (and concentration) of drug in the plasma, however, remains decreased.

This situation may mislead the physician into the belief that the dose of drug is too low when, in fact, the concentration of unbound drug is appropriate. Increasing the dose of the drug will elevate the concentration of unbound drug, often into the toxic range. The foremost example of this problem is phenytoin in renal failure. Phenytoin metabolism is not altered in renal disease, but phenytoin binding to albumin is decreased substan-

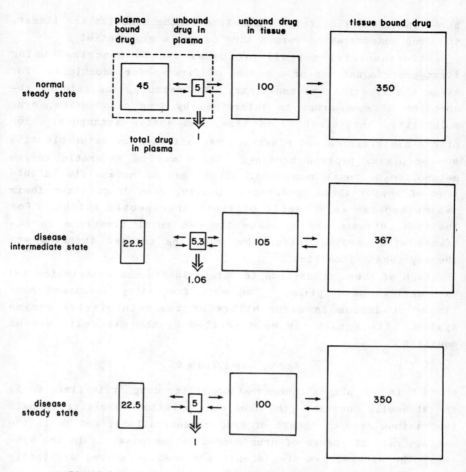

| plasma bound drug | unbound drug in plasma | unbound drug in tissue | tissue bound drug |

normal steady state — 45 ⇄ 5 ⇄ 100 ⇄ 350

total drug in plasma — 1

disease intermediate state — 22.5 ⇄ 5.3 ⇄ 105 ⇄ 367

1.06

disease steady state — 22.5 ⇄ 5 ⇄ 100 ⇄ 350

1

Fig 13-12   Example of the Protein Binding Relationship of a Drug in Health and Disease

tially. Patients who have their drug doses increased so as to achieve plasma concentrations of phenytoin within the therapeutic window frequently show toxic effects. Analogous situations arise for valproic acid in renal failure, for both phenytoin and valproic acid in hypoalbuminemia, and for warfarin when drugs that compete for binding sites on albumin are coadministered.

Nonlinear Kinetics

Many if not most drug processes are first order. Because the rate of change of drug concentration depends in a linear fashion upon the concentration of drug, first-order processes are said to have linear kinetics (note that although the kinetics are linear, the drug concentration versus time curve is exponential).

Unfortunately, not all processes can be described using first-order equations or a series of first-order equations. For these the kinetics are nonlinear. For example, the rate of absorption of some drugs is determined by drug dissolution, drug solubility, intestinal blood flow, and active transport. For others distribution and clearance are affected by saturable tissue or plasma protein binding. There may be saturable enzyme metabolism or renal secretion. There may be metabolite inhibition of any of these processes. Lastly, some drugs alter their own metabolism as a result of their therapeutic action. For instance, digoxin may increase its own renal clearance in patients with cardiac failure by improving cardiac function and thereby renal blood flow.

Each of these conditions is unique in its characteristics and mathematical description. The most frequently discussed nonlinear condition is saturability of the metabolizing enzyme system. Its result can be described by the Michaelis-Menten equation

$$-dC/dt = Vm \ C/(Km + C)$$

where C is the plasma concentration of the drug, t is time, Km is the Michaelis constant (the drug concentration resulting in half the maximum rate of change of drug concentration), and Vm is the maximum rate of change of drug concentration possible in the system. The Michaelis-Menten equation cannot be solved explicitly for plasma concentration as a function of time. To use this equation then, it must be simplified by making some assumptions. One may take two extreme conditions. If Km $\gg$ C, the equation reduces to

$$-dC/dt = (Vm/Km) \ C.$$

This is a first-order equation with the constant, Vm/Km, equal to the rate constant. If Km $\ll$ C, then

$$-dC/dt = Vm.$$

Here the rate of change of the plasma concentration is a constant, Vm. This is the equation of a zero-order process.

Reconciling these two conditions, if -dC/dt is plotted as a function of plasma concentration, -dC/dt increases linearly at first. As the concentration increases further, -dC/dt continues to increase but at a rate less than proportional to the concentration. As the concentration increases further, $-dC/dt$ approaches the asymptote, V_m.

There are important implications for therapeutic monitoring from this kind of kinetic behavior. Because the elimination rate is not constant, drug half-life can only be calculated at a defined plasma concentration. It follows then that the sum of four half-lives is unknown because each half-life is dependent on the plasma concentration in a complex way. Therefore, the time until steady state is indeterminate. Furthermore, since the elimination rate is dependent on the concentration, the steady-state plasma concentration is also indeterminate. Figure 13-13 represents the behavior of a drug with these characteristics. At low doses, curves A and B, the drug's kinetic behavior is linear. In this dose range the drug reaches steady state in the same

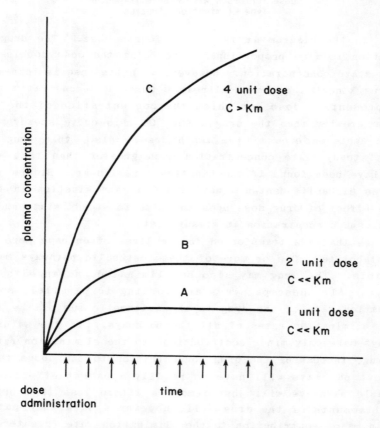

Fig 13-13   Influence of Drug Dose upon the Accumulation Curve
for a Drug with Michaelis-Menten Elimination Kinetics

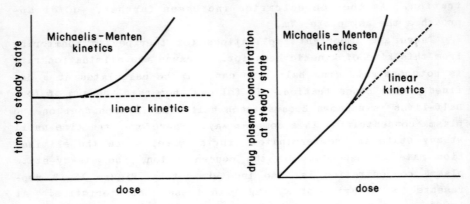

Fig 13-14   Dependence of the Time to Steady State
and the Steady State Plasma Concentration upon
Dose for Drugs with Michaelis-Menten
Type Elimination Kinetics

time. In the diagram it is at the fourth dose. The drug accumulation is also proportional: doubling the dose doubles the
steady-state concentration. However, when the dose is increased,
the drug kinetics become nonlinear. Curve C demonstrates this.
It represents a dose for which the concentration of the drug
becomes greater than the drug's Km. On this curve steady state
is not achieved even at the tenth dose. Also, this drug will
have a steady-state concentration much greater than that which
would have been found if the kinetics were linear. Figure 13-14
compares Michaelis-Menten kinetics and linear kinetics in terms
of the effect of drug dose upon the time to steady state and the
drug plasma concentration at steady state.

Drugs that are transformed in the liver often have more than
one metabolite. One or more of these metabolic pathways may be
saturable. The drug may also be eliminated unchanged by the
kidneys. All these pathways are working in parallel, so the
elimination rate of the drug is the arithmetic sum of the individual elimination rates of all the pathways. If the saturable
pathways make only minor contributions to the elimination rate of
the drug, increasing the drug concentration to one above the Km
of those pathways will have no readily apparent effect. The
saturable pathways will just remove a little less than proportional amounts of the drug. If, however a saturable pathway
makes a major contribution to the elimination rate (greater than
40%), the effect will be apparent because this relatively impor-

- 282 -

Table 13-1

Important Drugs Exhibiting Nonlinear Kinetics Within
or Near the Therapeutic Window

Aspirin

Disopyramide

Ethanol

Heparin

Hydralazine

Phenobarbital

Phenytoin

Propranolol

Theophylline

---

tant pathway will be operating less efficiently. The parallel
minor pathways will compensate by increasing their individual
elimination rates as the concentration rises, but they will not
be able to overcome the deficit completely. The drug concentration will rise disproportionately. Theoretically, all drugs
that are metabolized should demonstrate saturable properties if
the dose is high enough. However, only a few drugs demonstrate
it within or near the therapeutic window (Table 13-1).

Theophylline and phenobarbital are two drugs that cause
confusion because they usually exhibit nonlinear kinetics only at
concentrations above the therapeutic window. The confusion
arises in the setting of an overdose. In this situation the
half-life of the drug becomes prolonged because linear kinetics
no longer pertain. Calculations predicting the concentration of
the drug as a function of time based on published half-lives will
be in error. Figure 13-15 shows an example of this kinetic behavior. The curves for doses of 1 and 2 U represent the linear
kinetic situation near the therapeutic window. Here the concentrations are less than the Km, so the elimination curves are
parallel on a log-linear graph. The concentrations are also
proportional to the dose. But at the 15-U dose, these relationships change and the initial portion of the curve is bowed. The

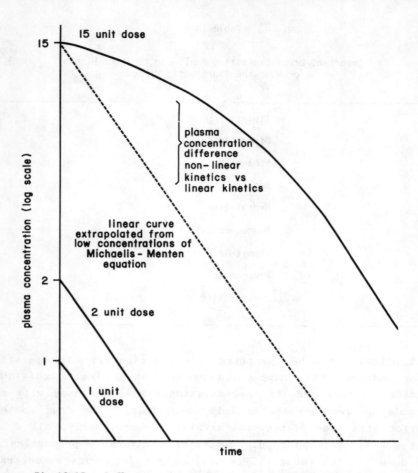

Fig 13-15   Influence of Drug Dose upon the Elimination Curve
of a Drug with Michaelis-Menten Type Elimination Kinetics

concentration falls at a much slower than anticipated rate. This
is the explanation for the fact that repeated drug concentration
determinations early in the course of a large overdose often do
not fall but appear to be level for long periods of time.   More
confusion is added by the fact that the analytical variation
usually becomes larger at concentrations above the range for
which the assay was designed.

When the concentration finally begins to fall, it will fall
at a greater and greater rate until it reaches those concentrations in which the metabolic pathway is not saturated.   This is
the portion of the curve that is parallel to those of the lower
doses. Notice the large difference between the actual drug concentrations at the 15-U dose and the concentration calculated if
one assumed linear kinetics.

A POTPOURRI OF PRACTICAL POINTS PROVIDING PARTICULARLY POIGNANT INFORMATION

The foregoing discussion has been very academic in the sense of outlining lofty principles. But the clinician cannot afford to be a medical aesthete. Much confounding is untangled by an awareness of what is happening at the bedside, of the way hospitals are run, and of human nature.

The interpretation of drug plasma concentrations requires attention to details. The clinician is advised <u>always</u> to check the nursing charts and notes, those unhallowed fonts of much surprising information. In the notes one can find descriptions of such fascinating observations as self-induced vomiting, pieces of capsules in the toilet, and the fact that the IV has been restarted three times during the shift. Sometimes the drug gets to the floor late or doesn't come up at all. The clinician often remembers to check the time since the previous dose but doesn't realize that the 2 a.m. dose was missed for some reason.

Nurses try to notify us about important matters. They know it's not the end of the world because a patient received his digoxin 1 hour late or because one dose of antibiotic was skipped. But if we are not aware of this we can easily draw erroneous conclusions with unpleasant, expensive, or embarrassing results. Perhaps a sampling from the Yarns of Dr. Karen Kumor, junior consultant, will illustrate this best.

Case 1.

I was called to consult on a mysterious case. The patient, a gentleman from the Orient, had seizures, schistosomiasis, and cancer. He was being treated with a new phase one drug (a drug the consultant had never heard of) to treat his schistosomiasis. He was also receiving phenytoin for his seizures, but for some reason the phenytoin concentrations were only in the vicinity of 5 µg/ml, despite large doses. Before seeing the patient I checked the chart briefly. The patient was vomiting and in no condition to talk, so I spoke to the house officer, a pleasant fellow. He gladly described increasing the dose of intravenous phenytoin and remarked upon how unusual it was that the concentrations had not increased. He suggested that perhaps the basis for the problem was a novel drug interaction with the new antibiotic.

Everything fell into place for me. I was assured a new publication outlining the novel interaction. Not a very important issue, perhaps, but still something for a junior faculty member

to publish. So it was that I was happily imagining the publication as I looked for the chart to check the doses on the medication sheets.

First, it was difficult to find the chart. Some other
equally unimportant consultant had squirreled the thing away
someplace. When I found it, the last page of the nursing notes
was missing. The dosing sheet was complete, indicating that the
drug was given on the schedule in a regular fashion. I was now
quite satisfied and ready to leave, my consultant sheet already
half filled out. But I hadn't seen those nursing notes. None of
the nurses were in the nursing station. I found one with her
patient and waited for her to finish. I asked for the notes
because in my training I was forced (the burn scars are barely
noticeable now) to be complete, to be compulsive. To be compulsive about being compulsive! It turned out that one of the
nurses had it because she was entering her latest note. There
nestled innocently amidst all sorts of minutiae was a note about
finding a phenytoin capsule in the vomitus. Hmm ... That was
interesting! The friendly house officer was nearby, so I asked
him about whether the phenytoin is being given by the intravenous
or oral route. He replied that he was sure he wrote an order for
intravenous drug days ago because the patient was vomiting a lot.
I showed him the nursing note and together we rechecked the medication sheet, which indicated that phenytoin was coming to the
floor as capsules. The house officer became angry and indignant.
He was certain that he had written orders for intravenous medication. I cautioned him to check on that before arranging for
the assassin's services. We relocated the chart (that pest
consultant from the other service was hogging it again) and found
his order:

5/16 10 a.m. phenytoin 200 mg bid P.O.

We were both quiet. He was embarrassed. I had lost my publication and wished I were somewhere else. Silently, I held
grateful thoughts about my compulsive mentors. I held up the
pink consultant's sheet from which the charges for my services
are made. I told the resident, "Let's forget about this, OK?"
He said, "Yeah, I wish we could forget about this." I tore up
the sheet. That is how I spent approximately 2 hours one sunny
afternoon.

Case 2.

I recall another afternoon, but it was cold and drafty in my office. Nice Dr. L.P. was on the phone with me. He was very upset. He was really angry. It seemed that my laboratory did not care about patient care and that nobody in the lab was doing his job.

He was taking care of a child recovering from <u>Haemophilus influenzae</u> meningitis. He had sent a sample for a chloramphenicol determination and needed the result desperately because the previous levels had been low and the dose had been increased. The determination had not been done in the 3 days since sending the specimen, and as it was Friday, it would not be performed until Monday.

I 'was at a loss because the laboratory should get the results out much quicker than that. I apologized to Dr. L.P., normally a nice guy. I wandered into the laboratory and asked some casual questions, like "What the heck is going on with the chloro levels!" (Reader, please note: I was in error in being disrespectful to the technologists, but I must tell the story the way it occurred.) The technologists explained the problem. The assay requires an enzyme and our batch was bad. The assay had been attempted on the Wednesday run, but the controls were out of acceptable limits. There was a problem again on Thursday. Friday they thawed some stored enzyme, but it didn't work either. We eventually decided to send the specimen to a reference laboratory.

The results received on the following Monday indicated low concentrations. This was followed by a second unpleasant phone call complaining about our poor service and the lousy assay (the good doctor wasn't aware we sent the specimen out). I asked him if he checked to see if there were other drugs that might change the clearance rate of chloramphenicol or whether he had checked other possibilities. He replied angrily that he knew what he was doing. Then I became angry. I went onto the ward and found the chart. The nursing notes were very interesting.

It happened that the child had been hospitalized for a long time. Her veins were very poor and keeping IV lines was very difficult. If the child's IV line came out near the time of her dose, the house officer ordered an oral dose and then put back in the IV line when he could. But in that hospital changing orders results in a significant delay in getting the drug to the floor. By the time the oral dose came, it was time for the next intravenous dose so the oral dose was dropped to avoid giving two doses together. And so for days the patient received only about half of her doses. The house officers and the attending physician were unaware of this persistent problem. The doses most often missed were those on the night shift when the delays in pharmacy service and in replacing the IV lines were greatest because the pharmacy and house staff were on skeleton shifts. Thus, because the samples for analysis were drawn in the morning after rounds, the effect of missing the 2:00 a.m. dose was great, even if the 8:00 a.m. dose was given. The child's drug concentrations were consistently low because she consistently received less drug than she should have.

I wrote Dr. L.P. a controlled but angry letter informing him, and we both decided not to bring the matter up again. We are still friendly and the child recovered uneventfully.

Those two stories are mostly about the bedside, the laboratory, and the pharmacy. The last anecdote is about the laboratory.

Case 3.

A 12-year-old boy was admitted in a semiconscious state. His parents related that he had what seemed to be hallucinations followed by seizures that morning. A drug overdose was suspected clinically, so blood and urine was sent to the laboratory for toxicologic analysis. The analyses were performed and were reported as negative for toxic substances.

The attending physician called me the next day and complained a little about the negative result and asked if we were sure phencyclidene (PCP) wasn't present in the urine sample. I checked in the laboratory and found out that PCP wasn't done because it wasn't requested. The remaining sample was then used to assay for PCP. It was not detected. The attending physician was puzzled and miffed and insisted that on clinical grounds the most likely diagnosis was a PCP overdose.

After several days the boy woke up and returned to normal. He denied drug use. Meanwhile, I was invited to discuss the case at Pediatric Grand Rounds. I'd like to believe that I was invited because I give insightful and interesting rounds full of wisdom, but I suspect differently. What could I say? There are a number of chemicals related to PCP that would not be positive in our assay system (or most anyone's for that matter). One of these substances could have been taken. Another possibility also existed. The urine taken from the child was collected about 18-24 hours after the estimated time of drug exposure the previous evening. The first hospital urine was sent for a urinalysis. The next was spilled onto the bed and the third got to the laboratory.

Despite the long duration of psychoactivity, the plasma half-life of PCP is relatively short. It is possible that at 18 hours after ingestion, the concentration found in the urine slipped under the detectable threshold in the laboratory. The reader may well guess where the PCP might have been. In this case, we shall never know.

This case demonstrates that the laboratory staff cannot read the clinician's mind; that the correct laboratory study cannot make up for the wrong sample; laboratory studies cannot replace clinical acumen and good judgment. In this case, the physicians caring for the patient performed excellently. They did not abandon the correct diagnosis because of the lack of laboratory confirmation. I believe, however, that the lack of laboratory support for the diagnosis cost them something psychologically and the parents financially, as the bill was surely higher because the lack of laboratory confirmation necessitated a further diagnostic search. Nevertheless, good judgment deserves to be revered, especially in a stressful situation.

EXERCISES

A 64-year-old woman with essential hypertension is being treated
with hydrochlorothiazide, potassium chloride, propranolol, hydralazine, and reserpine. Her blood pressure is 164/120 mmHg.

13-1. Are the drugs having the desired effect? How could you
       evaluate each one?

13-2. If there does not seem to be adequate drug effect, what
       diagnosis must be pursued before proceeding further? Why?

13-3. After ruling out this diagnosis, what would you do next?

You have a patient who has an arrhythmia that is difficult to
control. You start your patient on procainamide using routine
doses. Properly drawn blood samples show the plasma procainamide
plus N-acetylprocainamide concentrations to be 25 μg/ml. The
arrhythmia is abolished and the patient is comfortable on the
drug. The therapeutic window for procainamide plus its metabolite is about 8-16 μg/ml.

13-4. Should the dose be changed? Why?

13-5. If the drug were quinidine and the concentration were
       above the therapeutic window, would you change the dose?
       Why?

A 1-year-old child has been mistakenly overdosed with intravenous
theophylline over several days. She is being treated for asthma
and bronchiolitis and is desperately ill. The overdose is discovered after the child develops seizures. The serum theophylline concentration is 47 μg/ml (the therapeutic window is 10-20
μg/ml). The drug is stopped and hemodialysis is considered.
However, the child is small, making access for hemodialysis
difficult. The physicians hesitate, reasoning that the half-life
of theophylline in children is only about 4 hours, so therefore,
the drug concentration will decline rapidly. Six hours later the
theophylline concentration is 49 μg/ml and the child has continued to seize.

13-6. Why is the concentration of theophylline so high in the
       second specimen?

13-7. How can it be higher than the concentration 6 hours before
       it?

A 70-year-old man requires digoxin to treat his heart failure.
He weighs 65 kg. His serum creatinine is 1.3 mg/dl.

13-8. What is his GFR?

A sick patient is referred to you. You review the chart and find
several reported drug concentrations that do not generally correlate with the doses the patient was receiving.

13-9. What should you check?

The choices:

a. The standard curve, controls, and quality control for
the assay

b. Other drugs the patient has started or stopped recently

c. Weight gain

d. Nursing medication sheets

e. Malabsorption predisposition (vomiting, diarrhea, poor
IV line)

f. Changes in excretory and metabolic functions

g. Time of drug administration in relation to the time of
sampling

13-10. Which are the four most important items to check and why?

Mind-Expanding Exercises

A healthy young person (GFR = 125 ml/min) eliminates 35% of a
dose of digoxin in 24 hours. Fifteen percent is eliminated via
the liver. The remainder of the drug is eliminated in the urine.

13-11. What percent of our patient's drug dose is eliminated in
24 hours?

13-12. What is the correct maintenance dose for him if the appropriate loading dose is 1 mg?

13-13. What is the drug's elimination rate (K) in h^{-1}? What is
the half-life?

13-14. If the drug is given once daily starting October 1st at 9
a.m., what is the soonest date and time you should draw a
blood sample for evaluating the steady-state blood
concentrations?

REFERENCES

Blaschke, T.F.   Protein binding and kinetics of drugs in liver disease. Clin. Pharmacokinet. 2:32, 1977.

Chennarasin, P., Brater, D.C.   Nomograms for drug use in renal disease. Clin. Pharmacokinet. 6:193, 1981.

Dettli, L.   Elimination kinetics and dosage adjustment of drugs in patients with kidney disease. Prog. Pharmacol. 1:1-34, 1977.

Feinstein, A.R.   Clinical biostatistics. XII: On exorcizing the ghost of Gauss and the curse of Kelvin. Clin. Pharmacol. Ther. 12:1003, 1971.

Holford, N.H., Sheiner, L.B.   Understanding the dose-effect relationship: Clinical application of pharmacokinetic pharmacodynamic models. Clin. Pharmacokinet. 6:429, 1981.

Rowland, M., Tozer, T. Clinical Pharmacokinetics: Concepts and Applications. Lea & Febiger, Philadelphia, 1980.

Sheiner, L.B., Tozer, T.N.   Clinical pharmacokinetics: The use of plasma concentrations of drugs. In: Melmon, K., Morelli, H. (eds.) Clinical Pharmacology: Basic Principles in Therapeutics, 2nd ed.. Macmillan, New York, pp. 71-109, 1978.

Tognoni, G., Bellantuono, C., Bonata, M., et al. Clinical relevance of pharmacokinetics. Clin. Pharmacokinet. 5:105, 1980.

SUGGESTED READING

Eadie, M.J., Tyrer, J. Anticonvulsant Therapy: Pharmacological Basis and Practice, 2nd ed. Churchill Livingstone, New York, 1980.

Kucers, A., Bennett, N.M. The Use of Antibiotics. A Comprehensive Review with Clinical Emphasis, 3rd ed. J.B. Lippincott, Philadelphia, 1979.

Timing of Blood Collection for
Therapeutic Monitoring

The following table lists the time of blood collection for therapeutic monitoring for a number of drugs frequently measured in the clinical laboratory. The clinical indications for the use and monitoring of the drugs are specified.

Appendix Table 13-1

Timing of Blood Collection for Therapeutic Monitoring

Drug	Indication	Timing of blood collection
Aminoglycosides (Smith et al. 1977)	Infection	Infuse over 30 min. Obtain "peak" 1 hr after infusion complete. Obtain "peak" 1 hr post IM injection. Obtain "trough" for either dosing regimen shortly before next scheduled dose.
Carbamazepine (Eadie and Tyrer 1980)	Convulsions	Random sample after steady state achieved (oral dose).
Digoxin (Smith and Haber 1971)	Heart failure	Sample 8-12 hr after oral dose.
Digitoxin (Lukas 1971)	Heart failure	Sample 6-12 hr after oral dose.
Disopyramide (Hulting and Rosenhamer 1976; Ward and Kinghorn 1976)	Arrhythmias	Sample 2-3 hr following oral dose.
Ethosuximide (Sherwin 1982)	Convulsions	Random sample after steady state achieved (oral dose).
Lidocaine (Benowitz 1974)	Arrhythmias	Sample 1 or 2 levels at 6-12 hr after an infusion (when steady state expected). 10-120 min after IM injection.
Lithium (Prien et al. 1972)	Manic-depressive illness	Sample 8-12 hr after last dose.
Pentobarbital (Brodie et al. 1953)	Therapeutic coma	Sample >4 hr after IV dose or time infusion begun.
Phenobarbital (Eadie and Tyrer 1980)	Convulsions	Random sample after steady state achieved (oral dosing only).

Phenytoin (Eadie and Tyrer 1980)	Convulsions	Random sample after steady state achieved (oral dosing only).
Procainamide (Koch-Weser 1971,1974)	Arrhythmias	Sample "peak" 1-1.5 hr after oral dose. "Trough" shortly before next dose. Sample "peak" 20-30 min after IV infusion. Note: Patients with myocardial infarction have variable absorption rates.
Quinidine	Arrhythmias	Sample 3-8 hr after oral dose (sulfate only).
Salicylates	Rheumatic disease	Sample 2-4 hr after a dose.
Theophylline (Wolfe et al. 1978; Levy and Koysooko 1975)	Asthma	Sample 1-1.5 hr after completion of IV infusion. Sample 2 hr after oral dose.
Valproic acid (Schobben et al. 1975)	Convulsions	Sample 2 hr after oral dose.

APPENDIX REFERENCES

Benowitz, N.L. Clinical applications of the pharmacokinetics of lidocaine. Cardiovasc. Clin. 6:77, 1974.

Brodie, B.B., Burns, J.J., Mark, L.C., et al. The fate of pentobarbital in man and dog and a method for its estimation in biological material. J. Pharmacol. Exp. Ther. 109:26, 1953.

Eadie, M.J., Tyrer, J. Anticonvulsant Therapy: Pharmacological Basis and Practice. Churchill Livingstone, New York, 1980.

Hulting, J., Rosenhamer, G. Anti-arrhythmic and haemodynamic effects of intravenous and oral disopyramide in patients with ventricular arrhythmias. J. Int. Med. Res. 4 (suppl 1):90, 1976.

Koch-Weser, J. Pharmacokinetics of procainamide in man. Ann. N.Y. Acad. Sci. 179:370, 1971.

Koch-Weser, J. Clinical application of the pharmacokinetics of procainamide. Cardiovasc. Clin. 6:63, 1974.

Levy, G., Koysooko, R. Pharmacokinetic analysis of the effect of theophylline on pulmonary function in asthmatic children. J. Pediatr. 86:789, 1975.

Lukas, D.S. Some aspects of the distribution and disposition of digitoxin in man. Ann. N.Y. Acad. Sci. 179:338, 1971.

Prien, R.F., Caffey, E.M., Kluth, C.J. Relationship between serum lithium level and clinical response in acute mania treated with lithium. Br. J. Psychiatry 120:409, 1972.

Schobben, F., van der Kleijn, E., Gabreëls, F.J.M. Pharmaco-kinetics of di-n-propylacetate in epileptic patients. Eur. J. Clin. Pharmacol. 8:97, 1975.

Sherwin, A. Relationship of plasma concentration to seizure control. In: Woodbury, D.M., Penry, J.K., Pippenger, C.E. (eds.) Antiepileptic Drugs, 2nd ed. Raven Press, New York, pp. 637-646, 1982.

Smith, C.R., Baughman, K.L., Edwards, C.Q., et al. Controlled comparison of amikacin and gentamicin. N. Engl. J. Med. 296:349, 1977.

Smith, T.W., Haber, E. The clinical value of serum digitalis glycoside concentrations in the evaluation of drug toxicity. Ann. N.Y. Acad. Sci. 179:322, 1971.

Ward, J.W., Kinghorn, G.R. The pharmacokinetics of disopyramide following myocardial infarction with special reference to oral and intravenous dose regimens. J. Int. Med. Res. 4 (suppl 1):49, 1976.

Wolfe, J.D., Tashkin, D.P., Calvarese, B., Simmons, M. Broncho-dilator effects of terbutaline and aminophylline alone and in combination in asthmatic patients. N. Engl. J. Med. 298:363, 1978.

PART IV:

SELECTED ASPECTS OF LABORATORY PRACTICE

CHAPTER XV

SELECTED ASPECTS OF LABORATORY PRACTICE

Chapter 14

CLINICAL MICROBIOLOGY

James R. Carlson, Ph.D. and David G. Moore, Ph.D.

INTRODUCTION
(Lorian 1981)

Clinical microbiology is a continually changing area of laboratory medicine. In the laboratory, the older, classic methods for diagnosis coexist with newer, technically advanced methods that provide more rapid results. These new developments in the technology of medical microbiology, together with an evolving array of parasitic microbes that may produce disease, cause many physicians to be tenative or distant in their dealings with this area of the clinical laboratory. This circumstance should not exist. In fact, good communication between the medical microbiology staff and the physician is required to provide the highest quality service.

Techniques for the laboratory diagnosis of pathogenic microorganisms can be divided into two basic categories: 1) direct visualization or culture and 2) serologic detection of antibodies and antigens in body fluids.

DIRECT VISUALIZATION AND CULTURE OF PATHOGENIC MICROORGANISMS
(Washington 1981)

Direct visualization of a microbe in a clinical specimen often offers the clinician important clues to the etiology of an infectious process. The advantages presented by these techniques are the ease and speed at which they can be performed. Their chief disadvantages are that they lack sensitivity and depend upon subjective interpretations. Confidence and skill at interpretation can be gained, however, if competent instruction is followed by frequent practice.

Culturing a microbe from a clinical specimen, although time consuming, is sensitive, definitive, and offers the opportunity to perform in vitro antimicrobial sensitivity assays (Table 14-1).

Table 14-1

Time of Earliest Detection, Identification, and Antimicrobial Susceptibility
Testing of Certain Common Microbial Pathogens

Time	Detection	Identification	Antimicrobial[a] susceptibility
1 day	Streptococci Staphylococci Enterobacteriaceae[b] Pseudomonas aeruginosa	Streptococci Staphylococci	
2 days	Anaerobic bacteria[c] Herpes simplex virus (HSV) Yeasts[d] Molds[d] Chlamydia	Enterobacteriaceae P. aeruginosa HSV Chlamydia Yeast (Candida albicans)	Streptococci Staphylococci Enterobacteriaceae P. aeruginosa
3 days	Enterovirus[e] Coccidioides immitis		
5-7 days	Cytomegalovirus (CMV) Nocardia spp. Cryptococcus neoformans	Enterovirus Molds	
2-4 weeks	Mycobacterium tuberculosis	Molds	
>4 weeks	Histoplasma capsulatum Blastomyces dermatitidis	M. tuberculosis H. capsulatum B. dermatitidis	M. tuberculosis

[a] Data are being evaluated on the in vitro antimicrobial susceptibility testing of fungi. However, at present, antimicrobial susceptibility testing is usually only recommended for bacteria.
[b] The family Enterobacteriaceae includes the Gram-negative bacteria, Escherichia coli, Klebsiella spp., Citrobacter spp., Proteus spp., Enterobacter spp., Serratia spp., Salmonella spp., Shigella spp.
[c] Some common anaerobic bacteria are Bacteroides fragilis, Clostridium spp., Fusobacterium spp., and Propionibacterium acnes.
[d] Fungi pathogenic to man can be divided into two basic groups by vegatative growth forms: yeast and molds. Molds consist of those fungi that grow in filamentous form, whereas yeasts are unicellular and reproduce by budding.
[e] Enterovirus includes poliovirus, coxsackievirus, and echovirus.

Specimen Collection and Transport

As important as the proper laboratory techniques for direct visualization and culture are for diagnosis, many times the most critical steps in the identification of a pathogen occur before the specimen arrives in the laboratory, i.e., in the collection and transport of the specimen to the laboratory. The most well-equipped and well-staffed laboratory cannot overcome deficiencies introduced during the collection and transport of clinical specimens.

Specific techniques for the collection of specimens have been described in great detail elsewhere; however, the following comments can be used as a general guide. Blood, cerebrospinal fluid

(CSF), and other specimens taken by aspiration or under aseptic conditions at surgery are not normally contaminated by microbes other than the pathogenic agent (contamination does occur, however, when the correct specimen collection techniques are not followed, e.g., inadequate skin decontamination), whereas sputum, clean-catch urine, external wounds, and genital tract cultures are taken from areas of the body that are unavoidably associated with a resident bacterial population. This population is called the normal flora.

We all possess normal flora that exist for the most part as commensals, i.e., obtaining nutrients from the host but causing no harm. Therefore, the basic principle in specimen collection is to culture the active site of the lesion, avoiding the indigenous flora. This in reality is a difficult task because, for example, skin harbors approximately 10^5-10^7 bacteria/cm^2, mucous membranes support 10^7-10^8 bacteria/cm^2, and feces contain 10^{10}-10^{12} bacteria/g. Understandably, spurious results can arise when there is undue contamination of the specimen with the normal flora. Antisepsis and the use of invasive procedures are approaches that can be employed by the physician to eliminate or bypass the normal flora to obtain an uncontaminated specimen.

Iodine, soap, alcohol, or other agents can be used for antisepsis, e.g., skin preparation before needle aspiration or disinfection of the external genitalia before collection of a "clean catch" urine. Table 14-2 briefly describes the steps for proper disinfection before collection of the examples cited.

Transtracheal aspiration of sputum, suprapubic aspiration of urine, and needle and open lung biopsy are examples of techniques that may be used in extreme situations to aseptically "invade" the host to circumvent contamination by normal flora. It must be stated here that specimens obtained by invasive procedures must be treated with extreme care since a second specimen may be difficult or impossible to obtain. Prior notice to the laboratory will help assure proper and complete processing of the specimen.

The following techniques are used by the laboratory to eliminate or detect normal flora contamination: 1) specimen decontamination, e.g., sodium hydroxide treatment of sputum is used to selectively inhibit bacteria other than Mycobacterium tuberculosis; 2) use of selective and differential media, e.g., the medium used for the isolation of the diarrheal pathogens Salmonella and Shigella from feces contains inhibitory compounds for normal flora; 3) quantitative cultures, where the number of bacteria per

Table 14-2

Skin and External Genitalia Antisepsis
Before Specimen Collection

Skin antisepsis	External genitalia antisepsis	
	Females	Males
1. Select optimal site.	1. Wash hands, dry.	1. Wash hands, dry.
2. Cleanse site with 70% isoproponol.	2. With one hand hold labia apart until specimen is collected.	2. Retract foreskin.
3. Swab concentrically with 2% tincture of iodine.	3. Wash vulva with wet soaped sponge (5% tincture of green soap in water), front to back only. Discard, repeat 3 times.	3. Clean glans penis with wet soaped sponges.
4. Allow disinfectant to act for 1 minute.	4. Wash with warm sterile water.	4. Wash with warm sterile water.
5. Perform needle aspiration without hand contamination.	5. Void 20-25 ml and catch specimen in midstream in a sterile, wide-mouth urine container.	5. Void 20-25 ml and catch specimen in midstream.
	6. Avoid contact of container with legs, vulva, or clothing.	

milliliter or gram of specimen is determined (normal flora are present in low concentrations, pathogens in high concentrations); and 4) cytologic examination of sputum, exudates, and urine for the presence of squamous epithelial cells, which indicates contamination.

Attention must also be paid to the selection of the proper tool for collecting a microbiologic specimen. Swabs are convenient and economical to use, which probably explains their overuse in the clinical setting. In fact, swabs often provide inadequate amounts of specimen for complete laboratory analysis. At least 10^6 organisms must be present on a swab for their detection on a Gram-stained smear because the recovery of bacteria from swabs represents less than 10% of the original inoculum. Specific indications for the use of swabs include the collection of specimens from skin and mucous membranes (Table 14-3).

Needle aspiration should be used to collect pus or exudate and fluids obtained at surgery, whereas infected tissue should be biopsied (Table 14-3). For these specimens the phrase "more is better" certainly applies. Casual swabbing is pointedly discouraged.

After the specimen has been collected, it must be transported to the laboratory expeditiously. Drying, the presence of toxic fatty acids associated with cotton fibers, exposure to extremes of temperature, or exposure of anaerobic organisms to oxygen will result in decreased viability of fastidious organisms. When mixed flora are present in the specimen, a delay in transport may result in the true pathogen being obscured by an overgrowth of a nonpathogenic organism.

A variety of transport media has been developed to solve the above problems in a practical manner for bacteriology specimens. These media consist of non-nutritive substances that have been found to eliminate specimen drying and to maintain the original relative bacterial numbers by preventing the overgrowth of normal flora. Virus and Chlamydia transport media contain antibiotics to inhibit bacteria that may be present. The effectiveness of transport media decreases with time. Therefore, many laboratories require the recollection of specimens that are delayed in transport, e.g., for more than 2 hours.

Table 14-3

Indications for Use of Swabbing, Needle Aspiration, and Biopsy
for the Collection of Microbiologic Specimens

Methods	Specimens	Pathogens
Swabbing	Skin	Staphylococcus aureus Group A streptococci
	Genital	Trichomonas vaginalis Neisseria gonorrhoeae Chlamydia trachomatis Yeasts Herpes simplex virus
	Anal crypts	N. gonorrhoeae
	Rectum	Salmonella, Shigella
	Throat	Group A streptococci N. gonorrhoeae
Needle aspiration	Pus or exudates, fluids obtained at surgery, vesicular fluid	Anaerobic bacteria as well as all other pathogenic agents including mycobacteria and viruses
Biopsy	Infected tissue	Anaerobic bacteria as well as all other pathogenic agents including mycobacteria and fungi

- 303 -

Special treatment is required for specimens when the etiologic agent is thought to be anaerobic bacteria. The aspirate should be transported in a capped syringe, or a biopsy of deep tissue should be brought to the laboratory immediately after collection. If any delay is anticipated, the specimen should be placed into anaerobic transport media or into a container with reduced atmospheric oxygen.

The transport of urine for bacterial cultures also presents a problem in that urine will support the growth of bacteria. Since quantitative culture of urine is important in microbiologic diagnosis, it is imperative that the urine specimen be refrigerated if there is to be a delay in its transport.

All other specimens not transported in supportive media, especially spinal fluid and pus, must be transported and processed without delay to preserve the viability of the bacteria present in the specimen.

Direct Examination

Direct microscopic examination of clinical material can often provide a rapid presumptive identification and diagnosis of the etiologic agent in an infectious process. The Gram stain, acid-fast stain, potassium hydroxide (KOH) preparation, India ink preparation, and the direct wet mount are conventional techniques that are readily available to the physician (Table 14-4). Direc-

Table 14-4

Direct Microscopic Examination of Specimens by
Using Commonly Available Methods

Method	Pathogens
Gram stain	Bacteria, Nocardia spp., leukocytes
Acid-fast stain	Nocardia[a] spp., mycobacteria
KOH mount	Fungi
India ink stain	Cryptococcus neoformans
Wet mount	Trichomonas vaginalis Intestinal protozoa and helminths

[a] Nocardia are acid fast only when dilute acid in water is used for the decolorization step (termed "weak acid-fast stain"). Note: acid-alcohol is used for mycobacteria.

- 304 -

tions for the use of these techniques are listed in Table 14-5.
Concentration of the specimen by centrifugation is often helpful
to increase the sensitivity of direct visualization in certain
specimens, e.g., CSF.

Table 14-5

Procedures for Direct Visualization of Microorganisms
in Clinical Specimens

Procedure	Technique	Time	Results
Gram stain	Flood heat-fixed smear with crystal violet solution. Flood smear with iodine solution. Wash with tap water. Decolorize with solvent until reagent flows colorlessly off slide.[a] Counterstain with safranin.	1 min 1 min 5-30 sec 30 sec	Gram-positive bacteria are blue; Gram-negative bacteria are red.
Acid-fast stain	Flood heat-fixed smear with Kinyoun carbol-fuchsin. Decolorize with acid alcohol until reagent flows colorlessly off the slide.[a] Wash. Counterstain with methylene blue.	2 min 30 sec- 2 min 1 min	Acid-fast bacteria are red; the background and other organisms are blue.
KOH preparation	Mix pus, exudate, or tissue with an equal volume of 10% or 20% KOH. Cover with no. 2 coverslip and press to make a thin mount. Gentle warming may aid tissue clearing.	1 hr- overnight	Presence of fungal elements.
India ink preparation	Mix pus, exudate, sputum, or sediment from CSF with drop of India ink on a slide. Cover with no. 2 coverslip.	Immediate	Mucoid capsules of Cryptococcus appear as a clear halo that surrounds the yeast cell; the background is black.
Wet preparation	Mix specimen with sterile saline to a consistency where newspaper print can be read through the preparation after covering with no. 2 coverslip.	Immediate	Observe for motility, e.g., Entamoeba histolytica — progressive directional motility; Trichomonas spp. — jerky; Giardia lamblia — falling leaf in stream of water.

[a] The time for decolorization is dependent on the solvent used: 95% ethyl alcohol, slow; 100% acetone, fast; and acetone-alcohol, intermediate.

- 305 -

Table 14-6

Application of the Gram Stain to the
Diagnosis of Bacterial Infections

Disease	Specimen	Positive result	Indicators of poor specimen quality
Septicemia	Buffy coat skin lesion	Intra- or extracellular bacteria present	
Meningitis	Spinal fluid (centrifuged pellet)	Intra- or extracellular bacteria present; PMNs present[a]	
Wound infections	Tissue biopsy, aspirate	Bacteria present with pathogen in predominance; PMNs present	Squamous epithelial cells present
Pneumonia	Expectorated sputum	Bacteria present with pathogen in predominance; less than 10 squamous epithelial cells per low-power field	Mixed bacterial flora; greater than 10 squamous epithelial cells per low-power field
Urinary tract infections	Clean-catch urine (uncentrifuged)	Greater than 1 bacteria per oil-immersion field	Mixed bacterial flora; epithelial cells present
Genital tract infections	Swab	Intracellular Gram-negative diplococci; PMNs present.	Mixed bacterial flora; no PMNs

[a] PMNs, polymorphonuclear cells

The Gram stain is by far the stain most commonly used for the direct microscopic examination of clinical specimens and has been widely applied (Table 14-6). Not only is the method valuable for the morphologic characterization of bacteria, but it also detects characteristic structural differences in the cell envelope, i.e., Gram negativity versus Gram positivity, that are significant in determining the susceptibility of the microbe to antibiotic therapy. Leukocytes (which stain Gram negative) are also detected by Gram stain and are indicators of infectious processes. Polymorphonuclear leukocytes can be identified by their characteristic multilobed nucleus, whereas mononuclear cells cannot be further characterized by Gram stain and are termed round cells.

The Ziehl-Neelsen, Kinyoun, and auramine/rhodamine stains are used for the detection of acid-fast bacilli and __Nocardia__. Sputum, tissue suspensions, exudates and urine are all appropriate specimens for examination by acid-fast stains. The auramine/rhodamine stain is as specific as the Ziehl-Neelson and Kinyoun stains but is more sensitive since auramine/rhodamine-stained bacteria fluoresce and may be seen readily at a lower magnification than that for the other two stains. However, while these stains yield a rapid diagnosis, both false-positive and false-negative results occur.

KOH preparations of sputum, tissue suspensions, skin scrapings, and exudates will aid in the detection of fungal elements. Both hyphae and yeast cells may be better visualized after clearing tissue debris with the KOH. This method is useful for the diagnosis of vulvovaginitis caused by <u>Candida</u> <u>albicans</u> and for skin, lung, and other tissue infections caused by other fungi.

An India ink, wet mount preparation may be used on CSF from patients with chronic meningitis. If <u>Cryptococcus</u> <u>neoformans</u> is present, the encapsulated yeast cells can be visualized in this manner.

Wet mount preparations may be used to establish the diagnosis of vulvovaginitis caused by <u>Trichomonas</u> <u>vaginalis</u> by observing for the typical jerky motility of the organisms. Protozoan cysts and trophozoites and helminth eggs can be seen in wet preparations of stool specimens. The specific diagnosis of parasitic diseases should be left to experienced laboratory personnel, however.

In addition to the more or less standard battery of routine stains that have been described, other special stains may also be used to visualize certain pathogenic organisms in clinical material (Table 14-7). Paraffin sections of tissue can be stained with Gomori methenamine-silver stain for the detection of <u>Nocardia</u>, fungi, and <u>Pneumocystis</u> <u>carinii</u>. <u>P</u>. <u>carinii</u> can also be detected by touch preparations of lung tissue that are stained with toluidine blue or Giemsa. In addition, Giemsa can be used to stain <u>Plasmodium</u>, hemoflagellates, and microfilariae in blood smears and chlamydial inclusions in conjunctival scrapings. Trichrome stain is used to better visualize the nuclear and cytoplasmic character of protozoan parasites in order to confirm their identification. It is recommended that the above tests be performed and interpreted by skilled laboratory personnel.

Isolation by Culture

The growth of microorganisms in culture provides the opportunity for definitive identification and, for bacteria, antibiotic susceptibility testing. In addition, in vitro culture may be more sensitive than either direct visualization or antigen

Table 14-7

Direct Microscopic Examination of Specimens by
Using Special Stains

Stain	Pathogens
Gomori methenamine-silver	Nocardia, fungi, Pneumocystis carinii
Toluidine blue	P. carinii
Giemsa	P. carinii, Plasmodium, hemoflagellates, microfilariae, Chlamydia
	Herpes simplex virus
Trichrome	Protozoan cysts and trophozoites in stool
Dieterle silver	Legionella pneumophila; Legionella-like organisms

detection because of the multiplication of microbes in culture.
The disadvantage of in vitro cultivation is the prolonged time
interval between specimen collection and the isolation of the
microorganism. For example, 48 hours is usually the minimum time
necessary for complete identification and routine antibiotic
susceptibility testing for bacteria. Certain viruses, fungi, and
mycobacteria require considerably longer for their detection in
culture (Table 14-1).

Enriched, differential, and selective media in the form of
agar plates or tubed broth are used for the primary isolation of
bacteria and fungi from clinical material. Enriched broth media
is the most sensitive method for the culture of bacteria and is
used for specimens from sites that are not usually exposed to the
indigenous flora, e.g., blood cultures, where the isolation of a
single bacterial strain is expected. When enriched broth media
are contaminated with normal flora, overgrowth by these bacteria
would in all likelihood mask the presence of the pathogen.
Therefore, for specimens taken from mucous membranes or from the
gastrointestinal tract, selective and differential media have
been devised to isolate the pathogenic bacteria. These media
allow the bacteriologist to provide preliminary information about

the culture regarding the relative numbers of bacteria present and presumptive identification based on growth characteristics, colony morphology, and color changes. For example, MacConkey's agar selects for the enteric Gram-negative bacilli and differentiates the lactose and nonlactose (Salmonella and Shigella) fermenters within this group by media color change. Thayer-Martin media incorporate the antibiotics vancomycin, colistin, and nystatin in order to select for Neisseria gonorrhoeae.

Chlamydia and viruses are isolated in tissue cultures. The presumptive identification of viruses is based on the cytopathic effect (CPE), the time after inoculation that CPE is noted, and the predilection of the virus to specific cell culture varieties. Identification of Chlamydia is based on the detection by special staining of cytoplasmic inclusions in the tissue culture cells.

Antibiotic Sensitivity Testing

Isolated bacterial colonies may be tested for their susceptibility to antimicrobial agents. Two standard methods are used for susceptibility testing: the antimicrobial disc diffusion assay (Kirby-Bauer) and the broth or agar dilution determination of the minimum inhibitory concentration (MIC).

In the disc diffusion method, antibiotics diffuse out of drug-impregnated discs into media that have been streaked with a lawn of bacteria. The size of the zone of bacterial inhibition around the disc relates to the susceptibility of the isolate to the antibiotic. Antibiotic resistance will result in a narrow zone while susceptibility will be demonstrated by a wide zone. It is important to note that the resulting classification of organisms as sensitive (S) or resistant (R) correlates with levels of drug achievable in the blood only and do not, for example, take into account the increased concentration of certain drugs in urine or the exclusion of certain drugs from CSF.

The MIC is the determination of the minimum concentration of an antibiotic that will inhibit the growth of a patient's bacterial isolate. The MIC value that is generated must then be evaluated by the physician relative to the pharmacokinetics of the antibiotic. Although the MIC is a measure of bacterial growth inhibition by an antibiotic, it may also be important to determine the drug concentration that actually kills the bacteria, the minimum bactericidal concentration (MBC). The MIC and the MBC are usually equal or very close to the same dilution when bactericidal antibiotics are tested. However, certain strains,

particularly Staphylococcus aureus, may have a low MIC but a high
MBC. Thus the antibiotic concentration achieved in the patient
may inhibit but not kill the isolate. In this instance the resistant bacteria is called tolerant.

Antibiotic combination therapy can also be tested in vitro.
Drugs in combination can be synergistic, additive, or antago-
nistic in their actions.

SEROLOGIC DETECTION OF HOST ANTIBODIES AND MICROBIAL ANTIGENS IN BODY FLUIDS

Serologic tests have become an important tool in the diagnosis of certain infectious diseases. The principal advantage of
these methods is that they detect either antigen present in
various biologic fluids or specific antibody produced in response
to infection. Thus there is no requirement for the cultural isolation and biochemical identification of the infectious agent,
although confirmation of the rapid diagnosis by culture is desirable. In this light, serologic tests have become particularly
useful in cases in which the infectious agent has been cleared
from the patient by antimicrobial therapy, or under those circumstances in which the pathogen is difficult or impossible to
isolate by present cultural techniques, e.g., arboviruses,
Legionnaire's bacillus (Legionella pneumophila), and rickettsia.

The principal problem of serologic testing for serum antibodies stems from the fact that measurement of antibody levels at
a single point during the course of the disease is seldom useful
to confirm a diagnosis. An increase in antibody titer must be
observed between sera collected early (acute phase) and later
(convalescent phase) in the course of the disease. To establish
a diagnosis the difference in antibody titer should be at least a
fourfold rise, e.g., an acute phase serum dilution of 1:4 compared to a convalescent phase serum of 1:16 or greater. The
early and late sera should be assayed at the same time when
making this determination. An exception to this rule is in the
use of serology for the diagnosis of syphilis. A positive (any
titer) VDRL (Venereal Disease Research Laboratories) test or RPR
(rapid plasma reagin) test supported by a positive fluorescent
treponemal antibody absorption test is diagnostic of syphilis.
Another example of a single antibody titer being meaningful is a
rubella virus hemagglutination inhibition titer of 1:8 or greater
in the serum of a pregnant woman. Here any amount of antibody
indicates that the patient is immune to infection with rubella

virus and more importantly indicates that the offspring is not likely to be afflicted with congenital rubella infection.

Detection of Host Antibody in Body Fluids

Host antibody in serum can be detected by reacting the specimen with whole bacterial cells or with soluble microbial antigen, either attached to inert matrices or free in solution. Specific interaction of sera and suspensions of whole cells or antigen-coated carrier molecules is detected by clumping (agglutination) of the reactants into large insoluble aggregates. Mixing sera with soluble antigen results in precipitation of the antigen-antibody complexes. The interaction of some immunoglobulins with their specific antigens does not readily result in insoluble complexes. These antibodies can be detected by incubating the serum with microorganisms or specific antigens that have been attached to the surface of a solid support, such as a glass microscope slide or to the bottom of a well in a plastic tray. The patient's antibody bound to this antigen can be detected by the addition of antihuman immunoglobulin antibody that has been labeled with a fluorescent compound (immunofluorescence) or an enzyme (enzyme-linked immunosorbent assay or ELISA). The addition of patient serum to a specific virus preparation often results in viral inactivation (neutralization) that is manifested in failure of the virus to successfully infect tissue culture and produce the characteristic CPE. Similarly, certain bacterial toxins can be inactivated after incubation with patient serum. The toxin neutralization can be detected by the loss of the typical CPE or of a toxin-specific enzymatic reaction. The ability of certain antibodies to bind complement can also be used as a diagnostic aid. Free complement present in the assay mixture can be detected by lysis of red blood cells in conjunction with an antierythrocyte antibody (hemolysin). Table 14-8 lists some common microbial pathogens and the tests routinely used to detect antibody produced in response to infection with these organisms.

Detection of Microbial Antigen in Body Fluids

Detection of microbe-specific antigen directly in a patients' specimen is the most rapid method for the diagnosis of an infectious disease. The necessity for culturing the offending organism and waiting for the host to mount a detectable immune response is eliminated. The principal concern is the potential

Table 14-8

Methods for the Detection of Antibody Produced
in Response to Microbial Infection

Serologic reaction	Pathogens
Precipitation	Fungi
Agglutination	Leptospira Francisella tularensis Brucella sp. Treponema pallidum Entamoeba histolytica Epstein-Barr virus Rubella virus Rickettsia
Immunofluorescence	Legionella spp. T. pallidum Cytomegalovirus Herpes simplex virus Toxoplasma gondii
Neutralization	Group A streptococci Viruses Cytomegalovirus Herpes simplex virus Rubella virus T. gondii T. pallidum
Complement fixation	Fungi Herpes simplex Cytomegalovirus T. pallidum

for a false-positive result occurring from the interaction of antibody with crossreacting antigen.

Generally, immunoglobulin preparations made by immunization of a laboratory animal with the purified microbial antigen are incubated with the body fluid specimen, and the reaction mixture is examined for the evidence of a specific reaction, e.g., agglutination or precipitation. If a reaction is present, the specimen must contain the microbial antigen. Several detection systems are available. The simplest consists of latex beads coated with antigen-specific antibody. Mixing these beads with reactive antigen-containing specimens results in agglutination. The tendency of antigen and antibody to migrate in an electric current is utilized to detect antigen by counterimmunoelectrophoresis (CIE). Here the specimen and an antisera are placed in separate wells in an agar plate and an electric current is applied. The antigen in the specimen and the immunoglobulin in the antisera move toward each other, and where the zone of antigen-antibody equivalence is reached, a precipitin band forms. Table 14-9 lists common antigen detection methods, the micro-organisms identified, and the appropriate specimen.

Table 14-9

Methods for the Detection of Microbial Antigens

Antigen detection method	Microbial pathogens	Appropriate specimen
CIE	Streptococcus pneumoniae	CSF, serum, urine, sputum, and pleural and other body fluids
	Neisseria meningitidis	CSF, serum, urine
	Hemophilus influenzae type B	CSF, serum, urine
	Group B streptococci	CSF
Latex agglutination	H. influenzae type B, group B streptococci, S. pneumoniae, N. meningitidis, Cryptococcus neoformans	CSF, serum, urine
ELISA	Rotavirus	Stool
Immunofluorescence	Legionella	Lung
	Herpes simplex virus	Brain

Lorian, V. (ed.). Significance of Medical Microbiology in the Care of Patients. Williams and Wilkins, Baltimore, 1981.

Washington, J.A. (ed.). Laboratory Procedures in Clinical Microbiology. Springer-Verlag, New York, 1981.

Chapter 15

SPECIMEN COLLECTION PROCEDURES

INTRODUCTION

The goals of specimen collection are to 1) obtain an appropriate specimen of adequate volume and 2) limit the preanalytic component of measurement variability while 3) minimizing the pain and risk of complications for the patient. The collection methods described in this chapter have been designed with these goals in mind. But sound methods alone are not enough. The clinician must also develop technical skill in the performance of the procedures. To that end, guidance from an experienced teacher, practice, and more practice are needed.

VENIPUNCTURE
Equipment and Reagents

Antiseptic: 70% isopropanol is preferred. Disposable gauze wipes soaked in isopropanol are available.

Sterile cotton gauze pads: 2x2 inches is a convenient size.

Sterile syringe and plunger or vacuum tube holder: Disposable plastic syringes have replaced reusable glass syringes. A vacuum tube holder need not be sterile.

Disposable needle: The gauge of the needle should be appropriate to the size of the vessel to be entered. A "butterfly" needle (a short needle attached to a flexible plastic tube that ends in a syringe hub) may be used but is rarely available in smaller gauges. Two-sided needles are required when vacuum tube containers are used.

Tourniquet

Specimen tubes: Venous blood is always collected into tubes. Sealed vacuum tubes are a popular choice.

Sites

Preferred site: veins of the antecubital fossa

Alternate sites: lower arm veins, hand veins

<u>Procedure</u>

1. Have the patient sit or lie down.

2. Prepare the specimen tubes and the needle/holder/syringe assembly and place them beside the patient.

3. Select the arm to be used for the procedure. Position the arm so that it is straight, well supported, and comfortable. Position yourself so that you are comfortable and have ready access to the puncture site.

4. Place the tourniquet about 10 cm above the elbow to distend the veins. By palpation, identify a vein that is of adequate size, pliant, and well seated (visual inspection will not detect many excellent deeper veins.) If the veins are difficult to palpate, blood flow to the arm may be accentuated by wrapping the arm in a warm towel for 10 minutes prior to the procedure. Alternatively, <u>limited</u> forearm exercise (for example, making a fist) can be used in an effort to "bring out" a vein. Do not massage or slap the arm.

5. Release the tourniquet before proceeding.

6. Cleanse the puncture site with antiseptic and allow it to air dry or wipe it dry with a sterile gauze pad.

7. Reapply the tourniquet.

8. Hold the skin taut over the puncture site by applying downward tension on the forearm with the thumb of the free hand. The free hand is also often needed to provide additional support for the patient's arm.

9. Hold the needle/holder/syringe assembly in the line of the vein to be punctured at an angle approximately 30° with the arm. The bevel of the needle should be up, the cutting tip down.

10. Puncture the skin and underlying vein, using a steady, moderately fast movement. The needle should be advanced no deeper than the estimated distance needed to enter the lumen of the vein. A slight give can usually be felt when the vein is entered. Also blood can often be seen at the needle hub.

11. Apply negative pressure by puncturing the vacuum tube or by gently retracting the syringe plunger. Blood should flow freely into the tube or syringe. If the flow is irregular, rotate the needle to reposition the bevel. Sometimes the needle tip has passed through the vein — the lumen can be reentered by pulling the needle backward slightly.

12. Remove the tourniquet once blood is flowing into the tube or syringe to prevent venous stasis at the puncture site.

13. Once the specimen has been collected, remove the needle and immediately apply pressure to the site, using a sterile gauze pad until the bleeding stops. The patient may apply the pressure with his/her hand. Do not allow the patient to bend his/her arm as this reopens the defect in the vein.

14. Specimen tubes containing anticoagulants must be mixed promptly and may be inverted with one hand while applying pressure with the other.

15. A sterile adhesive bandage may be applied to the puncture site.

Sources of Variability

1. Increased capillary hydrostatic pressure causes water to shift from the intravascular into the interstitial space. Blood cells, plasma proteins, and protein-bound constituents will be present in increased concentrations in this setting because they will be distributed in a reduced volume of plasma water. This is called hemoconcentration. It can result from a systemic increase in capillary pressure such as is seen with prolonged standing or from local effects, most notably, a prolonged time of application of the tourniquet during venipuncture. Both the time of standing prior to venipuncture and the time of tourniquet application should be kept to a minimum.

2. Rapid flow through small-bore needles and exposure to large negative pressures lead to hemolysis with its accompanying contamination of the plasma portion of the blood specimen with red cell cytoplasmic constituents. Hemolysis is minimized by the use of large-bore needles, moderate flow rates, and moderate negative pressures. Invert specimen tubes gently to mix the blood with additives.

3. Blood specimen contamination with intravenous fluids is not uncommon. Blood should not be drawn from a site above an intravenous infusion, but must be obtained from a site on the patient's other arm or, if necessary, below the infusion site.

Medical Considerations

1. Local trauma from a venipuncture is usually minimal. If bleeding into the soft tissues or from the skin puncture site is noted during the procedure, the tourniquet should be removed immediately and direct pressure applied.
2. At the end of the venipuncture, direct pressure should always be applied to the puncture site until bleeding has ceased. This may take a long time in patients who are anticoagulated or who have a bleeding disorder.
3. Thrombosis and thrombophlebitis are rare complications.
4. Some patients become faint during venipuncture. The procedure should be terminated immediately and the patient should lie flat until he/she recovers.

ARTERIAL PUNCTURE

Equipment and Reagents

The necessary equipment for an arterial puncture is usually available as a packaged, sterilized "arterial blood gas set."

Antiseptic: Povidone-iodine is the preferred agent.

Local anesthetic: Lidocaine hydrochloride is the preferred agent.

Sodium heparin solution (1000 or 5000 U/ml)

Sterile cotton gauze pads: 2x2 inches is a convenient size.

Sterile syringes and plungers: Disposable plastic syringes or reusable glass syringes may be used. A disposable plastic syringe is used to administer the anesthetic.

Disposable needles: A 19-gauge needle is usually used when heparinizing the syringe, and a 25-gauge needle is used when administering the anesthetic. Medium-bore needles (e.g., 21 gauge) are usually used for the actual puncture.

Specimen containers: Specimens should be collected in the containers recommended by the hospital laboratory. Almost always the syringe itself will serve as the specimen container.

Sites

Preferred sites: brachial and radial arteries
(If using the radial artery, test for collateral blood supply via the ulnar artery.)

Alternate sites: Use of the femoral artery is discouraged.

Procedure

1. Using a large-bore needle, draw 1 ml of sodium heparin solution into the syringe and with it thoroughly lubricate the barrel. Test the plunger to assure easy mobility, then expel the heparin, leaving the dead space filled with residual heparin.

2. Identify the artery to be punctured by its pulsations.

3. Cleanse the skin over the puncture site, using the antiseptic.

4. The use of local anesthesia is not required but is encouraged. Infiltrate the skin and soft tissue at the puncture site with 1 ml of lidocaine hydrochloride.

5. If necessary, change the needle on the syringe. For puncture, the needle gauge should be appropriate to the caliber of the artery to be entered.

6. Position the arm so that it is well supported and comfortable. Dorsiflexion of the wrist may be required for the radial artery. Position yourself so that you are comfortable and have ready access to the puncture site.

7. Hold the needle/syringe parallel to the artery at an angle of 45°-60°. The bevel of the needle should be up, the cutting tip down.

8. Puncture the skin and underlying artery, using a steady, moderately fast movement. The needle should be advanced no further than the estimated distance needed to enter the lumen of the artery. A slight give can usually be felt when the artery is entered.

9. Once the specimen has been collected, withdraw the needle and immediately compress the puncture site for at least 5 minutes, using a sterile gauze.

10. If air has accidentally been aspirated into the syringe, expel it.

11. Remove the needle, place an airtight cap over the tip of the syringe, and place the syringe into ice.

12. Deliver the specimen to the laboratory immediately.

Sources of Variability

1. Contact with air, even as air bubbles within the syringe, will result in substantial alterations in the partial pressure of oxygen (P_{O2}) in the specimen. Because the P_{O2} of arterial blood is always subatmospheric in patients who are not receiving oxygen therapy, exposure to

air for even short periods will cause the P_{O2} to increase. Air bubbles should be expelled from the syringe, and the tip of the syringe should be capped securely.

2. Because carbon dioxide is readily absorbed into heparin solution, a large volume of heparin in the collection syringe (as can happen in small syringes with large dead spaces) will cause a decrease in the P_{CO2} of the specimen. Minimize the residual heparin in the syringe prior to obtaining the specimen.

3. Cellular respiration in a blood specimen leads to a decrease in its P_{O2}. Cooling the specimen to $0^{\circ}C$ by immersing it in ice water effectively slows this process. Immediate delivery and processing of the specimen further reduces the likelihood of significant oxygen consumption.

Medical Considerations

1. Local anesthesia can greatly reduce the discomfort experienced by the patient, so its use is encouraged.

2. Local trauma from an arterial puncture is usually minimal when arm arteries are used. In adults, femoral arteries are frequently atherosclerotic. Consequently, puncture of these arteries can lead to dislodgment of atherosclerotic material, with downstream embolism. In addition, hemostasis is much more difficult to achieve with an atherosclerotic vessel. This is especially problematic for the femoral arteries, which lie deep in the soft tissues of the groin where direct pressure cannot be applied effectively. Massive blood loss can occur. In consideration of these concerns, femoral artery punctures are discouraged.

3. At the end of the procedure, direct pressure must be applied to the puncture site until the bleeding has stopped. This takes at least 5 minutes. A much longer time will be required for patients who are anticoagulated or who have a bleeding disorder.

4. Thrombosis is an uncommon complication of arterial puncture. Nonetheless, collateral circulation to the hand via the ulnar artery must be confirmed prior to use of the radial artery as a puncture site.

5. When the brachial artery is used as a puncture site, care must be taken to avoid the underlying brachial nerve.

FINGERSTICK

(Meites and Levitt 1981)

Equipment and Reagents

Antiseptic: 70% isopropanol is preferred. Disposable gauze
wipes soaked in isopropanol are available.

Sterile cotton gauze pads: 2x2 inches is a convenient size.

Skin puncture lancet: Sterile disposable lancets should be
used.

Specimen containers: A variety of disposable microspecimen
containers are available. Specimens should be collected in
the container recommended by the hospital laboratory.

Sites

Palmar surface of the distal phalanx of the second, third, or
fourth fingers

Procedure

1. Choose a finger that is not cold, cyanotic, or swollen.
   Note: If the patient's hands are cold, wrap one of them
   in a towel warmed in hot water ($39^{\circ}-44^{\circ}C$) for 3-10 minutes before the puncture is performed.

2. Cleanse the puncture site with the antiseptic.

3. Wipe the site dry with a sterile gauze pad.

4. Remove the lancet from its protective paper without
   touching the tip.

5. Hold the patient's finger firmly with one hand and make a
   swift puncture with the lancet, halfway between the center of the ball of the finger and its side. The puncture
   should be 2-3 mm deep.

6. The cut should be made across the fingerprints to produce
   a large round drop of blood.

7. Wipe away the first drop of blood with a sterile gauze
   pad.

8. Ease and reapply the pressure on the proximal portion of
   the finger as drops of blood form and are collected. Do
   not massage the finger.

9. Collect the specimen.

10. Once the collection is complete, apply pressure to the
    site with a sterile gauze pad until bleeding stops.

11. A sterile adhesive bandage may be used.

Sources of Variability

1. Gentle pulsatile pressure on the finger in the manner described in the above procedure usually produces adequate capillary blood flow for a complete collection. In addition, traumatic hemolysis and contamination of the specimen with extracellular fluid is minimized. However, even when proper technique is employed, hemolysis is not uncommon.

2. Capillary blood differs in composition from arterial and venous blood. If the finger is properly warmed, capillary blood will resemble arterial blood closely. Still, when there is impaired peripheral perfusion, even a warm limb will yield capillary blood more similar to venous blood.

Medical Considerations

1. Local trauma from a fingerstick is minimal when a proper sized lancet is used and only gentle pressure is applied. Deep incisions or vigorous manipulation of the site lead to soft tissue bleeding and certainly to greater pain for the infant.

HEELSTICK

(Meites and Levitt 1981)

Equipment and Reagents

Antiseptic: 70% isopropanol is preferred. Disposable gauze wipes soaked in isopropanol are available.

Sterile cotton gauze pads: 2x2 inches is a convenient size.

Skin puncture lancet: Sterile, disposable lancets should be used. For neonates younger than 6 months, the lancet tip must be less than 2.5 mm in length.

Specimen containers: A variety of disposable microspecimen containers are available. Specimens for blood gas determinations should be collected in the containers recommended by the hospital laboratory.

Sites

The safe area for heelstick is indicated in Figure 15-1. Use only the areas shown in black.

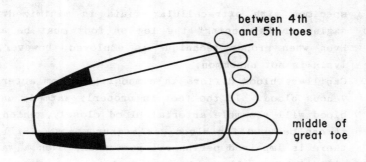

between 4th
and 5th toes

middle of
great toe

Fig 15-1   Safe Areas of an Infant's Foot
to Use for a Heelstick

Procedure

1. Warm the foot to be punctured. Wrap it in a towel soaked in hot tap water (39°-44°C) for 3-10 minutes before the puncture is performed.
2. Cleanse the puncture site with the antiseptic.
3. Wipe the site dry with a sterile gauze pad.
4. Remove the lancet from its protective paper without touching the tip.
5. Lay the infant down so that his or her foot is horizontal throughout the procedure. Hold the infant's heel firmly with the forefinger at the arch of the foot and with the thumb at the ankle.
6. Make a swift puncture with the lancet held perpendicular to the skin surface.
7. Wipe away the first drop of blood with a sterile gauze pad.
8. Ease and reapply pressure with the thumb as drops of blood form and are collected. Do not massage the foot or leg.
9. Collect the specimen.
10. Once the collection is complete, apply pressure to the site with a sterile gauze pad until bleeding stops.
11. Do not use adhesive bandages.

Sources of Variability

1. Gentle pulsatile pressure on the foot in the manner described in the above procedure usually produces adequate capillary blood flow for a complete collection. In addition, traumatic hemolysis and contamination of the

specimen with extracellular fluid is minimized. Massaging or "stripping" the leg or foot must be avoided. Even when proper technique is employed, however, hemolysis is not uncommon.

2. Capillary blood differs in composition from arterial and venous blood. If the foot is properly warmed, capillary blood will resemble arterial blood closely, which is why it can be used for blood gas measurements. Still, when there is impaired peripheral perfusion, even a warm limb will yield capillary blood more similar to venous blood.

Medical Considerations

1. The puncture must be made in the safe areas to avoid entering the calcaneus. Osteomyelitis of the cancaneus can occur if the bone is entered.
2. Local trauma from a heelstick is minimal when the proper sized lancet is used and only gentle pressure is applied. Deeper incisions or vigorous manipulation of the site lead to soft tissue bleeding and certainly to greater pain for the infant.

LUMBAR PUNCTURE

(Fishman 1980)

Equipment and Reagents

The necessary equipment for a lumbar puncture is usually available as a packaged, sterilized "lumbar puncture tray."

Antiseptic: Povidone-iodine solution is the preferred antiseptic agent.

Local anesthetic: Lidocaine hydrochloride is the preferred agent.

Sterile syringe and plunger: A 10-ml syringe is used to administer the anesthetic.

Disposable needles: 25- and 20-gauge needles are usually used when administering the anesthetic.

Spinal needle: This should be 20- or 22-gauge.

Three-way stopcock

Manometer

Specimen containers: Specimens should be collected in the containers recommended by the hospital laboratory.

Sterile adhesive bandage

Sites

The lowest usable spinal interspace possible: L3-L4, L4-L5, or L5-S1.

Procedure

1. Monitor the patient's cardiorespiratory status during and following the procedure.
2. Place the patient in the lateral recumbent position with the craniospinal axis parallel to the floor and the flat of the back perpendicular to the procedure table.
3. Place the patient in the flexed knee-chest position. An assistant is needed to aid the patient in maintaining this position.
4. Identify by the palpation the spinal processes and interspaces. The line connecting the tops of the two iliac crests usually crosses the L3-L4 interspace. Use interspace L3-L4, L4-L5, or L5-S1.
5. Cleanse the skin over the puncture site using the antiseptic. The remainder of the procedure is performed with sterilized equipment and sterile technique.
6. Local anesthesia is usually employed. Infiltrate the skin and soft tissue at the puncture site with 2-3 ml of lidocaine hydrochloride. Use the 25-gauge needle for the skin and the 20-gauge needle for the soft tissue.
7. Insert a 20- or 22-gauge spinal needle with stylet in the midsaggital line of the prepared interspace. Hold the needle perpendicular to the plane of the back.
8. Advance the needle through the longitudinal ligament into the subarachnoid space. A slight "give" is usually felt when the needle penetrates the dura.
9. Remove the stylet. If cerebrospinal fluid (CSF) appears, the space has been entered. If no fluid appears, replace the stylet and rotate the needle 90°. Again remove the stylet and check for CSF. If there is still no fluid, replace the stylet and advance the needle a few more millimeters. Feel for the give of the dura and check for fluid. If this fails, withdraw the needle until the tip is subcutaneous, then redirect it along a new midline path. Again check for CSF.
10. When fluid appears at the needle hub, quickly attach the three-way stopcock and manometer. Orient the manometer in the true vertical. CSF should flow freely into the

manometer. This can be tested by having the assistant apply, then release firm pressure to the abdomen. The CSF pressure should rapidly rise and fall in response to the maneuver. If the CSF flow is sluggish or unresponsive to abdominal pressure, rotate the needle or, if necessary, reposition it.

11. Record the "opening pressure" (millimeters CSF) once it has become steady. The patient should be relaxed during the measurement.

12. If the "opening pressure" is elevated (>200 mm) or if the pressure quickly falls, only 1-2 m of CSF should be removed. If the opening pressure is less than 200 mm, withdraw adequate fluid to preform the desired studies. (If more than 20-30 ml is removed rapidly, a mild transient postural headache is likely.)

13. After the CSF sample has been removed, record the volume of CSF obtained and the "closing pressure" (millimeters CSF).

14. Replace the stylet and remove the needle.

15. Apply a sterile adhesive bandage to the puncture site.

16. Have the patient rest in the prone position for at least 3 hours following the procedure.

Sources of Variability

1. The CSF pressure is raised in patients who are straining. The patient should be relaxed and quiet during the determination of the opening pressure.

2. Incision of a vessel in the ventral vertebral venous plexus can lead to contamination of the CSF specimen with blood. This is referred to as a traumatic tap. In order to distinguish a traumatic tap from a valid finding of bloody CSF, centrifuge the first and last specimen tubes collected. If the fractional volume of blood in the last tube collected is much less than that in the first, the blood probably comes from a traumatic tap. A xanthochromic supernatant following CSF centrifugation indicates prepuncture CSF blood.

3. Adequate fluid should be withdrawn to perform the requisite laboratory studies. It is not the volume of fluid removed at the time of puncture (about 10 ml), but the subsequent leakage of CSF through the dural defect that is usually responsible for the volume-related complications of the procedure.

<u>Medical Considerations</u>

1. There are three settings in which the performance of a
   lumbar puncture entails a significant risk of a life-
   threatening complication. These are:
   a. The patient with increased intracranial pressure.
      Complication: brain herniation.
   b. The patient who has a hemorrhagic diathesis.
      Complication: spinal subarachnoid, subdural, or
      epidural hematoma.
   c. The patient with an infection at the proposed site of
      the lumbar puncture.
      Complication: meningitis.
   Each of these settings is a <u>relative contraindication</u> for
   a lumbar puncture. The need for a CSF specimen must outweigh the risk involved if a lumbar puncture is performed
   in such cases.
2. Respiratory compromise, which can mimic ventilation failure from brain herniation, can develop in weak patients
   or patients with pulmonary disease who are held in a
   highly flexed position. Be certain that the patient can
   breathe comfortably while positioned for the procedure.
3. The most common complication of lumbar puncture is
   postural headache, which is often accompanied by back-
   ache. The incidence of headache depends upon the technique and can be as high as 20%. Headache is uncommon
   when small-bore spinal needles are used, when the number
   of punctures is minimized, and when patients remain prone
   at least 3 hours following the procedure.
4. Radicular symptoms following a lumbar puncture suggest
   spinal nerve root trauma. Incorrect technique is the
   most frequent explanation for this complication. Spinal
   nerves are displaced and stretched when the CSF specimen
   is obtained using plunger action or when the spinal needle stylet is not replaced prior to withdrawal of the
   needle.

THORACENTESIS
(Fraser and Pare 1977; Kovarik 1970)

<u>Equipment and Reagents</u>

The necessary equipment for a thoracentesis is usually available as a packaged, sterilized "thoracentesis tray."
Antiseptic: Povidone-iodine solution is the preferred antiseptic agent.

Local anesthetic: Lidocaine hydrochloride is the preferred
agent.
Sterile syringes and plungers: A 10-ml syringe is used to
administer the anesthetic.   A 30 to 50-ml syringe is used
for pleural fluid withdrawal.
Disposable needles: 25- and 20-gauge needles are usually
used when administering the anesthetic.
Thoracentesis needle: an 18- or 20-gauge spinal needle or
intravascular catheter with trocar
Three-way stopcock
Sterile tubing: 30-50 cm of tubing should be adequate.
Hemostat
Specimen containers: Specimens should be collected in the
containers recommended by the hospital laboratory.
Sterile adhesive bandage

Sites

The intercostal space at the site of maximum dullness to per-
cussion; usually in its posterolateral aspect.   Posteriorly
the site should be above the ninth rib, and laterally, above
the seventh rib.

Procedure

1. Place the patient in the sitting position, preferably
   with his or her legs over the side of the procedure
   table.   Support the patient's feet and rest his or her
   arms on a pillow on a tableside stand.
2. Place the patient's arm, on the side to undergo thoracentesis, across his or her chest with the hand resting
   on the opposite shoulder.
3. Cleanse the skin over the puncture site using the antiseptic.   An area incorporating three interspaces should
   be cleansed.   The remainder of the procedure is performed
   with sterilized equipment and sterile technique.
4. Infiltrate the skin and soft tissue at the puncture site
   with 5 ml of lidocaine hydrochloride.   Use the 25-gauge
   needle for the skin and the 20-gauge needle for the soft
   tissues.   Always advance the needle above the lower rib.
   The intercostal nerve and blood vessels located at the
   lower margin of the upper rib are thereby avoided.   The
   patient will usually complain of pain when the parietal
   pleura is touched.   Inject the bulk of the anesthetic

there. Reposition the needle a number of times to assure that a large area of pleura is anesthetized.

5. For the thoracentesis, use the thoracentesis needle and large syringe. If a large volume of fluid is to be removed, use an intravascular catheter as described below.

6. Insert the thoracentesis needle into the prepared interspace. While applying modest negative pressure with the plunger, advance the needle through the interspace, always staying just above the lower rib. Once the parietal pleura has been punctured and fluid can be aspirated, affix the hemostat to the needle flush with the skin to stabilize the needle's depth.

7. If no fluid appears after the thoracentesis needle has been inserted just beyond the parietal pleura, withdraw the needle until the tip is subcutaneous, then redirect it along a new path, always staying just above the lower rib.

8. With the needle secure, obtain adequate fluid to perform the desired studies.

9. To collect a large volume of pleural fluid, an intravascular catheter should be used. Insert the trocar with catheter into the prepared interspace and advance it on through the parietal pleura, always staying just above the lower rib. When fluid appears in the catheter tubing, remove the trocar while keeping the catheter in place. Attach the three-way stopcock to the hub and the syringe to the stopcock. Also attach the plastic tubing to the stopcock. The pleural fluid can be drained directly through the tubing, or the syringe can be used to obtain fluid, which then is expelled through the tubing.

10. Remove the needle or catheter. Apply direct pressure to the puncture site to seal the puncture track and prevent aspiration of air.

11. Apply a sterile adhesive bandage to the puncture site.

12. Monitor the patient's respiratory status. Obtain a radiograph of the chest following the procedure to check for a pneumothorax.

Sources of Variability

1. Incision of a vessel can lead to contamination of the pleural fluid specimen with blood. The volume of fluid is usually so large that such contamination has little

effect upon the laboratory studies. However, this possibility must be kept in mind if the study results are at variance with the clinical impression.

Medical Considerations

1. The most common complication of thoracentesis is pneumothorax due to puncture of the visceral pleura. This is usually small and does not produce symptoms. Larger pneumothoraces require prompt therapy. The risk of puncturing the visceral pleura is minimized by 1) avoiding those portions of the chest where pleural adhesions are known to exist, 2) advancing the thoracentesis needle only just beyond (less than 1 cm) the parietal pleura, and 3) using flexible, nonincising catheter tubing if a large volume of pleural fluid is to be removed.

2. Subcutaneous emphysema around the needle track is avoided by sealing the puncture site immediately after withdrawing the needle.

3. Hemorrhage into the intercostal space and the pleural cavity will occur if the intercostal vessels, especially the artery, are punctured. Significant acute blood loss and hemothorax can result. This complication is rare if the needle is advanced through the intercostal space, always staying just above the lower rib.

4. Puncture of the diaphragm and subdiaphragmatic organs is avoided by proper positioning of the puncture site. The site should not be below the ninth rib posteriorly or the seventh rib laterally.

ABDOMINAL PARACENTESIS

Equipment and Reagents

The necessary equipment for an abdominal paracentesis is usually available as a packaged, sterilized "paracentesis tray."

Antiseptic: Povidone-iodine solution is the preferred agent.

Local anesthetic: Lidocaine hydrochloride is the preferred agent.

Sterile syringes and plungers: A 10-ml syringe is used to administer the anesthetic. A 30 to 50-ml syringe is used for peritoneal fluid withdrawal.

Disposable needles: 25- and 20-gauge needles are usually used when administering the antiseptic.

Paracentesis needle: a 20-gauge spinal needle or intravascular catheter with trocar

Three-way stopcock

Sterile tubing: 30-50 cm of tubing should be adequate.

Specimen containers: Specimens should be collected in the
containers recommended by the hospital laboratory.

Sterile adhesive bandage

Sites

The avascular midline, through the linea alba, one-third of
the distance from the umbilicus to the symphysis, and the
lower quadrants, 1-2 cm lateral to the margin of rectus
sheaths, are the two preferred sites. The upper quadrants
can be used, but only after the location of the liver and
spleen are demonstrated. Avoid surgical scars.

Procedure

1. Have the patient empty his or her bladder.
2. Place the patient in the supine position on the procedure
   table.
3. Cleanse the skin over the puncture site(s) using the
   antiseptic. The remainder of the procedure is performed
   using sterilized equipment and sterile technique.
4. Infiltrate the skin and soft tissue at the puncture site
   with lidocaine hydrochloride (5-10 ml of anesthetic for
   each site). Use the 25-gauge needle for the skin and the
   20-gauge needle for the soft tissue.
5. Insert the paracentesis needle into the prepared site.
   Hold it perpendicular to the abdominal wall. If the
   linea alba is to be punctured, have the patient lift
   his or her head off the pillow to tense the rectus ab-
   dominis and its sheath. Before the peritoneal cavity is
   entered, tip the needle toward the pelvis to avoid entering the posterior abdominal vessels if the needle
   passes too far posteriorly.
6. If no fluid appears after the paracentesis needle has
   been inserted through the peritoneum, advance the needle
   a short distance (less than 2 cm) while applying modest
   negative pressure with the plunger. To reposition the
   needle, withdraw it until its tip is at the peritoneum,
   then slowly redirect it along a new path.
7. Once fluid can be aspirated, obtain adequate fluid to
   perform the desired studies.

8. To collect a large volume of peritoneal fluid, an intra-vascular catheter should be used. Insert the trocar with catheter into the prepared site and advance it through the peritoneum. When fluid appears in the catheter tubing, remove the trocar while keeping the catheter in place. Attach a three-way stopcock to the hub and the syringe to the stopcock. Also attach the plastic tubing to the stopcock. The fluid can be drained directly through the tubing or the syringe can be used to obtain fluid, which then is expelled through the tubing. Never withdraw more than 500 ml of fluid.

9. Remove the needle or catheter. Apply direct pressure to the puncture site.

10. Apply a sterile adhesive bandage to the puncture site.

11. Monitor the patient's renal status.

Sources of Variability

1. Incision of a vessel can lead to contamination of the peritoneal fluid specimen with blood. The volume of fluid is usually so large that such contamination has little effect upon the laboratory studies. However, this possibility must be kept in mind if the study values are at variance with the clinical impression.

Medical Considerations

1. The performance of an abdominal paracentesis in a patient with a hemorrhagic diathesis is associated with a significant risk of serious abdominal wall or intraperitoneal hemorrhage. Because of this risk, this setting is a relative contraindication for a paracentesis. The procedure can be made much safer by therapeutic correction of the bleeding disorder (if possible) and by using the linea alba puncture site only.

2. Perforation of bowel is unusual if the bowel is mobile. Even if punctured, the bowel usually does not leak its contents. Peritonitis can develop, however, so closely monitor any patient who suffers a bowel perforation during paracentesis. The chance of puncturing the bowel is minimized by 1) not selecting a puncture site near a surgical scar (intraperitoneal adhesions can tack the bowel to the anterior abdominal wall), 2) awaiting decompression of the bowel in patients with bowel distension,

and 3) using flexible, nonincising catheter tubing if a large volume of peritoneal fluid is to be removed.

3. Puncture of the bladder is avoided by making certain that the patient's bladder is empty. Keep medial to the gall bladder and liver when placing a puncture in the right upper quadrant and avoid the spleen in the left upper quadrant.

4. Peritoneal fluid may leak from puncture sites and may infiltrate along puncture tracks into the abdominal wall.

5. In patients with cirrhosis, the removal of a large volume of peritoneal fluid (more than 500 ml) can lead to a decrease in the circulating blood volume as the fluid rapidly reaccumulates. Oliguria and shock can result. Therefore, never withdraw more than 500 ml of fluid during a procedure.

URINE: RANDOM VOIDED SPECIMEN
(Free and Free 1975)

Equipment

Specimen container: The container should be chemically clean and sealable; disposable plastic cups are preferred.

Procedure

1. Random specimens may be collected at any time.

2. Instruct the patient to urinate into the specimen container.

3. Seal the container tightly and submit the specimen immediately.

Sources of Variability

1. The specimen container should be chemically clean. In particular, residues of the quaternary ammonium compounds used to clean reusable containers can cause falsely positive qualitative protein determinations.

2. Microscopy and routine chemical urinalysis should be performed immediately, that is, on fresh, warm urine. Delay will result in the disappearance of leukocytes, casts, and bilirubin; the appearance of crystals and crystal aggregates; and the proliferation of bacteria with resultant pH changes.

URINE: TIMED VOIDED SPECIMEN
(Free and Free 1975)

Equipment and Reagents

Specimen container: The container should be chemically clean and sealable; disposable plastic containers are preferred. The container should be large, usually 4 liters. The appropriate preservative should be placed into the container prior to the start of the collection. If the analyte to be assayed is light sensitive, a dark container is necessary.

Preservatives: the appropriate preservative is usually added by the laboratory.

Procedure

1. Patient cooperation is imperative for a successful timed urine collection, so carefully instruct the patient in the procedure and encourage his/her cooperation.

2. Warn the patient if the urine preservative is caustic.

3. Instruct the patient to <u>discard</u> a voiding and record the time. For 24-hour collections, it is usual to discard the first morning voiding.

4. Have the patient collect every subsequent voiding for the duration of the timed collection. The urine may be collected in a wide-mouthed, chemically clean container and then poured into the specimen container.

5. The specimen container should be kept refrigerated throughout the collection period.

6. The last urine collection should be a complete, forced voiding at the exact end of the timed period.

7. Seal the container tightly and submit the specimen immediately.

Sources of Variability

1. The specimen container should be chemically clean.

2. The analyte of interest must be preserved during the storage of the urine while the collection is in progress. Light-sensitive analytes should be shielded in dark bottles. Refrigeration is used to retard bacterial growth as well as to stabilize certain analytes. Acidification of the urine is necessary to assure stability of a large number of analytes. (Boric acid serves not only to acidify the urine but also to inhibit bacterial and cellular catabolism of analytes.)

3. Since the timed urine collection is used to calculate an excretory rate (i.e., amount of analyte excreted per unit time), it is imperative that the collection be complete and properly timed. Unfortunately, timed collections very frequently are incomplete, usually because of the forgetful discarding of a voiding(s) during the collection. Over-collection does happen but is much less common. In fact, variability in the completeness of the collection is by far the most important variable in timed collections. Consequently, care must be taken to instruct the patient or nursing staff in the importance of a proper collection.

REFERENCES

Fishman, R.A. Cerebrospinal Fluid in Diseases of the Nervous System. W.B. Saunders, Philadelphia, pp. 141-146, 1980.

Fraser, R.G., Pare, J.A.P. Diagnosis of Diseases of the Chest. 2nd ed. W.B. Saunders, Philadelphia, p. 301, 1977.

Free, A.H., Free, H.M. Urinalysis in Clinical Laboratory Practice. CRC Press, Boca Raton, FL, pp. 21-26, 1975.

Kovarik, J.L. Thoracentesis: a modified technique. Postgrad. Med. 48:96, 1970.

Meites, S., Levitt, M.J. Skin-puncture and blood collecting techniques for infants. In: Meites, S. (ed.) Pediatric Clinical Chemistry. American Association for Clinical Chemistry, Washington, D.C., pp. 13-25, 1981.

THE ANSWERS

Chapter 1

1-1. 145 mmol/L.

1-2. 5 meq/L.

1-3. 23.3 nkat/L.

1-4. The medical arguments in favor of using molar units rest upon their physiologic appropriateness. The electrochemical activity and osmolality of analytes and the capacity of binding proteins are all determined by their molar concentrations. In addition, the use of molar units preserves the quantitative relationships between metabolic precursors and end products. An argument against the use of molar units is that substance concentration expressed in equivalent units and ósmolar units, which are familiar units, is already in its physiologically appropriate form.

1-5. Her body surface area is 1.36 m^2 (DuBois and DuBois 1916) or 1.45 m^2 (Gehan and George 1970) so her normalized creatinine clearance is 140 or 131 ml/min per 1.73 m^2.

1-6. This is an example of a case in which measurement of the actual catalytic activity of the enzyme is desired. This is because C1 esterase inhibitor serves its physiologic role as an enzyme constituent of the plasma. Its functional, i.e., catalytic, concentration is reduced here, so the patient has a clinical deficiency. The normal mass concentration of the inhibitor, as measured immunologically, indicates that normal amounts of an antigenically identical but enzymatically dysfunctional protein are being synthesized.

1-7.   For example, this nomogram:

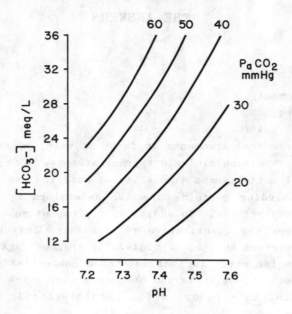

Chapter 2

2-1.   For example, these analytes:

Gender   Age

sex hormones   alkaline phosphatase
alpha-lipoprotein   cholesterol
calcium   albumin
creatinine   glucose

Diurnal rhythm   Analytic method

cortisol   enzymes
iron   bilirubin
uric acid

2-2.	Study value	Exhaustive frequency listing	Percentile listing
	5	0.03	0.03
	6	0.10	0.13
	7	0.17	0.30
	8	0.27	0.57
	9	0.23	0.80
	10	0.13	0.93
	11	0.04	0.97
	12	0.03	1.00

Mean = 8.27; standard deviation = 1.57.

2-3. The administration of insulin reverses the hyperkalemia of diabetes. The high potassium concentration in the second blood specimen is, therefore, an anomalous finding. Two explanations come immediately to mind, both of which must be investigated prior to additional therapeutic efforts. First, the patient may have received parenteral potassium with the insulin. Second, the laboratory value could be in error, the most likely cause being hemolysis in the specimen.

2-4. Both reference populations should consist of subjects who have clinical features that would prompt a physician to consider the diagnosis of acute myocardial infarction. This means that the subjects should have acute chest pain. Among subjects with an infarct the two most important considerations in terms of the spectrum of disease are variability in the size of the infarct and in the time since the onset of chest pain. Among the infarct-free subjects the whole variety of disorders that produce acute chest pain, other than myocardial infarction, should be represented.

2-5. Significant sources of interindividual variability for cholesterol include gender and age and, less so, race. Intraindividual sources of variability in cholesterol levels include a diurnal rhythm and possibly a seasonal cycle.

2-6. The following example of a percentile listing for plasma cholesterol concentration takes into account race (white), gender (men), age (years), and distribution among plasma lipoprotein transport forms (VLDL: very low density lipoprotein; LDL: low density lipoprotein; HDL: high density lipoprotein).

Age, years	VLDL, mg/dl		LDL, mg/dl		HDL, mg/dl	
	Mean	5th to 95th Percentile	Mean	5th to 95th Percentile	Mean	5th to 95th Percentile
<10	10	0–20	95	65–135	50	40–75
10–19	10	0–25	95	65–130	50	35–75
20–29	15	5–35	110	70–165	45	30–65
30–39	25	5–55	130	80–190	45	30–65
40–49	25	5–55	140	90–195	45	30–65
50–59	25	5–60	145	90–200	45	30–65
60–69	20	0–45	150	95–210	50	30–80
70+	20	0–40	145	90–195	50	30–80

* Data from Lipid Research Clinics Study of white North American males. The means and 5th and 95th percentiles from the original data have been rounded to the nearest 5 mg/dl.
SOURCE: The Lipid Research Clinics, Population Studies Data Book, vol. 1, visit II, 1980. Recalculation of data by 10-year age strata courtesy of Dr. Basil Rifkind, NHLBI.

(From Stanbury, J.B., Wyngaarden, J.B., Frederickson, D.S., et al. ed. The Metabolic Basis of Inherited Disease, 5th edition © 1983, McGraw-Hill Book Company, New York, p. 592.)

Chapter 3

3-1. In general, diagnostic studies perform less well when they are used in an unselected population. The sensitivity of the study might decrease because some iron deficient infants may not have been included in the screen-positive population. The specificity of the study might decrease because of the increased biologic variability to be found in the unscreened population. Some of these infants can be expected to have conditions that lower transferrin saturation despite normal iron stores, such as acute or chronic inflammatory states.

3-2. The predictive value of a positive result is 0.51. The predictive value of a negative result is 0.76. The efficacy is 0.67.

3-3.

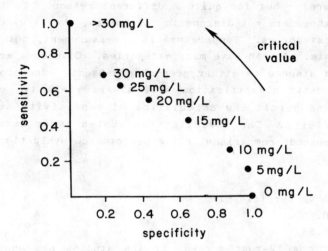

3-4. Transferrin saturation outperforms serum ferritin concentration. A side-by-side comparison of the performance characteristic curves readily demonstrates this. At similar levels of specificity, the sensitivity of transferrin saturation is greater, and at like levels of sensitivity, its specificity is greater. This is another use to which performance characteristic curves can be put — comparing study performances.

3-5. By definition:

true positive results = prevalence · number of subjects · sensitivity

false negative results = prevalence · number of subjects · (1-sensitivity)

true negative results = (1-prevalence) · number of subjects · specificity

false positive results = (1-prevalence) · number of subjects · (1-specificity)

Substitution of these expressions into the formulas confirms that the estimates of sensitivity and specificity are independent of the prevalence.

3-7. The example cited by Feinstein (1975) compares palpation to thermometry for measuring body temperature. A three-category scale is used for both: no fever, minor fever (38°-38.9°C), and major fever ($\geq 39^\circ$C). Feinstein argues that sensitivity and specificity cannot be computed readily because there are three rather than two diagnostic categories. Sensitivity and specificity cannot be measured — but for quite a different reason! It is because these are not diagnostic categories, they are measurement categories. Temperature is a measurement, not a diagnosis. It can have many categories. Diagnoses are binary, a disease is either present or absent. Therefore, diagnostic classification will always yield two categories and permit the calculation of sensitivity and specificity. The investigation quoted is an example of a methods comparison, not a performance evaluation.

Chapter 4

4-1.   5 µg ferritin/L.

4-2.   0.70.

4-3.   0.68.

4-5.   For a 12-test screen, if the studies are uncorrelated, the probability of two or more study results being outside of their reference intervals is

$$1 - (0.95)^{12} (0.05)^0 - 12(0.95)^{11} (0.05)^1 = 0.12 \quad .$$

probability of   *probability of*
no abnormal results   *one abnormal result*

4-6.   The slope of the line identifying the efficacy-maximizing point on the test series performance characteristic curve is -29. Using the following table:

Number of studies	Test series	
	sensitivity	specificity
4	0.079	0.996
5	0.042	0.999
6	0.022	0.9998
7	0.012	0.99994

the slopes of the lines <u>connecting</u> the performance points can be calculated. The slope from five studies to six is -25 and from six studies to seven is -71. Therefore the tangent line with slope -29 will pass through the performance pair corresponding to six studies in the series.

4-7. In the coordinate space formed by the logarithmic transforms of results, the line

$$log_{10}UH = 2 + 0.3\ log_{10}BP$$

separates result combinations in metastatic disease from those in osteoporosis. The discriminant function is

$$log_{10}UH - 0.3\ log_{10}BP.$$

Its antilogarithm is the discriminant diagnostic ratio

$$UH/BP^{0.3}.$$

The critical value of the discriminant diagnostic ratio is the antilogarithm of the critical value of the discriminant function

$$10^2 = 100.$$

4-8. 1.00.

4-9. Using a discriminant function of

$$log_{10}UH - log_{10}BP$$

i.e., that associated with the diagnostic ratio, the maximum efficiency is achieved with a critical value of 1.13. Efficiency = 0.84.

Chapter 5

5-1. 0.15.

5-2. Using the prevalence of SLE among patients of full-time rheumatologists as the estimate of prior disease likelihood, the posterior likelihood would be 0.93. This is the usual answer. Using the prevalence of SLE among women aged 15-64 years as the estimate of prior disease likelihood, the posterior likelihood would be 0.15. This is the correct answer.

5-3. The two disease estimates differ because they utilize vastly different estimates of the prior disease likelihood. The correct estimate is the one based upon the biologic attributes of the patient and her age and gender, not the one based upon the historic experience of rheumatologists. This distinction between the patient and the practitioner lies at the very heart of individualizing diagnoses.

5-4.   This is sound clinical advice but only because of the
        inexactitude of the word "uncommon." In speaking of an
        uncommon manifestation of a common condition, we mean a
        manifestation that is seen in perhaps 1 case in 10 or 20.
        An uncommon condition, on the other hand, may be found in
        1 case in 1,000 or 10,000. The Bayesian formula for com-
        peting diagnoses shows that the common condition should
        be diagnosed. For example, if the prior likelihood of
        the uncommon condition is 1/100 of the prior likelihood
        of the common condition, and if the relative frequency of
        the uncommon manifestation is 1/20 of that of the common
        manifestation (both of which are conservative numbers),
        the posterior likelihood of the common condition is 0.83,
        whereas that of uncommon condition is only 0.17.

5-7.   0.40.

5-8.   Multiple endocrine adenomatosis syndrome has to be con-
        sidered in this patient because of his provocative family
        history; therefore a plasma catecholamine determination
        is in order.

5-9.   Diamond and Forrester (1983) report that the 90% confi-
        dence interval is 0.05 to 0.64 with a mean likelihood of
        0.30.

Chapter 6

6-1.   The following studies have posterior likelihoods that
        exceed 0.075, given a prior likelihood of 0.01:

Test	Posterior likelihood
acid phosphatase - enzyme	0.09
urine cytology before massage	0.08
prostatic secretion cytology after massage	0.13
urine cytology after massage	0.10

        Therefore, they can be used to screen for prostate cancer
        in asymptomatic men.

6-2.   Most of the symptomatic patients free from prostate can-
       cer can be assumed to have prostatic hypertrophy. It is
       reasonable to expect that the specificity of the tests in
       such patients is less than that in asymptomatic men. In
       contrast, the sensitivity of the tests is likely to be
       greater in the symptomatic patients because, on average,
       their disease can be expected to be more advanced than
       that in the asymptomatic men.

6-3.   An excluding study must have performance characteristics
       that satisfy the inequality

       $$0.24 \text{ specificity} + \text{sensitivity} > 1 \ .$$

       None of the studies qualify. Only rectal examination
       comes close. This is because it is the study with the
       greatest sensitivity, and high sensitivity is required of
       excluding studies.

6-4.   A confirming study must have performance characteristics
       that satisfy the inequality

       $$0.33 \text{ sensitivity} + \text{specificity} > 1 \ .$$

       This is so for all the studies except acid phosphatase-
       RIA, lactic dehydrogenase V/I ratio, and leukocyte-
       adherence inhibition. Rectal examination would appear to
       be the preferred confirming study because it is the least
       expensive and is minimally invasive. However, prostatic-
       secretion cytology after massage is the most accurate
       study.

6-5.   A positive screening study result yields a disease like-
       lihood of 0.09. The best follow-up study would be one
       that could serve as both an excluding and a confirming
       study. Computation of the posterior likelihoods for
       positive and negative results for the listed studies
       reveals that two studies, prostatic-secretion cytology
       after massage and urine cytology after massage, have this

property. Prostatic-secretion cytology is the more accurate of the two and therefore to be preferred. A less tedious way to arrive at this conclusion is to identify the study that is the best classifier, using the performance characteristic curves for the studies, as shown below. The line identifying the best classifier has a slope of -10. Study 6 is prostatic-secretion cytology.

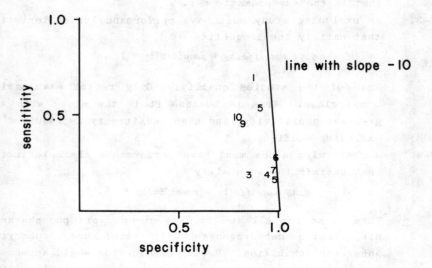

6-6.   A detailed discussion of the rationale for this recommendation is given in the article, "ACS Report on the Cancer-Related Health Checkup" (American Cancer Society, 1980).

Chapter 7
Things have their due measure; there are ultimately fixed limits, beyond which, or short of which, something must be wrong.
Satires, I.i.106.

7-1.   It would be expected that the plasma albumin concentration is decreased in cirrhosis because of reduced synthesis of albumin, but in fact, most cirrhotic patients have normal or even increased albumin synthetic rates. The liver has a tremendous synthetic reserve that can compensate for extensive hepatocyte loss (lesson: hepatic synthetic function as measured by albumin concentration is the product of cell number and average cell synthetic activity). It is often suggested that an increased volume of distribution explains the reduced plasma concentrations but as discussed in the text, steady-state concentrations are independent of the volume of distribution. Increases in the plasma clearance rate of albumin therefore must be the reason. Experimental evidence supports this conclusion.

7-2.   22 mmol/L.

7-3.   Blood P_{CO2} is the most important of the feedback signals in the regulation of pulmonary ventilation. Desirable characteristics for such a feedback marker include moderate responsiveness to changes in ventilation — too little responsiveness and the signal is missed; too much and profound metabolic changes will accompany even small ventilation changes — and equal sensitivity to increases and decreases in ventilation. These qualities are found at the genu of the clearance relationship.

7-4.   35 ml/minute.

7-5.   720 mg/24hours.

7-6.   Clearance differences may result from inaccuracy of the method used to estimate the creatinine synthetic rate in the patient and from variability in the measurement of the renal clearance rate. In addition, patients with moderate to severe renal impairment have appreciable extrarenal clearance of creatinine, so the plasma clearance rate will systematically overestimate the renal clearance rate.

7-7.   Using formula 1 from Table 7-4, the magnitude of a detectable change in creatinine concentration is 0.6 mg/dl. This is larger than the typical magnitude quoted in Table 7-5, i.e., 0.3 mg/dl. Using the individualized value the change in concentration is not significant, but using the typical value it is. An explanation for this difference is that it is inappropriate to use a typical magnitude defined in healthy individuals when evaluating a patient with renal disease. The measurement variability for creatinine concentration is larger in renal disease, so the magnitude of a significant concentration difference is greater.

7-8. Bile acids are good markers of liver plasma flow rate whereas bilirubin is not. If the hepatic plasma flow rate changes more than the intrinsic clearance rate in early disease, bile acids will be the superior disease marker. In addition, if bile acids have less measurement variability, they will be more sensitive markers.

7-9. Two kinds of clearance studies are described in this chapter. The first kind, steady-state clearance studies, use the measurement of the steady-state plasma concentration of endogenous substances or exogenous substances administered by continuous infusion. The second kind, nonsteady-state clearance studies, utilize the plasma clearance curve of exogenous substances administered by bolus intravenous injection or by gastrointestinal absorption. The postprandial bile acid study represents an example of a nonsteady-state clearance study using an endogenous substance. Approximately half of the bile acids secreted into the bile are sequestered in the gallbladder. Taking a meal stimulates the release of cholecystokinin, which causes gallbladder contraction and discharge of the sequestered bile acids into the duodenum. The subsequent ileal uptake of the bile acids produces the nonsteady-state, which can be monitored as the plasma clearance curve or as a one-sample clearance study.

7-10. The text's assertion that the extraction fraction decreases as the plasma flow rate increases is true as long as the intrinsic clearance rate of the organ is a constant. If the intrinsic clearance rate is not a constant, the statement will apply only as long as the intrinsic clearance rate increases less rapidly than the plasma flow rate. When discussing the relationship between plasma flow rate and extraction fraction among individuals, the same is true. The extraction fraction will be inversely related to the plasma flow rate if and only if the intrinsic clearance rate has a concave relationship to the flow rate. If the relationship is linear, the extraction fraction will be a constant. If it is convex, the extraction fraction will be directly related to the plasma flow rate. This is the case for the spleen. In rheumatic and hematologic diseases, spleen size corresponds to the intensity of phagocytic activity; larger, more active spleens have disproportionately more phagocytic cells than smaller, less active organs. What would be expected from an investigation using patients with portal hypertension due to cirrhosis?

Chapter 8

Harmony in discord. Epistles, I.xii.19.

8-1. Patients who have pheochromocytomas come to the hospital with symptoms referable to increased circulating catecholamines; catecholamine metabolites do not produce symptoms. Therefore tumors that predominantly or exclusively release active catecholamines will produce symptoms and be detected while they are still small. Tumors that release more catecholamine metabolites than active species will be much larger before they elaborate the active catecholamines at a rate leading to symptoms and clinical detection. In both cases the plasma catecholamine concentrations will be distinctly elevated, but only in the latter case will urinary metabolite excretion be markedly increased.

8-2. Epinephrine is synthesized in the adrenal medulla. Extra-adrenal paraganglionic tissue produces only norepinephrine. Pheochromocytomas arising in extra-adrenal sites, therefore, cause isolated elevations in plasma norepinephrine.

8-3. For example, these sources of variability:

Plasma catecholamines

patient stress
temperature and duration of sample storage

Urinary catecholamine metabolites

patient stress
drugs altering catecholamine metabolism (e.g., monoamine oxidase inhibitors)
drugs with catecholamine-like metabolites (e.g., alpha methyldopa)
dietary catecholamines

8-4. The feedback marker for renin is the urinary sodium excretion rate; primary hyperreninism is associated with high excretion rates (normally a suppression signal), and secondary hyperreninism with low excretion rates.

Note: Renin is an enzyme, so it is usually measured in terms of its catalytic activity, called plasma renin activity (PRA).

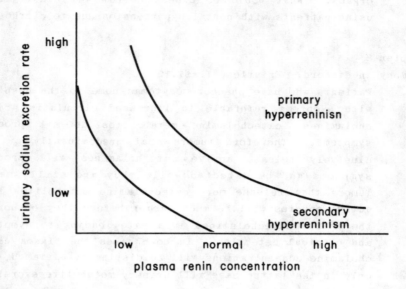

8-5.   Polydipsia and polyuria in a patient who is not experiencing an osmotic diuresis suggest the diagnosis of diabetes insipidus, i.e., deficient production of antidiuretic hormone (ADH). To confirm this diagnosis a stimulation test is needed. The preferred stimulus is dehydration, in the form of overnight water deprivation, and the function marker is urine osmolality. In patients with diabetes insipidus, urine osmolality will be low, even with profound dehydration. Patients with pituitary diabetes insipidus are distinguished from those with nephrogenic diabetes insipidus by their response to the administration of ADH. Urine osmolality will not increase in response to ADH in patients with effector tissue dysfunction.

8-6.   The plasma cortisol concentration will fall, which will cause release of ACTH from pituitary adenomas but not from the chronically suppressed pituitary glands of patients with cortisol-secreting adrenal neoplasms. Consequently, plasma 11-deoxycortisol levels will increase in patients with Cushing's disease but not in patients with primary adrenal tumors. In this way primary and secondary forms of Cushing's syndrome can be distinguished.

8-7. The anterior pituitary is a conglomeration of autonomously functioning hormone units. Individual units, e.g., the cells that secrete adrenocorticotrophic hormone, may hyperfunction but the organ as a whole does not. Evaluating pituitary hyperfunction therefore entails study of the functional status of the hormone unit of interest. Individual units may also hypofunction, causing selective pituitary hormone deficiencies. These should be evaluated selectively. However, the gland can hypofunction as a whole due to neoplastic compression or vascular compromise. Progressive loss of hormone unit function is frequently seen in this circumstance. Growth hormone deficiency is noted first, followed in order by deficiencies of the gonadotrophins, thyroid-stimulating hormone, and adrenocorticotrophic hormone. Thus growth hormone deficiency will be the most sensitive marker of panhypopituitarism. Demonstration of the deficiency of another of the hormones will distinguish panhypopituitarism from isolated growth hormone deficiency. Maximum sensitivity will be achieved if the gonadotrophins are used as the second marker. The functional reserve of the other pituitary hormones also will need to be evaluated concurrently or subsequently in order to plan replacement therapy. As with isolated deficiencies, the demonstration of combined deficiencies is best accomplished using a stimulation study. Table 8-3 indicates that concurrent provocation with insulin (to induce hypoglycemia) and gonadotrophin-releasing hormone will allow detection of growth hormone and gonadotrophin deficiency. Hypoglycemia also permits evaluation of the adrenocorticotrophic hormone reserve. Simultaneous administration of thyrotrophin releasing hormone allows concurrent measurement of the thyrotrophin reserve.

Chapter 9

9-1.   Increased: hypocalcemia, diabetes mellitus. Decreased: nephrotic syndrome, multiple myeloma. An increased anion gap may be caused by a decrease in the concentration of unmeasured strong cations (hypocalcemia) or an increase in the concentration of unmeasured strong anions (keto-anions in diabetes mellitus). A decreased anion gap may be caused by an increase in the concentration of unmeasured strong cations or a decrease in the net anionic change of the proteins (decreased anionic species in nephrotic syndrome and increased cationic species in multiple myeloma).

9-2.   The laboratory data indicate that this patient has an acidosis of metabolic origin with respiratory compensation. The acidosis can be further classified as a high anion gap type metabolic acidosis.

9-3.   Water loss equals the weight loss: approximately 4 L. Body water is typically distributed between extra- and intracellular water in a ratio of 2:3, so the extracellular loss is 1.6 L and the intracellular loss, 2.4 L.

9-4.   Body water content is decreased, so body sodium content is normal or decreased. If the sodium content were normal, the plasma sodium concentration would be increased due to the loss of extracellular water. It is decreased and thus body sodium content must be decreased, which indicates that there must be sodium loss in the urine. For this reason the text's formula for calculating the change in water content cannot be used in this patient. In addition, the increase in the osmolarity of the extracellular water caused by the increased glucose concentration has caused an intercompartment shift of water into the extracellular space. This has further lowered the plasma sodium concentration (approximately 0.3 meq sodium/L per mmol glucose/L). In this case the increase in plasma potassium concentration does not indicate increased body potassium content. There has been an intercompartmental shift of potassium into the extracellular space due to acidosis and insulin deficiency. In fact, there is probably some decrease in body potassium content due to urinary losses.

9-5.   The defect is at site 1, precursor uptake. Cellular
        glucose transport is impaired, so glucose accumulates in
        the extracellular fluids. The need for an alternate
        energy source for the cells is met by the activation of
        the fatty acid metabolic pathway, which produces keto-
        acids as end products. These reflux from the cells into
        the extracellular fluids.

9-6.   Decreased ferritin concentration and increased red cell
        volume heterogeneity. The mean red cell volume is not
        decreased, which is unusual for but does not exclude
        iron-deficiency anemia.

9-7.   The iron therapy has made the patient iron replete, as
        indicated by the normal ferritin concentration, but his
        anemia is not cured. In the iron-replete state the mean
        red cell volume is high and the volume heterogeneity is
        increased, so folate or vitamin B12 deficiency must be
        considered. Concurrent iron and folate/B12 deficiency
        would also explain the normal mean red cell volume found
        prior to the institution of iron therapy.

9-8.   Two features of deficiency states are 1) an increase in
        the plasma clearance rate of the trace metal due to
        increased rates of cellular uptake and 2) a reduction in
        the rate of synthesis and secretion of substances, which
        depend upon the availability of the trace metal. Both of
        these can be used as the basis of laboratory studies of
        body trace metal stores. In the first case the plasma
        clearance rate of administered substance can be measured:
        if the clearance rate is increased, a deficiency state
        can be inferred. Because the flux of trace metals is
        minute, even in deficiency states, the accuracy of mea-
        surement is greatly increased if radiolabeled metal is
        administered. In the second case the administration of
        physiologic or pharmacologic doses of the deficient metal
        will result in an increased rate of synthesis and secre-
        tion of the suppressed substance. An increase in the
        plasma concentration of the substance following the ad-
        ministration of the metal confirms the presence of a
        deficiency state. Such a study is called a therapeutic
        trial. What marker is monitored following a therapeutic
        trial of iron in presumed iron deficiency?

Chapter 10

10-1. 3.5 µg/dl.

10-2. 10 µg/dl.

10-3. Rearrangement of the equilibrium mass action equation yields

$$K_a = \frac{[bound\ hormone]}{[unbound\ hormone][free\ binding\ sites]} \ .$$

Here

$$K_a = 0.14\ (\mu g\ cortisol/dl)^{-1}.$$

10-4. Hormone production must equal hormone elimination in steady state. Therefore,

$$\genfrac{}{}{0pt}{}{production\ rate\ of}{hormone} = \binom{clearance\ rate\ of}{available\ hormone} \cdot \binom{concentration\ of}{available\ hormone}$$

which yields on rearrangement:

$$\genfrac{}{}{0pt}{}{concentration\ of}{available\ hormone} = \binom{production\ rate\ of}{hormone} \Big/ \binom{clearance\ rate\ of}{available\ hormone} \ .$$

Here clearance is halved while the production rate is unchanged, so the concentration in liver disease is twice that in health: 20 µg/dl.

10-5. The quadratic equation presented in the text may be used. Thus,

$$B = 10 - 20 + 7 = -3\ \mu g/dl$$
$$C = 20/0.14 = 143\ \mu g^2/dl^2.$$

The concentration of unbound cortisol is 13.5 µg/dl.

10-6. No. The concentration of cortisol available peripherally is homeostatically controlled by the hypothalamus and pituitary. The production of cortisol will be reduced to a level yielding the set-point concentration of available (i.e., unbound and albumin-bound) cortisol, which is 3.5 µg/dl.

10-7. Because the concentration of occupied binding sites equals the concentration of bound hormone, the equilibrium mass action equation can be rewritten as

$$\frac{[unbound\ hormone]}{[occupied\ binding\ sites]} = \frac{1}{K_a\ [free\ binding\ sites]}\ .$$

Also

$$[free\ binding\ sites] + [occupied\ binding\ sites] = [total\ binding\ sites]\ .$$

If the concentrations of unbound hormone and total binding sites are known, these two equations can be used to solve for the two unknowns: the concentrations of occupied and free binding sites.
Thus,

$$[unbound\ hormone] = 3.5\ \mu g/dl$$

$$[total\ binding\ sites] = 10\ \mu g\ cortisol/dl.$$

The concentration of occupied binding sites is 3.3 μg cortisol/dl. Again, because the concentration of occupied binding sites equals the concentration of bound hormone, the concentration of total hormone is 6.8 μg/dl.

10-8. No. Calcium complexing to the citrate present in high concentration in the administered blood can lower the concentration of ionic calcium to symptomatic levels despite normal total calcium levels. Direct measurement of ionic calcium is necessary.

10-9. The concentration of unbound thyroxine parallels, and therefore is a reliable marker for, the concentration of available hormone in clinical conditions characterized by changes in hormone production or TBG concentration. Changes in albumin concentration will alter the relationship between unbound and available thyroxine, but the effect is not profound.

Chapter 11

11-1. 6 hours to 2 days.

11-2. 1 day to 4.75 days.

11-3. The later appearance of lactate dehydrogenase (LD) is due to slower extracellular release of LD from infarcted tissue and slower uptake into the circulation. Both of these are attributable to the higher molecular weight of LD. The later disappearance of LD is due to slower plasma clearance and slow redistribution into the plasma from the other body tissues. An additional, intriguing possibility is that the breakdown of inflammatory cells at the site of the infarct may contribute LD for days following the injury.

11-4. For example, these conditions:

Creatine kinase	Lactate dehydrogenase
muscular dystrophy	muscular dystrophy
myopathies	hepatitis
muscle trauma	cirrhosis
myocarditis	pancreatitis
pericarditis	megaloblastic anemia

11-5. One reason is that the patient has recently experienced or is experiencing an extension of his myocardial infarct. Other considerations include a prolonged diagnostic window because of a large infarct (not likely in this patient), myocarditis or pericarditis instead of infarction, and release of creatine kinase from a skeletal muscle source due to trauma.

11-6. Three: H_2, MH, M_2.

11-7. Five: H_4, H_3L, H_2L_2, HL_3, L_4.

11-8. Aspartate aminotransferase is present within the cell cytosol and also within the mitochondria. Alanine aminotransferase is exclusively cytosolic. Severe hepatic injury will cause the release of mitochondrial as well as cytosolic enzymes, which will result in a disproportionate elevation in aspartate aminotransferase. Therefore the prognosis is worse when the ratio of aspartate to alanine aminotransferase is greater than 1.

11-9. The majority of the increase in the ESR is due to the anemia caused by the marrow infiltration by the myeloma. The increased plasma concentrations of immunoglobulin in myeloma by itself cause only a small increase in the ESR.

11-10. Three reasons have been suggested: 1) the patients are detected earlier in the course of their disease when the anemia is not yet severe; 2) unlike immunoglobulin G, immunoglobulin M does not accentuate red cell aggregation (which precedes sedimentation); and 3) the increased plasma viscosity due to immunoglobulin M myeloma slows the rate of red cell sedimentation.

11-11. Alkaline phosphatase and γ-glutamyl aminotransferase are located in the plasma membrane of hepatocytes, most densely near the canalicular complex. When there is intrahepatic biliary obstruction, it is likely that hepatocyte injury at the canalicular complex causes loss of membrane fragments into the bile. Subsequent reflux of bile into the space of Disse could explain the plasma appearance of conjugated bilirubin, bile acids, high-molecular-weight enzymes (membrane-bound enzyme fragments) and lipoprotein X (membrane fragment-bounded plasma vesicles). Alternately, both lipoprotein X and the lipid component of the high-molecular-weight enzymes may be novel biliary lipoproteins.

Chapter 12

12-1. The substance causing the urine coloration should be identified. Routine chemical urinalysis will distinguish red cells, hemoglobin, and myoglobin from food and drug pigments. Red cells, red cell casts, and red cell cast remnants, i.e., hemoglobin casts, are identified by microscopy. Subsequent cytopathologic study of urine is appropriate in this case.

12-2. Morphologic examination will permit classification of the tumor. In particular, for papillary lesions of the bladder, the histologic grade will be determined. The prognosis and therapeutic plan will be based on the grade assigned.

12-3. None. The papillary tumors of the bladder are diagnosed and classified using morphologic techniques: the local extent of disease is determined by cystoscopy, pelvic examination, and intravenous pyelography; and distant disease, i.e., metastases, is detected using radiographic techniques. If there is ureteral obstruction, residual renal function can be determined using the serum creatinine concentration.

12-4. Neoplasm, abscess, hematoma.

12-5. Determination of serum hCG and alpha-fetoprotein concentrations. If the lesion is a neoplasm, it will most likely be a germ cell tumor, and these assays will help in determining if trophoblastic elements are present. The therapeutic approach is different if there is trophoblastic differentiation. Levels will be needed as a baseline for comparison after orchiectomy.

12-6.   Studies should be directed at defining the nature of the
        suspected mass, which could be a hepatoma. Studies
        should include determination of the serum alpha-fetopro-
        tein concentration, which is highly specific for hepatoma
        in this clinical setting. In addition, attention should
        be directed toward the problem of blood in the stool.
        Although this can be explained on the basis of varices
        secondary to the patient's cirrhosis, carcinoma of the
        intestinal tract must be considered, as well as benign
        ulcer disease.

Chapter 13

13-1.   No. Her blood pressure is markedly abnormal. Potassium
        chloride is evaluated by measuring the serum potassium
        concentration. Diuretics such as hydrochlorothiazide
        almost always have an antihypertensive effect, but quan-
        titation of the effect is not possible in the presence of
        other antihypertensive medications. The diuretic effect
        of hydrochlorothiazide can be evaluated crudely by moni-
        toring urine output and weight loss. Propranolol can be
        evaluated by observing the heart rate before and after
        light exercise or upon standing. A blunted response
        indicates the drug is active. The effect of hydralazine
        is difficult to evaluate. It does cause vasodilation
        that can be observed peripherally (warm skin, nasal con-
        gestion, and retinal artery dilation), but it is not
        clear if these signs are reliable indicators of its anti-
        hypertensive action. Reserpine is known to cause ortho-
        static hypotension as a consequence of its postganglionic
        adrenergic blockade. Therefore measurement of the blood
        pressure at rest and after standing can be a bedside test
        to monitor its effect.

13-2.   Patient compliance. It is important to rule out noncom-
        pliance because the patient could be harmed by sudden
        administration of effective doses of all of these drugs.

13-3.   One method would be to hospitalize the patient and remove
        all medications under close observation. The blood
        pressure could be controlled with nitroprusside, if
        necessary, while the drugs were added back one at a time.
        Each drug could then be evaluated for its antihyperten-
        sive effect.

13-4.   Yes, probably. Procainamide is known to cause a lupus
         syndrome. This syndrome occurs more frequently with
         chronically high concentrations of the drug and among
         patients who are slow drug acetylators. The dose might
         be decreased slightly to determine if the arrhythmia
         could be controlled with a smaller dose. Other options
         include switching drugs or treating with this dose while
         monitoring for lupus.

13-5.   The dose need not be changed because it results in the
         desired control of the arrhythmia and has no side ef-
         fects.

13-6.   Theophylline has nonlinear kinetics above the therapeutic
         window. At very high concentrations the elimination rate
         becomes dose dependent so the theophylline plasma half-
         life will be much longer than at usual therapeutic con-
         centrations. Consequently, the plasma clearance curve
         will be very flat.

13-7.   There are two possible explanations: continued drug
         treatment between the collection of the first specimen
         and the second, and measurement variability. The ana-
         lytic variability of the assay at concentrations above
         the therapeutic window is usually greater than within it.
         The result of 49 µg/ml may well have a standard deviation
         of ± 2 µg/ml. Then the magnitude of a significant dif-
         ference will be 5.5 µg/ml. Thus 47 µg/ml and 49 µg/ml
         are not significantly different from one another.

13-8.   50 ml/min (Siersbaek-Nielsen et al. 1971).

13-9.   All of the choices.

13-10.   d, e, f, g. These choices are most important because
         they are the most frequent causes of interpretive
         problems.

13-11.   23%. This is found by substituting the known values into
         the equation:

$$K_{total} = K_{renal} + K_{liver} + K_{other}$$

and solving for K_{renal}. Here

$$K_{renal} = 20\%/24 hours \ .$$

The K_{renal} will be proportional to renal function. This
patient has a lower than normal GFR. Therefore the new
K_{renal} will equal K_{renal} in the normal circumstance

multiplied by the fraction of the normal GFR the patient possesses, 50/125 or 0.4. Then

$$0.4 \cdot 20\%/24hours = 8\%/24 \ hours.$$

Substituting into the equation for the total elimination rate yields

$$K_{total} = (8\% + 15\% + 0\%)/24hours$$
$$= 23\%/24hours \ .$$

13-12. 0.23 mg or, rounded to the nearest tablet size, 0.25 mg. The total body load of digoxin is about 1 mg. Since 23% is lost daily, we must replace 23% of 1 mg in order to maintain a steady state.

13-13. 0.0096 h^{-1}. The half-life is 72 hours. This is calculated from the equation

$$t_{1/2} = 0.693/K.$$

13-14. Oct 12th at 1500 hours. The date is four times the half-life and the time is taken from the rule listed in the Appendix.

GLOSSARY

Bayes' formula: the formula for the calculation of a posterior likelihood

classification correlation: the tendency for diagnostic studies applied to the same patient to yield the same diagnostic classification

clearance rate: the constant of proportionality between the concentration of a substance in a fluid compartment and the synthetic rate of the substance

clinical algorithm: a set of step-by-step instructions designed to direct a clinical activity, such as making a diagnosis

confirming study: a laboratory study used to confirm a specific diagnosis in a symptomatic patient

critical value: the diagnostic study result that separates results indicating the presence of a specific disease from those indicating its absence. **optimal critical value:** the critical value that maximizes the clinical usefulness of a diagnostic study in a given clinical population

diagnostic ratio: the ratio of the results of two studies; may be used as the basis of a bivariate positivity rule

diagnostic-review bias: in performance evaluations, a bias in reference diagnostic classification in favor of agreement with known study results

diagnostic window: the interval of time following an episode of injury during which measurement of a specific marker substance will demonstrate the occurrence of the injury

efficacy: the overall frequency of correct classification for a diagnostic study in a given clinical setting

evidential study: a laboratory study used as a source of diagnostic information but not possessing the performance characteristics required of a confirming or excluding study

excluding study: a laboratory study used to exclude a specific diagnosis in a symptomatic patient

frequency distribution: the compilation of the frequency of occurrence of each possible result of a laboratory study. **reference frequency distribution:** the frequency distribution of a defined laboratory study performed upon a sample from a defined (reference) population

imprecision: random error in measurement

inaccuracy: systematic error in measurement

intrinsic substance clearance rate: the maximum substance clearance rate of which an organ is capable

isopleth: line of equal measure, e.g., an isobar is an isopleth of barometric pressure

joint frequency: the frequency of a result combination

likelihood ratio: the ratio of the frequency of a study result in persons with a specific disease to the frequency of the result in persons free of the disease. **conditional likelihood ratio:** the likelihood ratio based upon the result frequencies for persons in the reference populations who have identical results for the preceding studies. **joint likelihood ratio:** the likelihood ratio based upon the frequencies of a result combination

logistic function: a mathematical formula used to express the relationship between the values of and the associated likelihood ratios of a multivariate discriminant function

marker substance: a substance that marks or indicates a physiologic process even though it is separated from the process by distance and time

measurement variability: the differences in the magnitude of a quantity when measured in many individuals or many times in the same individual

model: a description of the relationship between a physiologic process and certain quantities measured by laboratory studies

multivariate discriminant function: a formula for combining study results with the property that the reference frequency distributions arising from it show maximal separation of the diagnostic classes; may be used as the basis of a multivariate positivity rule

net expected value: the sum of the expected benefit (the product of the magnitude of the benefit times its likelihood) and the expected cost (the product of the magnitude of the cost times its likelihood) of a decision

nomogram: graphic representation of an equation

normalization: elimination of a known source of measurement variability by a specific adjustment and rescaling of measured values

normal range: the frequency distribution of results of a laboratory study performed upon normal individuals

performance characteristic curve: the graphic form of a performance characteristic function

performance characteristic function: the set of sensitivity and specificity pairs generated by considering every possible critical value for a diagnostic study

plasma clearance curve: the time course of the plasma concentration of a substance during and following its administration

positivity rule: in multiple testing, the rule used to distinguish study result combinations indicating the presence of a specific disease from those indicating its absence. **multivariate positivity rule:** in combination testing, a positivity rule based upon the multivariate result frequency distributions

posterior likelihood of disease: the estimate of the likelihood of a specific disease based upon the prior likelihood of the disease and the result of a diagnostic study

prevalence: the fraction of persons in a given clinical population who suffer from a specific disease

predictive value of a study result: the frequency with which a study result yields a correct diagnostic classification

prior likelihood of disease: the estimate of the likelihood of a specific disease arrived at prior to the performance of diagnostic studies

protective factor: a patient characteristic associated with a less than average disease prevalence

qualitative study: a laboratory study that uses a binary scale of measurement

quality assurance program: a program of surveillance and testing of the precision and accuracy of analytical methods

quantitative study: a laboratory study that uses a scale of measurement graduated into regular divisions called units

quantity: a measurable characteristic. **base quantities:** a set of dimensionally independent quantities. **secondary quantities:** quantities based upon integral powers of a single base quantity. **derived quantities:** quantities based upon products of integral powers of base quantities

receiver operating characteristic curve: synonym for performance characteristic curve

reference interval: the set of study results that gives rise to a specified, usually central, fraction of a reference frequency distribution. **multivariate reference space:** the set of result combinations that give rise to a specified, usually central, fraction of a reference multivariate frequency distribution

result correlation: the tendency for a result of one diagnostic study to be associated with a particular result of another diagnostic study when both studies are performed upon the same patient

risk factor: a patient characteristic associated with a greater than average disease prevalence

screening study: a laboratory study used to detect a specific disease in asymptomatic individuals

semiquantitative study: a laboratory study that uses a scale of measurement divided into grades or categories

sensitivity: the frequency with which a laboratory study yields the correct diagnosis in persons with a specific disease

serial correlation: the tendency for one result of a laboratory study to be similar to the previous result of the same study

specificity: the frequency with which a laboratory study yields the correct diagnosis in persons who do not suffer from a specific disease

steady state: the physiologic state in which the plasma concentration of a substance is constant over time

stimulation study: a laboratory study used to improve the diagnostic separation of the functional classes of an endocrine gland by determination of the response of the gland to the administration of its trophic hormone or to a stimulatory level of its feedback signal

suppression study: a laboratory study used to improve the diagnostic separation of the functional classes of an endocrine gland by determining the response of the gland to a suppressive level of its feedback signal

synthetic rate: the rate at which a secretory product enters the plasma

test-review bias: in performance evaluations, a bias in the reporting of laboratory study results in favor of agreement with a known diagnosis

therapeutic window: the range of drug plasma concentrations that maximizes the percent of the patient population deriving a therapeutic effect while minimizing the percentage having adverse effects

threshold likelihood for accepting a diagnosis: the likelihood of disease at which, for the patient, the net expected value of accepting the diagnosis is zero

threshold likelihood for rejecting a diagnosis: the likelihood of disease at which, for the patient, the net expected value of rejecting the diagnosis is zero

unit: reference magnitude of a quantity

volume of distribution: the constant of proportionality between the concentration of a substance in a fluid compartment and the amount of substance in the compartment

work-up bias: in performance evaluations, a bias in the selection of study subjects that favors subjects with high prior likelihoods of having the disease of interest

INDEX

A

abdominal paracentesis   330-333
acid-base balance   177-187
acid-base disorders   179-181
  diagnostic classification   186-187
acid-fast stains   304-307
acidosis   179-182
  metabolic versus respiratory   186-187
acid phosphatase   246
active form   188, 190-191
acute phase proteins   229-232
acute phase response   229-232
adrenal glands   161-162
adrenocorticotrophic hormone   162, 268, 247
adverse response   261-264
age   19, 26, 42, 80, 116-119, 266
alanine aminotransferase   222, 226, 277
albumin   26, 148, 153, 191, 204-205, 208-214, 230-232, 277-279
aldosterone   162, 168, 203-204, 208-209, 214
alkaline phosphatase   222-223, 226, 246
  leukocyte   246
  Regan isozyme   246
alkalosis   179-182
  metabolic versus respiratory   186-187
all-tests-positive positivity rule   68-71
αamylase   221-223
αfetoprotein   245, 254
α_1 acid glycoprotein   208, 230, 277
α_1 antitrypsin   194, 230
americium scan   111-116
aminoglycosides   277, 293
ammonia   140
amyloid A protein   230
anaerobic bacteria   300
androgens   162
anemia   193
anion gap   185-187
antibiotic sensitivity testing   309-310
antibodies   310-312
antidiuretic hormone   162, 168, 247
antisepsis   301-302
antithrombin III   194-268
any-test-positive positivity rule   68-71
APUD system   247-248, 252
arboviruses   310
arterial puncture   318-320
aspartate aminotransferase   222-223, 226, 277
aspirin   283
association constant   206
availability of protein-bound substances   160, 211-216

B

basal body weight   175
Bayes' formula   83
  for multiple diagnostic alternatives   96
  for multiple study results   98
  nomogram   86
believe-the-negative positivity rule   65-68, 118
believe-the-positive positivity rule   65-68, 118
Bence-Jones protein   249
bile acids   140-142
biliary tract injury   222, 246
bilirubin   139-142, 153, 203-204, 277
binding proteins   201-212
  affinity   206
  and drugs   277-279
  capacity   8, 206
biopsy   250-251, 302-303
Blastomyces dermatitidis   300
blood cells   152-153, 191-193
  in the acute phase response   229-232
blood flow rate   140-142
body size   19, 26
body surface area   see surface area
bone
  cancer   246
  disease   222, 246
  enzymes   222
Brucella   312
buffer function   202-203, 205-212

C

calcitonin   247
calcium   8, 153, 162, 172-173, 175-177, 203-204, 213-214
calcium gluconate   270-271
Candida albicans   300, 307
carbamazepine   293
carbon dioxide   140, 153, 177-187
carcinoembryonic antigen   244-245, 254
carcinoid tumor   248
catecholamines   102-103, 161, 168
ceruloplasmin   191, 194, 230
cervical cancer   240-241
cesium scan   111-116
chi-square test   46
Chlamydia   300, 303, 308-309
chloramphenicol   272
chloride   178
chorionic gonadotrophin   246, 254
chromatography   215
classification correlation   67-71
clearance rate   131-134
  of exogenous substances   142-147
  organ   137-147
clearance study   142-147
  one-sample   145-147
  sampling schedules   144-145
clinical algorithm   101-103
clinical conversation   58-61, 91-93

clotting factors   194
cobalamin   see vitamin B12
Coccidioides immitis   300
colorectal cancer   241, 244-245, 254
combination testing   68-71
complement   194
computed tomography   242
confidence interval   46
  nomogram   47
confirming study   109-116
  performance characteristics for
    112-113
consequences of clinical actions   94
convalescent phase   310
copper   190-191, 203-205
coronary artery disease   80-85, 94-95,
  116-117, 119
cortisol   162, 168, 203-204, 208-209,
  211, 214-215
cortisol-binding globulin   204, 208-
  210
cost   90
  containment   123
C-protein   161
C-reactive protein   230-232
creatine kinase   45, 222-223, 226
  MB isoenzyme   222
creatinine   140, 153
creatinine clearance rate   138
  nomogram   276
  normalization   11-12
critical value   34
  optimal   55-63
  suboptimal   63-64
cryoglobulin   249
Cryptococcus neoformans   300, 304,
  307, 313
culture of microorganisms   307-309
  media   308-309
  quantitative   301-302
cytomegalovirus   300, 312
cytopathology   241, 251

D

data-base ordering   122
delivery function   201-203
detectable change in measurement   148-
  153, 223-225
  rules for calculation   151
  typical magnitudes   153, 226
diagnostic ratio   73-74
diagnostic-review bias   42
  effect on performance estimates   43
diagnostic window   223-225
digitoxin   293
digoxin   268-270, 280, 293
disopyramide   283, 293
distribution of drug   268-274
  equilibrium phase   269-272
dye contrast studies   242

E

ectopic hormone production   247-248
effector tissue   157-158
  disorders of   163-164
efficacy   36-38, 46-48
  maximizing   55-57
electrocardiographic exercise test
  82-85, 94-95
electrochemical activity   7
electron microscopy   252
endocrine glands   157-158
  function studies   160-161
  primary versus secondary dysfunction
    159, 161-162
  tumors   246-248
Entamoeba histolytica   312
Enterobacteriaceae   300
enteroglucagon   247
enterovirus   300
enzymes
  as tissue injury markers   219-223
  as tumor markers   245-246
  catalytic activity   8
  isozymes   221
  saturation   280-284
epinephrine   270-271
Epstein-Barr virus   312
equilibrium dialysis   215
errors
  laboratory   22-23
  in performance evaluation   43, 49
erythrocyte sedimentation rate   232,
  244
estradiol   203-204, 208-209, 211, 214
estrogens   162
ethosuximide   293
evidential study   120-121
excluding study   109-116
  performance characteristics for   114
expected benefit   87-90
expected cost   87-90

F

feedback marker   158, 161-162
ferritin   44, 68-71, 191
fever   229-230
fibrinogen   230, 232
fingerstick   321-322
first-order process   265, 272
Fisher exact test   46
folic acid   190-193, 203-204
follicle-stimulating hormone   162, 163
Francisella tularensis   312
free fatty acids   203-204
free thyroxine index   216
free triiodothyronine index   216
frequency distribution   23-27
  presentation   24
  reference   24-28, 44-46
fungi   300, 304, 307, 312

G

gallium scan 112-115
γglutamyltransferase 222, 226
gender 19, 26, 42, 80, 116-118
genital tract injury 222
gentamicin 272
germ cell tumor 245-246, 254
glucagon 158, 247
glucose 153
Gram stain 304-306
growth hormone 168

H

half-life 136, 265-268
haptoglobin 204, 230
heart injury 222
heavy chain disease 249
heelstick 322-324
helminths 304
hematocrit 153
hematoxylin and eosin stain 251
heme 203-204
hemoflagellates 307-308
hemoglobin 153, 203-205, 221-222
hemolysis 222
hemopexin 204
Hemophilus influenzae 313
Henderson-Hasselbach equation 12, 183
  nomogram 184
heparin 268, 283
herpes simplex virus 300, 308, 312-313
heterogeneity of a cellular characteristic 192
  of red cell volume 193
histamine 247
histopathology 249-252
Histoplasma capsulatum 300
homeostasis 157-158, 209-211
hormones as tumor markers 246-248
hydralazine 283
hydrogen ion concentration 177-181, 186
  compensatory mechanisms 182
  nomogram 180

I

immunoglobulins 153, 194, 232
  as tumor markers 248-249
immunohistology 251-252
imprecision 21
inaccuracy 21
inborn errors of metabolism 118-119, 194-196, 213
India ink preparation 304-307
injury versus death 220-221
insulin 161, 168, 247
Interleukin-1 229-230
interpretive reporting 9
intestinal injury 222

intrinsic substance clearance rate 141
iron 190-193, 203-205
islets of Langerhans 252
isotopic scanning 242-243
isozymes 221

J

joint frequency 98

K

ketoanions 178, 186
kidney
  as endocrine organ 161-162
  disease 275-279
  function studies 138, 140, 142, 144
  injury 222
kinetic radioimmunoassay 215
Kolmogorov-Smirnov statistic 46

L

lactate 178, 186
lactate dehydrogenase 222-223, 226, 245-246
  isozyme 1 222
lanthanic 116
Legionella pneumophila 308, 310, 312-313
Leptospira 312
lidocaine 270-271, 293
light miscroscopy 251-252
likelihood of a diagnosis 79-86
  prior 80-82, 97
  posterior 82-86, 94-98
likelihood ratio 83
  conditional 98
  joint 98
lithium 293
liver
  cancer 245
  disease 277
  function studies 139-142, 144, 148
  injury 222-223
lipase 221-222
logistic function 100-101
lumbar puncture 324-327
lung
  function studies 140
luteinizing hormone 162, 168
lymphoproliferative disorders 248-249, 252

M

macrocytosis   193
magnesium   172, 175, 176-178, 203-204,
    213
magnitude of tissue injury   225-229
  one-sample estimation   227-229
marker substance   129-130
  of body content   175-177
  of body stores   189-193
  of endocrine gland function   160-161
  of neoplasia   244-249
  of organ function   137-147
  of tissue injury   219-229
mean capillary transit time   211-212
mean red cell hemoglobin content   193
mean red cell volume   44, 68-71, 193
measurement variability   19
  analytic   21-22, 40-41
  biologic   19-21
  interindividual   19-20
  intraindividual   19-20
  postanalytic   22
  preanalytic   21
metabolic disease   194-196
metastases   253-254
Michaelis-Menten equation   280
microbial antigens   311-313
microcytosis   193
microfilariae   307-308
minimum bactericidal concentration
    309-310
minimum inhibitory concentration
    309-310
model   129-130
  of endocrine homeostasis   158
  of intracellular substance release
    219
  of metabolic fluxes   195
  of trace metal and vitamin dynamics
    188
  of water and abundant metal dynamics
    171
  parallel tube   141
monitoring   147-149, 223-225, 262-284
  strategies   149, 265-268, 271-275
morphine   260
multiphasic health screen   71
multivariate discriminant function
    72-73, 99-101
multivariate reference space   72
mycobacteria   304, 306
Mycobacterium tuberculosis   300-301,
    306
myeloma   249

N

needle aspiration   302-303
  fine needle   111-116, 251
Neisseria meningitidis   309, 313
net expected value   87-90
Nocardia   300, 304, 306-308
nomogram   12
  for Bayes formula   86
  for confidence intervals   47
  for creatinine clearance rate   276
  for Henderson-Hasselbach equation
    184
  for hydrogen ion concentration   180
  for surface area   13, 14
nonlinear kinetics   279-284
normal flora   301-302
normal   27-28
normalizing data   10-12
normal range   27-28
nuclear magnetic resonance   243

O

oat cell carcinoma   248
occult   116, 253
oncofetal antigens as tumor markers
    244-245
one-sample clearance studies   145-147
one-sample estimation of injury magni-
    tude   227-229
ordering studies   121-123
osmolality   7, 162, 175-176
ovaries   161-162

P

pancreatic injury   221-223
paraneoplastic syndromes   244, 247-249
parathormone   162, 247
parathyroid glands   161
pathologic examination as a reference
    method   41, 249-250
PCO2   see carbon dioxide
peak drug concentration   272, 275
pentobarbital   293
percentiles   24
performance characteristic function
    34-36, 45-46
performance evaluation   39-49
phenobarbital   271, 283, 293
phenytoin   278-279, 283, 294
pheochromocytoma   102-103, 161
phosphate   178, 185
phosphorus   153
pituitary, anterior   252
pituitary, posterior   161-162
plasma clearance curve   143
plasma proteins   177-186, 193-194,
    201-202

<u>Plasmodium</u>   307–308
<u>Pneumocystis carinii</u>   307–308
polyamines as tumor markers   245
positivity rules   64–71
  multivariate   72–73
potassium   7, 171–177
potassium hydroxide preparation   304–307
prealbumin   148, 204–205
predictive value   38–39, 46–48
prevalence   36, 43–48
probability distribution functions   24
procainamide   294
progesterone   203–204, 208–209, 214
prolactin   168
propranolol   283
prostatic cancer   246
protective factor   81
prothrombin time   277
protozoa   304, 307–308
<u>Pseudomonas aeruginosa</u>   300
putrescine   245

Q

quality assurance program   22–23
  clinician's role   22–23
quantities   4–6
quinidine   294

R

race   19, 80, 118
radiography   242
  computed tomography   242
  dye contrast studies   242
radioiodine   242–243
rate constant   265, 267
receiver operating characteristic curve
    see performance characteristic
    curve
receptor-mediated endocytosis   202
red cell culling   140, 144
red cell protoporphyrin   44, 68–71
reference interval   64
reference method   25, 41–43
  pathologic examination   41, 249–250
reference population   25, 42–43
relative exchange value scale   58–62
renin   162
repeat testing   65–68
resin T3 uptake   216
result correlation   98
retinol   see vitamin A
retinol-binding globulin   204–205
<u>Rickettsia</u>   310, 312
risk factor   81
rotavirus   313
rubella virus   310–312

S

salicylates   294
salivary gland injury   222
<u>Salmonella</u>   301, 309
screening study   116–120
  for neoplasia   240–241
  interval   118–120
  performance characteristics for   116
sensitivity   31–33
serial correlation   152
serological methods   310–313
serotonin   247
<u>Shigella</u>   301, 309
sign   80
skeletal muscle injury   222
sodium   7, 162, 171–177
soft tissue tumors   252
somatostatin   247
special stains   251, 307
specificity   31–33
  of multiphasic health screens   71
spectrum of biologic variability   25–26, 42–43
spermidine   245
spermine   245
spleen function studies   140, 144
staging of malignancies   253–254
staphylococci   300
steady state   131, 263–268
  time to achieve   265–268, 281–282
stimulation study   164–167
storage form   187–191
storage function   201–202, 205
streptococci   300, 313
strong ions   177–178
  difference   177–186
subclinical stage of disease   119–120
sulfate   178, 185
suppression study   164–167
surface area
  formulas   12, 14
  nomograms   13, 14
swabs   302–303
symptoms   80
synthetic rate   131–132, 193–194
  organ   137
syphilis   310

Système International d'Unités (SI)   5–6

  conversion between common units
    and SI units   18

T

temperature 231–232
testes 161–162
testosterone 203–204, 208–209, 214
testosterone-bonding globulin 204, 208–210
test-review bias 40
  effect on performance estimates 43
thallium scan 111–116
theophylline 272, 283, 294
therapeutic goal 257–258
therapeutic monitoring 258–260, also see monitoring
therapeutic response 261–261, 268–270
therapeutic window 261–262
thoracentesis 327–330
threshold likelihood 86–94, 96
  for accepting a diagnosis 87–90
  for rejecting a diagnosis 87–90
thyroid gland 161–162
  nodule 110–116
  tumor 242–243
thyroid hormone suppression test 112–115
thyroid-stimulating hormone 162, 168
thyroxine 162, 203–204, 208, 214, 216
thyroxine-binding globulin 204, 208, 210
timing of blood collection for therapeutic monitoring 293–294
tissue specificity of injury markers 221–223
Toxoplasma gondii 312
trace metals
  deficiency 188
  excess 188–189
  stores 188–193
transcobalamin I 191
transcobalamin II 191, 204
transferrin 191, 204, 230–231
transferrin saturation 31–32, 35–36, 44, 55–57, 62–63, 74
transport form 188–190
transport media 303
transport proteins 188, 190
Treponema pallidum 310, 312
Trichimonas vaginalis 304, 307
triiodothyronine 162, 203–204, 208, 211, 214, 216
trophic hormone 158, 161–162
trough drug concentrations 274–275
tumor location 240–241, 250–251, 253

U

ultrafiltration 215
ultrasound 243
unidirectional dissociation rate 211–212
units 3, 5–6
  conversion 10
  conversion between common and SI 18
  magnitude prefixes for 6
urea nitrogen 140, 153
urine collection 333–335

V

valproic acid 279, 294
value 57
  maximizing 57–63, 116
variance 150–152
vehicle function 201
venipuncture 315–318
viruses 309
viscosity 232
vitamin A 203–205
vitamin B12 190–193, 203–204
vitamin D 203–204
vitamin D-binding globulin 204
vitamins 187–193
volume of distribution 134–136, 146–147

W

Waldenström's macroglobulinemia 249
warfarin 279
water 171–177
  deficit 173–174
  distribution 172–175
  excess 173–174
wet mount preparation 304–307
work-up bias 42
  effect on performance estimates 43

YZ

yarns 285–289
zinc 190–191, 203–205
  metalloenzymes 191

DATE DUE

GAYLORD			PRINTED IN U.S.A.